This volume provides a timely and useful introduction to the theory and practical application of image analysis in histology. This powerful research technique can be used to detect not only stored products in a cell (immunocytochemistry) but the synthetic machinery and the factors that control it (*in situ* hybridization), as well as the specific binding sites that act as receptors for a molecule following its release (*in vitro* autoradiography).

The book provides a good introduction for beginners before looking in greater detail at more advanced material in selected areas. The volume highlights the importance of technique in gathering quantitative information. The book is divided into four parts: introductory material, image acquisition, image processing, and applications. The applications covered include quantitative pathology, neurobiology and immunocytochemistry as well as approaches to the important automation of quantification.

Image analysis in histology: conventional and confocal microscopy

POSTGRADUATE MEDICAL SCIENCE

This important new series is based on the successful and internationally well-regarded specialist training programme at the Royal Postgraduate Medical School in London. Each volume provides an integrated and self-contained account of a key area of medical science, developed in conjunction with the course organisers and including contributions from specially invited authorities.

The aim of the series is to provide biomedical and clinical scientists with a reliable introduction to the theory and to the technical and clinical applications of each topic.

The volumes will be a valuable resource and guide for trainees in the medical and biomedical sciences, and for laboratory-based scientists.

Titles in the series

Radiation protection of patients edited by R. Wootton

Monoclonal antibodies edited by Mary A. Ritter and Heather M. Ladyman

Molecular neuropathology edited by Gareth W. Roberts and Julia M. Polak

POSTGRADUATE MEDICAL SCIENCE

Image analysis in histology: conventional and confocal microscopy

EDITED BY

R. WOOTTON, D. R. SPRINGALL & J.M. POLAK

Published in association with
The Royal Postgraduate Medical School
University of London by

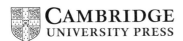

CAMBRIDGE
UNIVERSITY PRESS

Published by the Press Syndicate of the University of Cambridge
The Pitt Building, Trumpington Street, Cambridge CB2 1RP
40 West 20th Street, New York, NY 10011-4211, USA
10 Stamford Road, Oakleigh, Melbourne 3166, Australia

First published in 1995

Printed in Great Britain at the University Press, Cambridge

A catalogue for this book is available from the British Library

Library of Congress cataloguing in publication data

Image analysis in histology : conventional and confocal microscopy / edited by R. Wootton, D.R. Springall, & J.M. Polack.
    p.   cm. – (Postgraduate medical science)
ISBN 0-521-43482-3 (hc)
    1. Histology—Data processing. 2. Image processing—Digital techniques. 3. Microscopy—Technique. I. Wootton, R. (Richard) II. Springall, D.R. (David R.) III. Polak, Julia M. IV. Series.
    [DNLM: 1. Image Processing, Computer-Assisted. 2. Histological Techniques. 3. Microscopy—methods. QS 26.5 I31 1995]
QL807.I4 1995
574.8'24'028—dc20   94-18188 CIP

ISBN 0 521 43482 3 hardback

Contents

List of contributors   ix

Foreword   xi

Acknowledgements   xii

Abbreviations   xiii

Part I Basics

1   Introduction to histological image processing   3
    R. Wootton

2   Hardware and software for image processing   19
    M.E. Sherrington

3   Image input and display   33
    J.G. Weymes

4   Image file formats in biological image analysis   55
    D-C. Abrams

5   Basic image processing operations on the digitized image   69
    S. Bradbury

6   Study design   87
    P.K. Clark

7   Principles of stereology   96
    M.A. Browne, C.V. Howard and G.D. Jolleys

Part II Image acquisition

8   Samples and preparation methods   123
    D.R. Springall and J.M. Polak

9   Light microscopy   134
    P.J. Evennett

10 Confocal optical microscopy   151
    A. Boyde

11 Transmission electron microscopy   197
    F. Gracia-Navarro, A. Ruiz-Navarro, S. García-Navarro and J. Castaño

12   Television cameras and scanners   211
     P.M. Gaffney

     Part III Image processing

13   Segmentation   227
     A.K.C. Wong

14   Edge detection in microscope images   241
     M.Y. Jaisimha and R.M. Haralick

15   Image registration   262
     J.R. Jagoe

16   Computational haze removal   288
     N.F. Clinch and V.A. Moss

17   Computer based 3-D models of biological structures   300
     M.J. Cookson and W.F. Whimster

18   Three-dimensional visualization   313
     M.J. Cookson, R.A. Reynolds and D-C. Abrams

     Part IV Applications

19   Quantitative immunocytochemistry   339
     J.T. McBride

20   Quantification of nerves and neurotransmitters using image analysis 355
     T. Cowen

21   Automated grain counting as applied to *in situ* hybridization histochemi- 381
     stry
     J.A. Chowen

22   New interpretation techniques to aid automatic quantification of patho- 397
     logy
     J. Aldridge

23   Quantitative pathology   403
     D.R. Springall, S.M. Gentleman, G. Terenghi and J.M. Polak

Index   414

Plate section   between 208 and 209

Contributors

Mr D-C. Abrams	Department of Medical Physics, Royal Postgraduate Medical School, DuCane Road, London W12 0NN, UK
Dr J. Aldridge	Seescan plc, Unit 9, 25 Gwydir Street, Cambridge CB1 2LG, UK
Dr S. Bradbury	Pembroke College, Oxford, OX1 1DW, UK
Professor A. Boyde	Department of Anatomy and Developmental Biology, University College London, Gower Street, London WC1E 6BT, UK
Dr M.A. Browne	Confocal Technologies Ltd, South Harrington Building, Sefton Street, Liverpool L3 4BQ, UK
Dr J. Castaño	Departamento de Biologia Celular, Universidad de Cordoba, Avda. San Alberto Magno, 14004 Cordoba, Spain
Dr J.A. Chowen	CSIC, Instituto Cajal, Avenida Doctor Arce, 37, 28002 Madrid, Spain
Mr P.K. Clark	International Statistics and Data Management Department, Bldg 90, Wellcome Research, Langley, South Eden Park Road, Beckenham BE3 3BS, UK
Dr N. Clinch	Fairfield Imaging, Ashdown Court, The Square, Forest Row, East Sussex RH18 5EZ, UK
Dr M.J. Cookson	Hill Centre, The London Hospital Medical College, Turner Street, London E1 2AD, UK
Dr T. Cowen	Department of Anatomy and Developmental Biology, Royal Free Hospital School of Medicine, Rowland Hill Street, London NW3 2PF, UK
Dr P.J. Evennett	Department of Pure and Applied Biology, Leeds University, Leeds LS2 9JT, UK
Dr P.M. Gaffney	Seescan plc, Unit 9, 25 Gwydir Street, Cambridge CB1 2LG, UK
Dr S.M. Gentleman	Department of Psychiatry, Charing Cross Hospital, Fulham Palace Road, London W6 8RF, UK
Dr S. García-Navarro	Departamento de Biologia Celular, Universidad de Cordoba, Avda. San Alberto Magno, 14004 Cordoba, Spain

Dr F. Gracia-Navarro	Departamento de Biologia Celular, Universidad de Cordoba, Avda. San Alberto Magno, 14004 Cordoba, Spain
Professor R.M. Haralick	Department of Electrical Engineering, University of Washington, Seattle WA 98195, USA
Dr C.V. Howard	Department of Infant and Fetal Pathology, The University of Liverpool, P.O. Box 147, Liverpool L69 3BX, UK
Mr J.R. Jagoe	Department of Medical Physics, Royal Postgraduate Medical School, DuCane Road, London W12 0NN, UK
Dr M.Y. Jaisimha	Department of Electrical Engineering, University of Washington, Seattle WA 98195, USA
Mr G.D. Jolleys	Confocal Technologies Ltd, South Harrington Building, Sefton Street, Liverpool L3 4BQ, UK
Dr J.T. McBride	Pulmonary Division, Department of Pediatrics, University of Rochester Medical Center, 601 Elmwood Avenue, Box 667, Rochester, New York 14642, USA
Dr V.A. Moss	Fairfield Imaging, Ashdown Court, The Square, Forest Row, East Sussex RH18 5EZ, UK
Dr J.M. Polak	Department of Histochemistry, Royal Postgraduate Medical School, DuCane Road, London W12 0NN, UK
Dr R.A. Reynolds	Department of Diagnostic Radiology, Royal Postgraduate Medical School, DuCane Road, London W12 0NN, UK
Dr A. Ruiz-Navarro	Departamento de Biologia Celular, Universidad de Cordoba, Avda. San Alberto Magno, 14004 Cordoba, Spain
Dr M.E. Sherrington	Department of Medical Physics, Royal Postgraduate Medical School, DuCane Road, London W12 0NN, UK
Dr D.R. Springall	Department of Histochemistry, Royal Postgraduate Medical School, DuCane Road, London W12 0NN, UK
Dr G. Terenghi	Blood McIndoe Centre, Queen Victoria Hospital, East Grinstead, Sussex RH19 3DZ, UK
Mr J.G. Weymes	Department of Medical Physics, Royal Postgraduate Medical School, DuCane Road, London W12 0NN, UK
Professor W.F. Whimster	Department of Histopathology, King's College School of Medicine and Dentistry, Denmark Hill, London SE5 8RX, UK
Dr A.K.C. Wong	Department of Systems Design, University of Waterloo, Waterloo, Ontario N2L 3G1, Canada
Professor R. Wootton	Department of Medical Physics, Royal Postgraduate Medical School, DuCane Road, London W12 0NN, UK

Foreword

Modern microscopy is dramatically changing the classical concepts of cell biology and pathology. Both these sciences can now be performed quantitatively, making possible the analysis of biochemical events at the cellular level. This permits the study of these processes on a measurable basis, not only in individual cell types but also in relation to other tissue constituents at the microscopical level.

Image analysis allows pictorial information to be improved for qualitative human interpretation and offers the possibility of extracting quantitative data as well. It is not surprising, therefore, that the combination of modern microscopy with advanced image analysis is rapidly permeating all areas of basic and applied science.

Exciting new avenues for simple and reliable image analysis, as applied to histology and pathology, became evident while we were organizing the current teaching programmes of the Departments of Medical Physics (image analysis) and Histochemistry (modern pathology). It became clear that a single publication gathering together the growing areas of research in the field was not available and that a book of this kind was increasingly in demand, in particular for the MSc course, entitled 'Image Analysis in Histology', taught by the two Departments. This book contains contributions from an impressive list of contributors, many of whom have taught on the MSc course at Hammersmith. It provides both medical and non-medical scientists alike with a comprehensive view of the current problems in image analysis in microscopy.

Julia M. Polak, MD, DSc, FRCPath
Professor and Director of Histochemistry,
Royal Postgraduate Medical School

Acknowledgements

It is a pleasure to acknowledge the help and cooperation of a number of colleagues during the preparation of this text. In particular, I am grateful to Mr Doig Simmonds, the retired Head of Medical Illustration at the Royal Postgraduate Medical School, for his assistance with the artwork.

R.W.

Abbreviations

1-D	One-dimensional
2-D	Two-dimensional
$2\frac{1}{2}$-D	Two and a half-dimensional
3-D	Three-dimensional
4-D	Four-dimensional
5-HT	5-hydroxytryptamine or serotonin
1sTSM	CSLM using one side of one aperture disc
A–D	Analogue to digital
ABC	Avidin–biotin complex
ADC	Analogue to digital convertor
ALU	Arithmetic and logic unit
AOD	Acousto-optic deflection
ASCII	American standard code for information interchange
BHK	Baby hamster kidney
BSP	Binary space partitioning
CCD	Charge coupled device
cDNA	Complementary DNA
CD-ROM	Compact disk, read only memory
CGRP	Calcitonin gene-related peptide
CMY	Cyan, magenta and yellow
CMYK	Cyan, magenta, yellow and black
CPU	Central processing unit
cRNA	Complementary RNA
CRT	Cathode ray tube
CSLM	Confocal scanning laser microscope
CT	Computed tomography
DAC	Digital to analogue convertor
DHT	Dihydrotestosterone
DMA	Direct memory access
DSC	Deterministic similarity criteria
EGA	Enhanced (video) graphics adaptor
ET-1	Endothelin-1
FFT	Fast Fourier transform
FIF	Formaldehyde-induced fluorescence
FITC	Fluoroscein isothiocyanate

FWHM	Full width, half maximum
GIF	Graphics interchange format
GUI	Graphical user interface
HDTV	High definition television
HSV	Hue, saturation and value
IAD	Illuminated aperture diaphragm
IFD	Illuminated field diaphragm
IUR	Isotropic, uniform random
LCD	Liquid crystal display
LCS	Liquid crystal shutter
MIMD	Multiple instruction, multiple datastreams
MISD	Multiple instruction, single datastream
MRI	Magnetic resonance imaging
mRNA	Messenger RNA
MTF	Modulation transfer function
NA	Numerical aperture
NNA	Nearest-neighbour algorithm
NTSC	National Television Systems Commission
PAL	Phase alternating line
PAP	Peroxidase–antiperoxidase
PAS	Periodic acid–Schiff
PBS	Phosphate-buffered saline
PC	Personal computer
PeN	Periventricular nucleus
PET	Positron emission tomography
PK	Proteinase K
PMMA	Polymethylmethacrylate
POMC	Pro-opiomelanocortin
PSF	Point spread function
RAM	Random access memory
RGB	Red, green and blue
RIA	Radioimmunoassay
RISC	Reduced instruction set chip
RLE	Run-length encoding
RMS	Royal Microscopical Society
SA	Specific activity
SCSI	Small computer systems interface
SECAM	Séquential couleur á mémoire
SEM	Scanning electron microscopy
SIMD	Single instruction, multiple datastreams
SISD	Single instruction, single datastream
SIT	Silicon intensified target
SNR	Signal-to-noise ratio
SS	Somatostatin
SSC	Stochastic similarity criteria
SVGA	Super VGA
TEM	Transmission electron microscope
TGA	Targa image format
TH	Tyrosine hydroxylase
TIFF	Tag image file format
TV	Television
TSM	Transmission scanning microscope

USF	Unbiased sampling frame
UTP	Uridine-5′-triphosphate
VGA	Video graphics adaptor
VFF	Visualization file format
VRCSLM	Video rate, confocal scanning laser microscope
WORM	Write once, read many

PART I

Basics

1

Introduction to histological image processing

R. WOOTTON

Introduction

Image processing is a term without exact definition. In the context of histology it usually means the extraction of quantitative information from image data, which often necessitates the prior manipulation of images in a quantitative way. Digital image processing of this kind has been feasible on any real scale only following the availability of cheap and powerful computers during the last 20 years or so. This is evinced by the number of publications in the medical literature concerned with image processing. For example, the total number of publications indexed by the Medline database has risen approximately linearly for the last two decades, roughly doubling in that time to the present rate of nearly 400 000 per year (Fig. 1(a)). The number of publications which include the terms 'image processing' or 'image analysis' has risen exponentially in the same period, and now accounts for about 0.5% of all publications (Fig. 1(b)). Image processing publications concerned with histology (those including the term 'microscopy' or 'histology') have shown a similar inexorable rise: about one-third of all image processing publications in the medical literature now relate to histological work. Whatever the scientific quality of these publications – and as shown below quantitative image processing is more difficult than it first appears – the subject is increasingly popular.

Basic elements

Given the vast choice of computers currently available, it is a pertinent question to enquire what kind of computer is required for image processing? Such a system must comprise elements for:

1 Image input.
2 Image storage.
3 Image manipulation (i.e. processing).
4 Image output.

This configuration is not fundamentally different from that of any more general

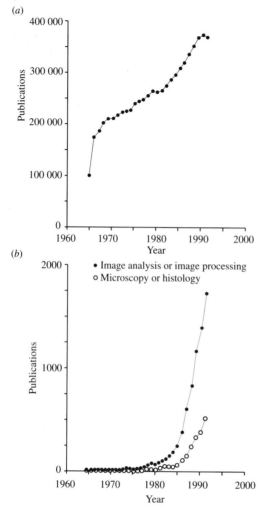

Fig. 1. Number of publications in the medical literature indexed by the Medline database. (*a*) All publications. The apparent plateau during the 1990s is an artefact due to the finite time required before publications appear in the database. (*b*) Publications containing the terms 'image processing' or 'image analysis' and also those containing in addition the terms 'microscopy' or 'histology'.

computer system (for 'image' above, read 'data') but the characteristics of the units in which the data are processed, in particular the sizes of the images, have implications for both the hardware and the software required. Until relatively recently it was usual to design special purpose hardware for the purposes of image processing. However, the continuing increase in computer power, together with the continuing fall in costs, now makes it possible to use a fairly standard digital computer for image processing work. The evolution of the ContextVision computer system illustrates this process very well. The Context-Vision GOP 300 system was launched in the early 1980s. It had a multi-processor architecture, being optimized for image processing, and the design incorporated some novel hardware to give it the necessary speed. Within a few years the company was able to replace certain of the internal processors with industry standard components (actually Sun computers) and at the time of writing the majority of the ContextVision image processing operations can be carried out using a standard Sun computer and software emulation.

This illustrates a second important point, that the hardware and software of computers in general, and image processing systems in particular, are in the course of rapid evolution. It is therefore extremely difficult for the prudent buyer, intent on the purchase of a system whose design is sufficiently mature that technological teething problems will not occur after installation, to obtain a system which will not rapidly become obsolescent. At the present rate of progress, computer systems installed for image processing are often obsolescent within three years and obsolete within five.

Image input

The first stage of any image processing operation is to convert the picture into electrical signals suitable for input into the computer. The image input device may work in real time, performing the conversion on live images, or it may work relatively slowly. Examples of real time devices include television (TV) cameras, and examples of slower devices include scanners that digitize the picture one line at a time in a manner similar to an office facsimile machine. Image capture may take place in monochrome or in colour. For devices such as TV cameras, a device called a framegrabber is used to assemble the image in an intermediate storage area, or frame buffer, from which it can be transmitted to the image processing computer. This avoids problems of synchronization between the camera and the computer.

Whatever the form of the image input device, the choice is heavily influenced by the required image resolution.

Digital image representation

When an image is converted into suitable signals and input to the computer, it is stored as an array of values which represent the original picture. That is, the original picture is decomposed into small picture elements (pixels) and a value representing some characteristic of the image at each element is stored. Fig. 2 shows an example. Although the array of values is almost always rectangular or square, there are certain circumstances when other patterns, such as hexagonal, may be advantageous.

There are two key parameters of the digital representation of an image. The first is the spatial resolution, i.e. the fineness of the mesh into which the image is divided, which controls the fineness with which spatial variations in the image are represented. The second is the corresponding parameter that describes the image at each point. For a monochrome image this is usually called

(a)

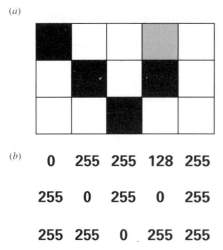

(b)   **0   255   255   128   255**

    255   0   255   0   255

    255   255   0   255   255

Fig. 2. (*a*) A portion of a simple image and (*b*) its digital representation. Black areas in the image are represented by the value zero and white areas by the value 255. Grey areas have intermediate values.

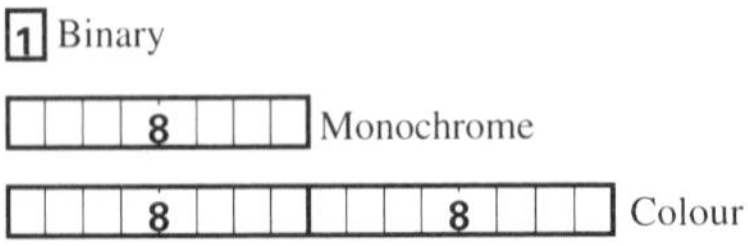

☐ Binary

☐☐☐☐☐ 8 ☐☐☐☐ Monochrome

☐☐☐ 8 ☐☐☐☐☐☐ 8 ☐☐☐ Colour

Fig. 3. Storage requirements for different pixel representations. Binary images require least storage space and, in general, colour images require most.

the greylevel resolution or quantization, i.e. it is the number of greylevels which represent the change from pure black to pure white. For a colour image, account has also to be taken of the spectral properties of the image.

Fig. 3 shows various ways in which each pixel can be represented in the computer. The simplest descriptor of a pixel is to classify it as either black or white, forming a binary image. Each pixel therefore requires a single bit of storage space. More complex, monochrome images are composed from pixels which are various shades of grey ranging from pure black to pure white. Such greyscale images are often quantized to eight bits, a convenient digital storage unit since generally eight bits form a single computer Byte. Colour images require most storage. Some systems represent three colour components, such as the red, green and blue intensities, as three consecutive units of five bits and pack them into a two Byte (or 16-bit) storage unit. Others store the three colour components as consecutive eight-bit Bytes, thus requiring 24 bits in total.

Spatial resolution

Fig. 4 shows the effect of altering the spatial resolution of a monochrome image. The example image is unrecognizable at a spatial resolution of 8×8

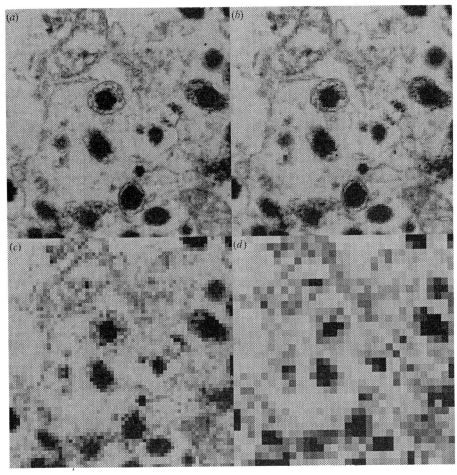

Fig. 4. Effects of altering the spatial resolution. The greylevel image is displayed in (*a*) with 256 × 256 pixels, in (*b*) with 128 × 128, in (*c*) with 64 × 64, and in (*d*) with 32 × 32 pixels.

pixels, but becomes recognizable at about 128 × 128 pixels. This confirms the power of the human eye and brain as an image processing system. For biological work, a resolution of about 512 × 512 pixels is usually adequate, although 1024 × 1024 is preferable. Higher resolutions such as 2048 × 2048 are necessary for more demanding applications such as digital radiography (Takahashi *et al.*, 1992), but have obvious cost implications.

Quantization

Fig. 5 shows the effect on the resulting image of altering quantization levels at a given spatial resolution. For monochrome images in biological work, about 256 greylevels (which can be represented in eight bits) are generally adequate.

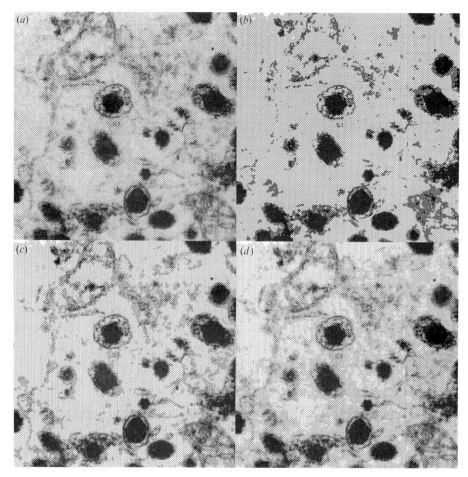

Fig. 5. Effects of altering the quantization or greylevels. The greylevel image is displayed in (a) with 256 greylevels, in (b) with 4, in (c) with 8, and in (d) with 16 greylevels.

More demanding applications such as digital radiography require ten bits (Takahashi *et al.*, 1992), even though the human eye does not have the ability to distinguish such a large number of greylevels.

Image quality

The examples above of the effects on image quality of varying the spatial resolution and quantization treat each parameter in isolation. As might be expected, however, image quality is affected by both parameters, the 'best' images being obtained by combinations of the higher resolutions and quantizations. The notion of image 'quality' is itself not easy to define, and also depends to some extent on the use to which the image is being put (Sharp, 1990). Experiments show that for images with a large amount of detail, relatively few greylevels are required in comparison with less detailed images (Gonzalez & Wintz, 1987; Hillman *et al.*, 1990). For histological work in monochrome, images of 512×512 pixels and 256 greylevels are generally satisfactory.

Image storage

In principle any device which can be used for storing computer data can be used for storing images. However, digital images are often fairly large in conventional computing terms. For example, an image of 1024×1024 pixels, each of 16 bits, will require 2 MBytes of storage space; 50 such images, e.g. from a confocal microscope dataset, would require 100 MBytes. The choice of device is therefore dictated by the total storage space required (i.e. principally by cost) and also the required access speed. Magnetic tape, which is extremely cheap per unit of information stored, is little used because of the length of time required to access information on the tape. Access to information stored in solid state memory, or RAM, is virtually instantaneous, but on the other hand it is the most expensive storage medium. Fig. 6 illustrates the point. In practice, disk technology is most often chosen as a reasonable compromise.

Image processing

In general terms, the choice of hardware for image processing is not particularly important: a more expensive processor is simply likely to perform faster than a cheaper model. What is crucial is the choice of software. This is because it is extremely unusual to be able to operate an image processing system in practice without resort to programming it. The manufacturer's supplied software almost inevitably needs alterations of either minor or major nature to suit the local conditions. It is important therefore that such programming can be carried out easily.

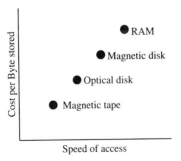

Fig. 6. Price and performance for various image storage devices.

Image output

An image processing system requires at least one device for image output, usually a TV-type display, known as a monitor. Some method for producing 'hard copy', for example a printer, is also common. Such output devices may be monochrome or colour, the choice not being especially critical in most applications, but being dictated largely by considerations of cost.

Monitors may be capable of displaying images in monochrome or colour, although for histological work the latter is more common. A typical display screen resolution is 512×512 pixels, although 1024×1024 and intermediate sizes based on personal computer (PC) standards, are increasingly being used. Both monochrome and colour images are usually displayed by use of a software lookup table. This is simply an area of computer memory in which a conversion table is stored for the purposes of translating the value of each pixel in real time as it is being displayed. The process of display is thus to convert each pixel value according to the lookup table, before feeding the converted value (through a digital to analogue converter) to the appropriate colour gun of the display tube. This is a much more efficient method of applying transformations to an image than changing the pixel values themselves. For example, alterations to the brightness or contrast of an image only require a new lookup table, rather than computation of a complete new image.

Human vision

The purpose of much of image processing is to assist the observer in interpreting the content of an image, very often in a quantitative way. An understanding of the basic visual-perception process is therefore helpful. In terms of image acquisition, the human eye is far superior to any camera yet developed. It can adapt to a range of light intensities spanning ten orders of magnitude, from the scotopic threshold at the low end to the glare limit at the high end. This huge dynamic range is far greater than that of any camera. However, the human visual system cannot operate over the entire range simultaneously and at any given ambient brightness level actually has a more limited range. This is called brightness adaptation.

The lens at the front of the eye serves to focus an image of the outside scene onto the retina at the back of the eye. The retina contains two classes of photoreceptor cells, called cones and rods. The cones are responsible for bright vision and there are six or seven million of them, located principally in the central region of the retina known as the fovea. Each cone is connected to the brain by its own nerve. The cones are highly sensitive to colour. Cone vision is known as photopic or bright level vision.

The rods are sensitive to light intensity, but not to colour. They have nerve endings and serve to give an overall picture of the image. There are many more rods than cones, perhaps 100 million or so, and they are distributed across the whole retina. In dim light, when the cones do not operate, the rods produce a monochromatic, greylevel image. This is known as scotopic, or dim light vision. The rods are so exquisitely sensitive that they can signal the absorption of a single photon.

The brightness perceived by the eye is a logarithmic function of intensity. A small increase at low light levels is therefore perceived as equal to a large increase in bright intensity.

Colour

Histological images are commonly acquired in colour. Human colour perception is extremely complex and as yet incompletely understood. It appears, however, that the cones are of three types which preferentially absorb light in one region of the visible spectrum, either at long, medium or short wavelengths. This is because the cones contain light sensitive pigments which respond either to red, green or blue light. Absence of one or more of the pigments results in colour blindness: red-blindness, for example, affects the ability to distinguish red and green.

Similar methods allow good colour images to be produced by computers. Such colour images are often produced by the superimposition of three primary images, one displayed in red, one in green and one in blue. This is the so-called RGB system. As is well known, almost all possible colours can be produced in this way.

RGB technology is common, because of its wide use in TV cameras and monitors. Processing colour information stored in the form of RGB images is not, however, the most efficient method. There can be significant computational gains in processing images stored in other formats, such as the HSV (hue, saturation and value) form – see Chapter 3.

Principal steps

The principal steps in the analysis of an image are usually considered to be:

1 Image capture.
2 Segmentation.
3 Measurement.

Image acquisition has been dealt with above. Segmentation is discussed briefly below, and in more detail in Chapter 13. Image measurements are also discussed briefly below, while Chapter 5 covers the subject more thoroughly.

Segmentation

Segmentation is the process of dividing an image into meaningful regions. In a simple case, one may wish to separate the object of interest from the image background. In a more general case, such as that shown in Fig. 7, there may be several objects of interest. An elementary technique for carrying out this separation is thresholding, which, in a monochrome image, is based on the greylevel information.

In an ideal case (Fig. 8(a)), a histogram of the greylevels in an image will show two well-separated peaks, corresponding to the greylevels in the object and the background. It is then a straightforward matter to choose a threshold value such that pixels below it can be considered to represent the background and those above it to represent the object of interest. In real life, however (Fig. 8(b)), there is almost always overlap and more sophisticated methods are required (see, for example, Niblack, 1986; Boyle & Thomas, 1988). Such

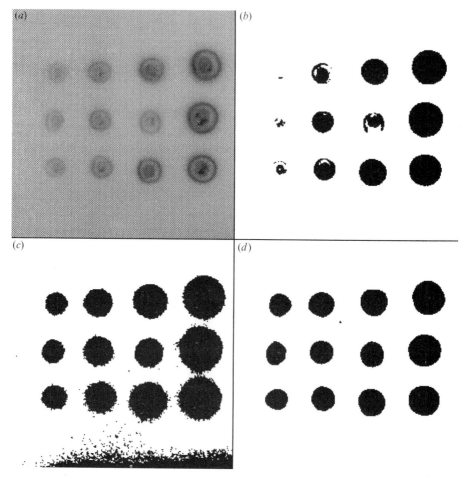

Fig. 7. Separation of objects of interest from the background. The original image is shown in (a). The result of applying a high threshold (173) is shown in (b) and a lower threshold (147) in (c). In order to delineate the features of interest more accurately, a more complex procedure than simple thresholding is required. The result of applying an edge-based detection procedure is shown in (d). Data courtesy of J.R. Jagoe.

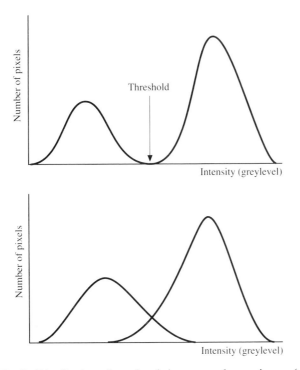

Fig. 8. Distribution of greylevels in a monochrome image (*a*) idealised (*b*) reality.

methods may depend, for example, on identifying certain features in the objects of interest, such as their edges (see Chapter 14).

Measurement and classification

Quantitative measurement is usually the ultimate goal of histological image processing. Once the image has been segmented into objects of interest, measurements can be made on the objects. Examples of measurements commonly made include:

1 Area, A.
2 Perimeter, P.
3 Compactness, often known as *P2A*. This is defined as $P^2/(4\pi A)$. A perfectly circular object has a *P2A* value of 1; as the shape of the object departs from circularity, *P2A* increases.
4 Length of the object when projected onto either x or y axes.
5 Diameter of the circle of equivalent area.
6 Centre of gravity, i.e. if the object were cut from a sheet of thin card, the point at which it would balance.
7 Moment of inertia.

Given such measurements a further stage is sometimes to use them for classification. For example, Fig. 9(*a*) shows six types of object which the

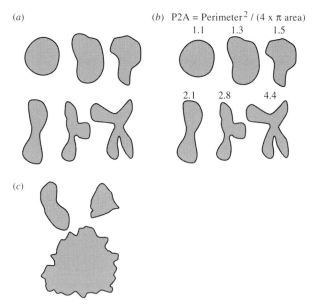

Fig. 9. Classification. (a) Six different objects, for example the boundaries of six different types of cell. (b) The result of measuring *P2A*. (c) Three unknown objects for classification. Although they are of fairly different shape, they all have the same value of *P2A*.

human might consider to be different. They might perhaps represent the boundaries of six different types of cells. Can suitable measurements be made which will differentiate them? It is important to realise that an infinity of possible measurements exists, so that the answer must be yes. In this case a very simple measure such as the ratio of the perimeter to the area (*P2A*) will separate them adequately (Fig. 9(*b*)).

This is an example of retrospective classification. More usually, one is interested in the question whether, having identified a suitable measurement it can be used prospectively to classify an unknown object. This is a much more difficult matter. Fig. 9(*c*) shows three objects of apparently different shape, yet all have identical *P2A* values and would therefore be classified as members of the same type of cells. The selection of the appropriate measure is therefore crucial. Fig. 10(*a*) shows a deceptively simple case in which only two classes exist, normal and abnormal. The aim is to assign the unknown object to the category to which it most closely belongs. Unfortunately, depending on which measurement is chosen, it is possible to allocate the unknown object to either class (Fig. 10(*b*)).

Measurement of stained area

A common, and apparently simple, requirement in histological image processing is the measurement of stained area. Fig. 11 shows two images. There are

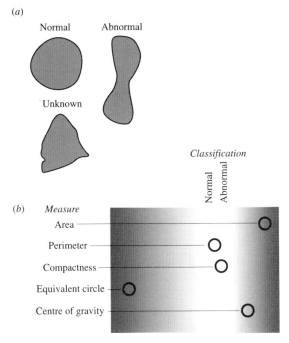

Fig. 10. Classification. (*a*) The normal and abnormal objects with an unknown to be allocated to the category to which it most closely belongs. (*b*) Results of classifying the unknown object by different measures. Depending on which measure is chosen, the object can be considered to be normal, or extremely abnormal.

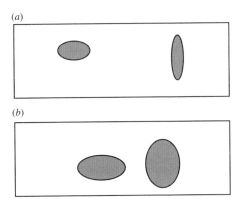

Fig. 11. Measurement of stained area. Within image measurements may be required (*a*), or between image comparisons (*a* and *b*).

two cases: one may wish to measure the area stained in a single image as a percentage of the total area of the image, i.e. to make a within image measurement; or one may wish to compare the area stained in the two images, i.e. to make a between image measurement. Unfortunately this is not as straightforward as it first appears, since there are a large number of factors which can affect the measurement. These include:

1 Thickness and uniformity of the sections. Clearly a change in the thickness of a section will alter the light transmitted through it, and thus the greylevels recorded by the image input system. Section thickness should therefore be constant within a given section, and should also be the same for all sections involved in a given measurement.

2 Colour and uniformity of the stain. Similarly, the characteristics of the staining must be constant: colour changes must not occur within or between sections.

3 Uniformity and stability of the illumination. Unless active steps are taken to prevent it occurring, there may be quite marked variations in the overall level of illumination of a given section due to fluctuations in mains power. The solution is a stabilized power supply for the light source. In addition, the illumination may be uneven across a given image. A microscope field with variations in illumination of up to 50% from one side to another can appear quite uniform to the human eye; differences of this magnitude will cause major problems for an image processing system. Finally, many TV cameras are extremely sensitive to infra-red radiation, so that blocking filters should be used to avoid artefacts in the image due to the lamp.

4 Image noise. Noise in the image may be due to various factors. For example, dust on the lens of the image capture device may degrade the image. This can be almost imperceptible to the human observer, yet create major problems for subsequent computer processing.

5 Precision and accuracy of the input digitization. The 'quality' of the images captured must be sufficient for the required measurements to be feasible.

6 Image magnification. A between image comparison must be made at the same magnification or, if this is not possible, an appropriate correction must be made.

Measurement of stained area is a deceptively simple image processing operation. In fact, there are a number of potential pitfalls. As is the case in radioactive work therefore, it is preferable to try to make relative measurements where possible, rather than attempting to make absolute measurements. A key principle, which underlies any image processing measurement, is that a method for validating the results by some independent technique should always be attempted.

Common pitfalls

Experience shows that there are a number of common pitfalls in histological image analysis. These can be summarized as follows:

1 If the human eye cannot see the feature of interest in the image, then the computer is most unlikely to be able to detect it. That is, no amount of computer processing will elicit information which is not present in the original image to start with.

2 Image 'analysis' is really a misnomer in practice. A term that better describes what computers can do in the present state of the art is image 'processing', since commercial systems for histological work cannot yet deliver any significant degree of artificial intelligence.

3 When purchasing an image processing computer system a large image store should be specified. In practice, images expand to fill (or overfill) the storage space available.

4 Despite what salespeople say, there is no such thing as a 'turnkey' system. Purchase of an image processing system should therefore be made with a view to ease of the subsequent programming that will inevitably be required to tailor it for real images.

5 Apparently quantitative image processing is almost always to some extent subjective. For example, for any given operation there are a very large number of possible algorithms to choose from and no definitive criteria on which to base a choice.

6 Absolute measurements on an image are difficult to make. It is preferable to make measurements relative to a standard. Absolute measurements involving colour images are especially difficult and require careful choice of camera and attention to calibration and quality control.

Advantages of image processing

Despite the rather negative tone of much of the foregoing, there can be significant advantages in image processing. These include:

1 Enhancement. If suitable measurements have been made it is often possible to compensate for deficiencies in the images, due, for example to variations in staining or illumination where these are unavoidable.

2 Quantification. When used properly, the techniques of image processing are capable of yielding accurate quantitative results from images.

3 Consistency. Any computer based technique is likely *a priori* to be more consistent in operation than one depending on human judgement. Image processing is no exception and careful measurements show that variability between human observers can be far higher than other sources of variation in histological image processing (Jagoe *et al.*, 1991).

4 Speed of operation. In principle, measurement by computer should be much faster than making the same measurements by hand. In practice, it is sometimes difficult to realise the potential speed advantage of computerised image processing, because of the length of time software development requires, and because of the difficulties of automating image selection procedures.

5 Non-stop operation. One virtue of machines in comparison with humans is their potential for continuous operation. However, in order to realize this potential in histological image processing, it is necessary to understand that producing the requisite software is only one of the steps. Systems for automatically presenting large numbers of slides for analysis, and for their automatic focussing, are still relatively crude and relatively expensive.

References

Boyle, R. D. & Thomas, R. C. (1988). *Computer Vision. A First Course*. Oxford: Blackwell Scientific Publications.

Gonzalez, R. C. & Wintz, P. (1987). *Digital Image Processing*. Reading, MA: Addison-Wesley.

Hillman, D. E., Llinas, R. R., Canaday, M. & Mahoney G. (1990). Concepts and methods of image acquisition, frame processing, and image data presentation. In *Three-Dimensional Neuroimaging*, ed. A. W. Toga, pp. 3–38. New York: Raven Press.

Jagoe, R., Steel, J. H., Vucicevic, V, Alexander, N., Van Noorden, S., Wootton, R. & Polak, J. M. (1991). Observer variation in quantification of immunocytochemistry by image analysis. *Histochemical Journal*, **23**, 541–547.

Niblack, W. (1986). *An Introduction to Digital Image Processing*. London: Prentice Hall International.

Sharp, P. F. (1990). Quantifying image quality. *Clinical Physics and Physiological Measurement*, **11** (Supplement A), 21–26.

Takahashi, M., Ueno, S., Tsuchigame, T., Higashida, Y., Hirata, Y., Moribe, N., Takada, T., Kamiya, M. & Koike, K. (1992). Development of a 2,048 × 2,048 pixel image intensifier-TV digital radiography system. Basic imaging properties and clinical application. *Investigative Radiology*, **27**, 898–907.

2

Hardware and software for image processing

M. E. SHERRINGTON

Introduction

The term image processing is often misleading and in many cases image databasing would be more accurate. That is, the processing actually comprises the routine acquisition and the indexing or linking of images, with a minimal degree of processing proper in between.

The majority of image processing computer systems are variations on a common generic model, as illustrated in Fig. 1. Most designers have opted for

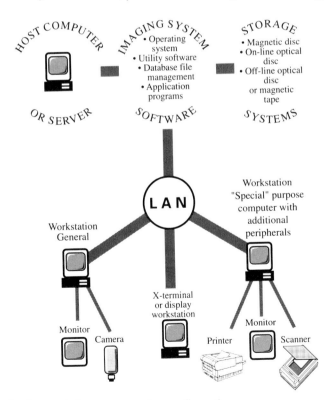

Fig. 1. A generic image processing configuration.

an 'open architecture', where in principle the components of the system are interchangeable. In practice this interchangeability is less than perfect, but the ability to mix elements from different vendors is marked compared with conventional data processing systems. This is due in part to the simplicity of the generic configuration and its elemental components.

Workstations

Image processing workstations hardly differ from their data processing equivalents. The principal difference, at least for workstations which are used for image acquisition, is the addition of a framegrabber board attached to a camera or scanner. Another difference is the presence of larger display monitors to accommodate the images. In IBM style personal computers (PCs), ordinary monitors of video graphics adaptor (VGA) or enhanced graphics adaptor (EGA) standard are often used. Unix workstations tend to be supplied with 19-inch monitors giving typical resolutions of 1200 pixels by 800 lines. In addition the PC or workstation used for image processing is likely to require extra memory (RAM), in order to manipulate images without the need to store them temporarily on magnetic disk.

Storage

Until recently, large image files were stored on optical disk, most of which were 30 cm in diameter, holding up to 1 GigaByte (GByte) of data. Early disk systems were only capable of write-once storage, so that, although data files could be rewritten, the disk space originally occupied by them was not recoverable. With current optical disks, image files can be erased and the space reclaimed. On-line access to large image datasets can be achieved via a jukebox containing as many as 50 disks in a carousel arrangement. In principle there is no reason why similar systems could not be made available using the smaller CD-ROMs, but other commercial considerations are currently preventing the sale of writable CDs.

At the time of writing, large conventional magnetic Winchester disks are being introduced (in excess of 2 GBytes capacity) that may herald the demise of optical disk storage. It now seems likely that the dramatic reductions in the prices of PCs and workstations that have occurred in the last few years are to be mirrored in the prices of magnetic disks.

Servers

Many systems are supported by relatively large central processors that function as fileservers. These may contain large quantities of rewritable disk storage (10–20 GBytes) that are available to all image processing workstations simultaneously. A consequence of such an arrangement is that the users may work on different computers on the network at various times and still be able to access any and all of their image data.

Networks

Local area network technologies such as ethernet and token ring require little modification for an image processing environment. However, where large amounts of data are frequently transmitted over the network the overall bandwidth and network topology needs careful consideration. It is possible to convert from copper to optical fibre as the transmission medium, but in small installations this may be an expensive option. Advances expected in the near future are likely to be in the speed and capacity of wide area networks, so that eventually an image workstation in the UK will be able to access image databases stored in Europe and the USA at rates little different from those of the local network.

Software

Software for routine image acquisition, indexing and access has been all but perfected and most of it will link easily with applications software to meet the particular requirements of a user. In essence it is the applications software and the problems to which this is to be directed that differentiate one type of image processing system from another, and this is the question addressed next.

Image processing classification

After the acquisition of a digital image it is normally necessary to perform some kind of analysis on it in order to glean the information sought. The type of analysis and the ability to perform it automatically, semi-automatically or (largely) manually dictates the class of image processing that can be performed. As yet, surprisingly few problems can be tackled without some manual intervention on the part of the user. The current challenge to image processing systems is to extend this class, as well as to break into the relatively uncharted area of computer vision.

By convention image processing problems are classified according to 'level', being termed low level or high level largely on the basis of the analysis required.

Low level image processing

Low level image processing is concerned with operations on individual picture elements (pixels) in order to improve overall the quality of the image. Such operations are now well understood and the algorithmic approach has been extensively researched (Rosenfeld & Kak, 1982; Niblack, 1986; Gonzalez &

Wintz, 1987; Schalkoff, 1989; Low, 1991). The tasks normally possess the following features:

1 The size of the output (processed) image is the same as the size of the input image.
2 Identical operations are applied to all pixels of the input image.
3 The computation involves only those pixels in the local neighbourhood of each individual pixel.

Typical problems in this area are noise removal, edge detection, geometric correction, feature extraction and object segmentation.

Noise removal

Removing noise from an image can often be achieved by making some simple assumptions about the character of the noise and the nature of the uncorrupted image. For instance, it is often reasonable to assume that the noise is distributed with zero mean so that pixel greylevel values are distorted randomly above and below their true values.

Simple smoothing techniques based on weighted averages within a neighbourhood of the pixel suffice to provide noise reduction (Gonzalez & Wintz, 1987; Huang *et al.*, 1979). In other cases, noise may manifest itself as spikes, i.e. very small areas, perhaps only one pixel in extent, which are significantly corrupt. This is termed speckle. Use of smoothing to remove speckle results in too great a loss of contrast. Speckle removal is normally carried out by applying a frequency domain approach to produce a low pass filter (Dainty, 1975). Computationally this is a much more demanding process than simple windowing.

Edge detection

Primitive edge detection attempts to determine whether an edge (a component of a boundary in the image) passes through or near to a given pixel. This can be done by examining the rate of change of intensity near the pixel, sharp changes being evidence of an edge and slow changes suggesting the converse. Methods due to Roberts (1965), Sobel (Davis, 1975) and Prewitt (1970) are typical of this approach.

The search for reliable edge detectors still remains an active area for research (Pratt, 1972), being a necessary prerequisite to a more detailed analysis of the information contained within an image.

Geometric correction

The acquisition system employed in image capture frequently introduces distortions. This can often be neglected when dealing with an individual image.

However, in the case of a set of images that correspond either to an individual scene captured a number of times or to several slices through a three-dimensional (3-D) volume, it is often necessary to apply corrections to over-come geometric distortion. These methods usually rely on the existence of known tie points in the images that are to be overlaid, since they are considered fixed relative to each other (Pratt, 1972; Karara, 1989). These tie points are placed in the same positions for each image. Processing is then necessary to recalculate all the other pixel greylevels by interpolation; this can be an extremely computationally intensive task.

Feature extraction

A feature is any type of measurement in an image that can be used in characterization or classification. The human eye is capable of detecting features such as texture, connectivity, parity and subtle degrees of contrast in an image, and is capable of filtering out extraneous information in accessing such features. This is also the aim of feature extraction.

A variety of approaches apply to the normal image and to its transform in the frequency domain (Brigham, 1974; Chen, 1982; Banks, 1990; Low, 1991). The results are normally expressed as a frequency vector which serves to parameterize the image by deriving a set of values for any quantifiable aspects. It is assumed that images with similar frequency vectors may be categorized together.

Object segmentation

In the process of segmentation, pixels are grouped to form higher level regional structures in an image. The simplest methods employ the greylevel histogram and thresholding techniques (Chow & Kaneko, 1972). Other approaches are based on edge detection (Canny, 1986) or on regional approaches (Tuceran, Jain & Lee, 1988) that attempt segmentation of the image through regional similarities, such as texture. A good quantitative summary is to be found in Zenzo (1983). Especially difficult cases arise when one object partially masks a second. Whereas the human observer has little difficulty in segmenting such an image, computer systems are unable to do so with anything approaching the same facility.

High level image processing

The example above illustrates some of the problems confronting researchers in attempting to extend the scope of image processing to domains where human intervention is currently required. This work is termed high level image processing or computer/machine vision.

In computer vision the aim is to 'make sense' of the overall image in a fashion that mirrors the way in which humans perceive the world. Low level techniques for object segmentation are obviously essential but computer vision is more than merely recognition: it is necessary to build meaningful and explicit descriptions of the types of objects detected in an image and to allow for the fact that the actual object seen will be a specific instance of a general type. For example we have a concept of the type 'chair' based on certain attributes, which allows us to say that a certain object is a chair immediately on sighting it.

A vision system therefore needs to possess a basic knowledge system to apply to the kinds of objects it sees. In addition it must be able to make inferences using the knowledge base to achieve an understanding of the scene being processed. This poses problems both in the way that the knowledge is stored and retrieved and in the processing power required by such a system in order to reach meaningful conclusions at speeds approaching real time. Indeed Lighthill's report on artificial intelligence (Lighthill, 1973) pointed out the difficulties that would arise from the use of sequential computation; it is only now that these difficulties are being confronted.

The essential difference between low level and high level processing is that in the latter the image is no longer considered merely as a collection of pixels. More convenient data structures need to be sought to represent the features of an image as a set of parametric measures.

Since the early 1980s growth in machine vision research has been rapid (Winston, 1975; Boyle & Thomas, 1988; Freeman, 1988; Schalkoff, 1989; Low, 1991). This is partly due to work on the following topics:

1 Certain problems in computing are hard to solve by current means even though they are simple for a human.
2 A large number of problems in the field of image processing are, in this sense, difficult.

Examples include filling in missing information in a scene, recognizing handwriting, and detecting the connectivity or parity of an object. To tackle such problems radical changes in the way that computers are designed, operated and programmed are necessary. Recent developments in computer hardware indicate that such new approaches will in fact be possible in the future and are considered further at the end of this chapter.

Major system components

Returning to current conventional, digital image processing systems, the basic components that are necessary in all systems can be summarized as follows:

1 A means of acquiring images from a variety of sources.
2 A means of converting image data into a computable form and a means of storing it.
3 A means of processing acquired data with the host computer or special peripheral processors.

4 Software for the processors.

5 A means of displaying the images.

6 Other specialist devices, such as those for producing hardcopies of images.

The first four components merit further discussion as they can significantly affect the choice and performance of the image processing system. The last two components, being on the downstream side of the processing, affect only the results; they can normally therefore be upgraded at a later stage if required.

Image acquisition

One measure of the information contained in an image is its definition. The number of lines per frame is important but so too is the rate at which the intensity can vary along each line. A third factor which needs to be considered is the range of intensity levels that an image can take at any pixel. Image acquisition usually takes place via a video camera or digitizer. Cameras fall into two broad classes: thermionic and solid state (see Chapter 3).

A cheap and effective thermionic device is the vidicon tube (van Wezel, 1987). This consists of an evacuated glass tube, one end of which (the target) is coated internally with a photosensitive layer. Inherent in such device are several distorting factors:

1 The target has a tendency to suffer from image persistence.

2 The target does not have a linear performance over the entire spectrum, certain colours producing brighter images than others.

3 The image can become permanently burnt onto the target.

4 Spatial accuracy can be impaired because the deflection coils do not produce a completely linear scan of the target.

These problems can be solved by using more costly devices such as the image orthicon tube, but cameras based on solid state technology such as the charge coupled device (CCD) are now preferred (see Chapter 3).

Charge coupled devices consist of a two-dimensional (2-D) array of photo-sensitive elements each of which produces an analogue output proportional to the amount of light incident on it. The elements act like a shift register of capacitors, each holding a charge proportional to the incident light upon it. CCDs have advantages over thermionic devices in all the areas mentioned above as well as in power consumption and sensitivity.

In addition to image acquisition by video cameras, an increasing number of mechanical scanners are becoming available. These generally have the properties of being able to capture a large, flat, static image with considerable accuracy. Mechanical scanners may be handheld or fixed, with the paper being fed through the body of the scanner or the scanner moving over the paper. Resolution varies from 100–1000 dots per inch (4–40 dots/mm). Some scanners have a single row of CCDs (typically 2048) that can collect intensity values without any internal movement for a single row of pixels. Other scanners have a single photosensitive device that mechanically scans the paper.

The main problems associated with scanners are that only a still image can be captured and that, because of their mechanical operation, reliability is inevitably forfeited. Nevertheless, as the office facsimile machine shows, scanning is in certain circumstances a cheap and accurate alternative to image capture by still camera.

Digitization techniques

The output from a camera conforms to a video standard, typically being a composite video or RGB signal. This is acquired by a device called a framegrabber, which converts the analogue electrical signals to a frame of digital pixels. The framegrabber usually comprises a single integrated circuit (or chip) with a number of associated memory chips to store the captured frame. Some of the cheaper framegrabbers use the memory of the computer to hold the frame; others contain sufficient memory of their own to hold a series of frames.

The memory in which a frame is stored is called the frame buffer. A frame buffer should be large enough to store at least one digitized image. This is usually 512×512 or 1024×1024 pixels. The frame buffer can be updated in real time and its contents transferred to the memory of the host computer at any chosen instant. In addition, the memory of the frame buffer can be used to drive a display monitor.

Digitization in real time (i.e. at video rate) is possible with a framegrabber given appropriate hardware. Any study involving motion in images will require real time digitization. For static images it is possible to digitize vertical slices of the field and transfer them directly to the host computer memory via a parallel connection.

The host computer system

The trend to cheaper host computers has been accelerating recently with the introduction of ever more powerful hardware chips at low cost coupled with dramatic reductions in memory prices. At the low end, IBM-standard PCs based on Intel 486/50 processors with Super VGA (SVGA) displays are an especially attractive option, particularly because of the variety of third party hardware available for the PC. The workstation market is now dominated by the reduced instruction set (RISC) processor, with the newly emerging super-scalar chips appearing likely to have a dramatic impact. The common factor in virtually all the commercially available systems is that they are based on the so-called 'von Neumann' architecture which has dominated computer design since the 1950s. This is now termed the SISD (single instruction, single datastream) architecture to differentiate it from other architectures which are discussed below.

The SISD machines include those of all the leading manufacturers, IBM (PC), Apple (Macintosh), DEC (VAX), Sun and SGI (Unix workstations) etc. More exotic architectures are available only in essentially research based systems. However, it is to be expected that systems based on these technologies will be introduced commercially in the near future.

The choice of host computer for an image processing system involves numerous decisions. In practice it will almost always be necessary to compromise. For example, it is necessary to decide whether the system is essentially for research or for production use, and whether it is to be dedicated to a few specific tasks or to several general ones. Also it has to be decided whether the system is required to support both batch and interactive modes of processing, whether it will be used to process largely 2-D or 3-D datasets and whether high speed graphics are required. Because it is almost always necessary to compromise, the *absolute* requirements should be specified at the outset, to ensure that these, at least, are met. Some features that should be considered are listed in the next section.

Software

It is often said that software sells hardware, although nowadays the trend to portability between different hardware platforms has made this less true than in the past. However there is little point in investing in an expensive system if you cannot get the required software to run on it.

In assessing the merits of any software package the following questions are important:

1 Functionality.
   - does it possess a wide range of processing operations?
   - are these sufficient for the tasks to be performed?
   - are morphological processes supported?
   - is colour processing/lookup table manipulation supported?
2 Flexibility.
   - how well does the package integrate with other software?
   - can commands be strung together as 'macros'?
   - is there a learning method to record macros?
   - can the software support a wide variety of image formats?
   - can data be processed in both real and complex format?
3 Extendability.
   - if a particular function is absent, can the package be extended to include it?
   - is it possible to customize the menu systems (if any)?
   - is the system likely to evolve to take account of current trends?
   - is there an extensive library of software?
   - how easy is software development going to be?

4 Hardware support.
   — what peripherals can be attached to the system?
   — can it interact with image capture devices?
   — can it drive devices such as plotters and postscript printers?
5 User interface.
   — is the user interface logical and consistent?
   — is it command oriented, menu driven or a hybrid?
   — does it operate under a Graphical User Interface (GUI)?
   — is help information available on line?
6 Documentation.
   — what is the standard of the user documentation?
   — are technical manuals available?

Deciding between different image processing software

It is a truism that all image processing software appears to be excellent when demonstrated by a salesperson. If this is not the case then the software should definitely not be purchased. If an expensive software package is seriously being considered, how should you proceed? Below are a few simple rules:

1 Ask for an evaluation copy or, better still, visit the vendor and try out the system in person.
2 See if you are left alone to your attempts and how well you are able to proceed using the documentation provided.
3 Take some of your own images along. Never rely on the supposedly typical images provided by the vendor.
4 Find out how long the product has been available, what is its current revision level and how often it is revised.
5 Find out how large the customer base is and ask for details of installations in your area.
6 Do not be over-impressed by what software can do. The chances are that competitive products can do the same.

What you must try to assess is whether this particular software can do it better, quicker, etc. In addition you must judge if it fits in with the way your image processing group operates and whether you feel you will get good support from the vendor. If the package is satisfactory in all respects, and you can afford to do so, then buy it!

Exotic architectures

The von Neumann (SISD) model of computers has no concept of parallel processing: all operations are carried out in a series of sequential steps. Other than building even faster processors, another means for increasing CPU performance must be found. This involves distributing the computational load between several processors. Until recently increasing the performance of SISD machines has been relatively cheap due to rapidly developing technologies. However fundamental physical limits are now being reached and this makes the development of multi-processor systems much more attractive.

Many low level image processing tasks are highly parallel. Owing to their spatial nature they can be implemented on machines with massively parallel, spatially orientated architecture (Unger, 1958). However, intermediate and high level computer vision tasks are not wholly spatially orientated and scepticism has been expressed about the use of such machines for solving low level image processing problems.

Massively parallel computers may have many thousands of individual processors. Examples of this class of machines are University College London's cellular logic image processors (CLIP) (Duff, 1978; Fountain, Matthews & Duff, 1988), AMT's distributed array processors (DAP) (Reddaway, 1979), Goodyear's massive parallel processor (MPP) (Batcher, 1980; Potter, 1985) and Thinking Machine's Connection Machine (CM) (Hillis, 1985).

Various classification systems have been proposed for the recent proliferation of parallel processing technologies. Flynn (1972) categorizes computers into four major types:

1 SISD. Single instruction, single datastream. As previously stated this is the traditional von Neumann computer architecture.
2 SIMD. Single instruction, multiple datastreams. Processors act synchronously to execute instruction on their local data. This includes the 'spatially' orientated processors mentioned above such as CLIP, DAP and MPP.
3 MISD. Multiple instruction, single datastream. Multiple processors act autonomously, executing different instructions on the same datum. There is speculation whether such an architecture is realizable in practice (Hwang & Briggs, 1985) but developments in superscalar, pipeline processors fit closest to this classification.
4 MIMD. Multiple instruction, multiple datastreams. Multiple processors act autonomously, each executing a different set of instructions on their own local data. Synchronization between processors is achieved by passing messages via an interconnection network or by accessing data in a shared memory area (Pease, 1977; Feldman, 1985).

For a full discussion of image processing on parallel machines the reader is referred to the comprehensive text by Hussain (1991).

Artificial neural networks

The emergence of parallel computers poses the question how such machines are to be programmed. Current programming languages were developed for the SISD architecture and in general fit easily on the new computing engines.

While some hope is offered by the development of more intricate multitasking operating systems and by the introduction of new languages such as OCCAM (May, 1983), the means to program these computers efficiently is still far from clear.

It is often argued that to tackle computationally difficult problems, including those involving vision systems, it is necessary not only to emulate the parallelism within the brain at the hardware level but also to mimic the computational processes that are performed in biological systems. This has given rise to a renewed interest in developing systems that can be taught rather than programmed. Many workers claim that these are the only practical way to make real progress in the field of high level computer vision. Such systems are termed artificial neural networks. Initial work in the 1960s led to the development of systems based on the Perceptron (Rosenblatt, 1958), but this was discredited by Minsky and Papert (1969) who showed that such a network would not be able to distinguish between many simple patterns. Work effectively ceased for 15 years until Hinton, Ackley & Sejnowski (1984) introduced the concept of the Boltzmann machine. Recent Perceptron-like devices such as WISARD have been shown to be good at pattern discrimination (Aleksander, Thomas & Bowden, 1984).

Work on artificial neural networks requires a multidisciplinary approach, combining elements of mathematics, computing and neuropsychology. Both the PDP group (Rumelhart & McClelland, 1986), and Steven Grossberg and co-workers (Grossberg, 1988; Carpenter & Grossberg, 1989) have been especially productive in this area. Also worthy of mention is the work by Kohonen on associative memory (Kohonen, 1988). For an introduction to neural computing the reader is referred to the text by Aleksander and Morton (1990).

Conclusions

In assessing where image processing stands at present it is perhaps pertinent to ask where it will be going in the near future. Progress in image processing will depend on developments in three areas:

1 Semiconductor technology.
2 Computer architecture.
3 Artificial intelligence techniques and algorithms.

After 30 years of research and development the question should be addressed: what are the major problems still to be solved to produce more varied and robust applications? Indeed, progress in image processing has been slow compared to other branches of computational science such as hardware design, compiler technology and computer graphics. Advances have been the result of developments in support technologies rather than developments in the image processing field itself. In essence the same type of operations are being performed as 10 years ago, only somewhat more quickly and more cheaply.

Arguably what is required is a general purpose computer vision system; certainly it cannot be built at present.

References

Aleksander, I. & Morton H. (1990). *An Introduction to Neural Computing*. London: Chapman and Hall.

Aleksander, I., Thomas, W. & Bowden P. (1984). WISARD, a radical new step forward in image recognition. *Sensor Reviews*, 120–4.

Banks, S. (1990). *Signal Processing, Image Processing & Pattern Recognition*. New York: Prentice-Hall.

Batcher, K. E. (1980). Design of a massively parallel processor. *IEEE Transactions on Computers*, C-29(9), 836–40.

Boyle, R. D. & Thomas, R. C. (1988). *Computer Vision. A First Course*. Oxford: Blackwell Scientific.

Brigham, E. O. (1974). *The Fast Fourier Transform*. Englewood Cliffs: Prentice-Hall.

Canny, J. (1986). A computational approach to edge detection. *IEEE Transactions on Pattern Analysis and Machine Intelligence*, PAMI 8(6) 679–98.

Carpenter, G. A. & Grossberg, S. (1989). Neural networks for pattern recognition and associative memory. *Neural Networks*, 2, 243–57.

Chen, C. H. (1982). A study of texture classifications using spectral features. *Proceedings 6th International Conference on Pattern Recognition*, Munich, pp. 1064–7.

Chow, C. K. & Kaneko, T. (1972). Automatic boundary detection of the left ventricle from cineangiograms. *Computers and Biomedical Research*, 5, 388–410.

Dainty, J. C. (1975). Laser speckle and related phenomena. *Topics in Applied Physics*, 9.

Davis, S. L. (1975). A survey of edge detection techniques. *Computer Graphics and Image Processing*, 4, 1–32.

Duff, M. J. B. (1978). Review of the CLIP image processing system. *Proceedings of the National Computer Conference*, 1055–60.

Feldman, J. A. (1985). Connectionist models and parallelism in high level vision. *Computer Vision, Graphics and Image Processing*, 31, 178–200.

Flynn, M. J. (1972). Some computer organisations and their effectiveness. *IEEE Transactions on Computers*, C-21, 948.

Fountain, T. J., Matthews, K. N. & Duff, M. J. B. (1988). The CLIP7A Image Processor. *IEEE Transactions on Pattern Analysis and Machine Intelligence*, PAMI-10, 310–310.

Freeman, H. (1988). *Machine Vision: Algorithms, Architectures and Structures*. New York: Academic Press.

Gonzalez, R. C. & Wintz, P. (1987). *Digital Image Processing* (2nd edition). Massachussetts: Addison Wesley.

Grossberg, S. (1988). *Neural Networks and Natural Intelligence*. Cambridge: MIT Press.

Hillis, W. D. (1985). *The Connection Machine*. Cambridge: MIT Press.

Hinton, G., Ackley, D. & Sejnowski, T. (1984). Boltzmann machines: constraint satisfaction networks that learn. *Technical Report No. CMU-CS-84-119*, Carnegie–Mellon University, Pittsburgh, PA.

Huang, T. S. et al. (1979). A fast two-dimensional median filtering algorithm. *IEEE Transactions on Acoustics, Speech and Signal Processing*, ASSP-27, pp. 13-18.

Hussain, Z. (1991). *Digital Image Processing: Practical Applications of Parallel Processing Techniques*. New York: Ellis Horwood.

Hwang, K. & Briggs, F. A. (1985). *Computer Architecture and Parallel Processing*. New York: McGraw-Hill.

Karara, H. M. (1989). Non-metric cameras. In *Developments in Close-Range Photogrammetry*, ed. K. B. Atkinson. London: Applied Science Publishers.

Kohonen, T. (1988). *Self-Organisation and Associative Memory* (2nd edition). Heidelberg: Springer-Verlag.

Lighthill, J. (1973). *A Report on Artificial Intelligence*. UK Science and Engineering Research Council.

Low, A. (1991). *Introductory Computer Vision and Image Processing*. London: McGraw-Hill.

May, D. (1983). Occam. SIGPLAN Not. *Journal of the ACM*, **18**, 69–79.

Minsky, M. & Papert, S. (1969). *Perceptrons: An Introduction to Computation Geometry*. Cambridge: MIT Press.

Niblack, W. (1986). *An Introduction to Digital Image Processing*. Englewood Cliffs: Prentice-Hall.

Pease, M. C. (1977). The indirect binary n-cube microprocessor array. *IEEE Transactions on Computing*, **C-26**, 458–73.

Potter, D. J. (1985). Computer-assisted analysis of two-dimensional electrophoresis images using an array processor. *Computers and Biomedical Research*, **18**, 347–62.

Pratt, W. (1972). *Digital Image Processing*. New York: Wiley.

Prewitt, J. M. S. (1970). Object enhancement and extraction. In *Picture Processing and Psychopictorics*, ed. B. S. Lipkin & A. Rosenfeld. New York: Academic Press.

Reddaway, S. F. (1979). The DAP approach. *Infotech State of the Art Report on Supercomputers*, **2**, 309–29.

Roberts, L. G. (1965). Machine perception of three dimensional solids. In *Optical and Electro-optical Information Processing*, ed. J. P. Tipper. Cambridge: MIT Press.

Rosenblatt, F. (1958). The perceptron: a probabilistic model for information storage and organisation in the brain. *Psychological Review*, **65**, 386–408.

Rosenfeld, A. & Kak, A. C. (1982). *Digital Picture Processing* (2nd edition). New York: Academic Press.

Rumelhart, D. E. & McClelland, J. L. (1986). *Parallel Distributed Processing*, vols. 1 and 2. Cambridge: MIT Press.

Schalkoff, R. J. (1989). *Digital Image Processing and Computer Vision*. New York: Wiley.

Tuceran, M., Jain, A. K. & Lee, Y. (1988). Texture segmentation using Voroni polygons. *Proceedings of the Computer Vision and Pattern Recognition Conference*, University of Michigan.

Unger, S. H. (1958). A computer orientated to spatial problems. *Proceedings of the Institute of Radio Engineers*, **46**, 1744–50.

van Wezel, R. (1987). *Video Handbook* (2nd edition). London: Heinemann.

Winston, P. H. (1975). *The Psychology of Computer Vision*. New York: McGraw-Hill.

Zenzo, S. D. (1983). Advances in image segmentation. *Image and Vision Computation*, **1**, 196–210.

3

Image input and display

J. G. WEYMES

Introduction

In order to store an image in a computer, the image must undergo a process of analogue to digital conversion. The image is then represented by a number of picture elements (pixels), each referring to a different position on the image. An image might be converted into an array of 2048 rows by 2048 columns of pixels, for example. The image is not only discretized by spatial position, but also by the brightness or colour content of each pixel. For instance, each pixel in a monochrome image might be described by one of 1024 possible values (quantization levels), each value representing a different shade of grey. By convention black is denoted by zero and white by 1023.

Obviously the quality of the stored picture will depend both on the number of pixels and the number of quantization levels used. An increase in either will require additional computer memory and probably a more expensive camera and associated electronics as well. In histological work, a realistic resolution for colour image capture is 2048×2048 pixels, at 1024 quantization levels per colour component.

Image input devices

There are two distinct categories of image input device: the scanner and the camera. A scanner involves movement of the object, the lens, or a sensor in order to scan the image, line by line. In comparison, cameras do not use physical movement to scan images.

Two kinds of cameras can be distinguished. These are vacuum tube cameras and solid state cameras. The former, also known as photoconductive cameras, use a raster scan technique to capture an image line by line. Solid state or charge coupled device (CCD) cameras, use a matrix of light-sensitive cells to capture an entire image in one operation. The photoconductive camera is now almost obsolete as an image analysis tool, the CCD camera being superior in every respect. Nevertheless, the photoconductive camera is described briefly below, because such cameras are still in use and because current video standards and terminology are related to their characteristics.

Scanners

A camera used in conjuction with appropriate electronics is an inexpensive way to obtain a moderate resolution raster image. In cases where this is not sufficient, perhaps for high quality publication work, a photo scanner can be used. The photograph is mounted on a rotating drum and a finely collimated light beam is directed at the photograph. The reflected light is measured by a photocell and as the drum rotates the light source moves from one end to the other, scanning the entire photograph. For coloured images, multiple passes are made using filters in front of the photocell to separate the different colours.

A second class of scanner uses a long strip of CCDs as the sensor. The photograph is digitized by passing it under the CCD array, incrementing the movement to the desired resolution. A single pass is sufficient to digitize a large image. Resolution is typically 8–40 pixels/mm (200–1000 pixels/inch), which is less than that of the photoscanner.

Photoconductive cameras

The generic name for the photoconductive type of video camera is the vidicon. Other names arise mainly from the use of different target materials (Fig. 1).

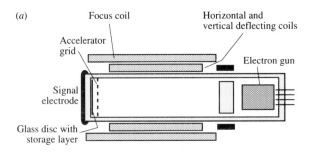

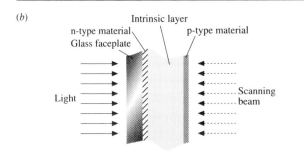

Fig. 1. Vacuum tube cameras. (*a*) The vidicon, (*b*) the plumbicon: detail of photosensitive target layer.

The electron gun, accelerating grids and the target are all contained in an evacuated glass envelope. The image is focussed onto the front of a target which is positioned behind a glass faceplate. The target consists of a thin transparent layer of tin oxide and a layer of light sensitive semiconductor. The semiconductor has a low resistance in light conditions and in the absence of light has a very high resistance. Where the image on the faceplate is bright, the potential difference across the target is reduced.

The electron gun fires a narrow beam of electrons towards the target. The direction of the beam is controlled by vertical and horizontal deflection coils, which are positioned along the camera tube. The beam performs a raster scan of the target, where it restores each picture element to the cathode potential. The quantity of charge (i.e. the current) required to restore the potential difference is directly related to the brightness of the image at this position.

Vidicon cameras suffer from geometrical distortions, variable sensitivity, poor signal-to-noise ratio (SNR), blooming (bright areas appear to be larger than they really are) and poor sensitivity. They are also rather bulky, are fragile and require high voltage deflection coils. Plumbicon and saticon cameras are improved versions of the vidicon, using different target materials for improved sensitivity and noise performance (Fink & Christiansen, 1989).

CCD cameras

In a CCD camera the image is focussed directly on a semiconductor surface of about $1 \, cm^2$ in area, which is made up of millions of sensing cells. Light impinging on a sensor cell increases its stored charge. After a set period, the image is saved by moving the charges held by the sensing cells to storage cells. The two most common architectures for CCD arrays are shown in Fig. 2. The difference between frame transfer and interline transfer devices is that in the latter the storage cells are adjacent to the sense cells. While the next image is being captured by the sensing cells the stored image is being moved from storage cell to storage cell towards the output, in 'bucket brigade' fashion.

Some designs of CCD semiconductors suffer from having too much dead-space between sensing elements. The deadspace is needed for gates and interline structures that help to remove the unwanted charge, which otherwise gets trapped on the surface. In addition, the charge transfer structures must be covered by an opaque mask. These factors combined can reduce the utilization of the incident light by 30–50%. One technique to increase the amount of light reaching the sensors is to use a layer of miniature lenses above the semiconductor, each of which directs the light from one pixel region to the sensor cell. The latest generation of CCD devices have full utilization of the incident light with the use of thin substrate devices illuminated from the rear. Light levels as low as individual photons can be detected (Prettyjohns & Schumacher, 1992).

Current CCD semiconductors can have up to four million pixels, although

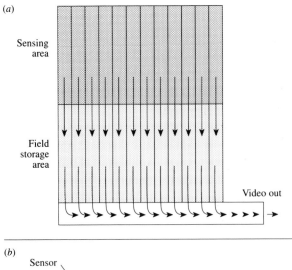

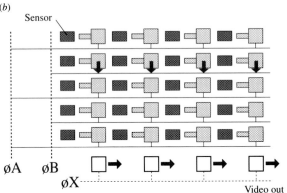

Fig. 2. Solid state cameras. Two architectures for the CCD arrays. (*a*) Frame transfer type, (*b*) interline transfer type.

this limit is likely to be exceeded in future. To increase the resolution further, a stepper motor is used to move the whole semiconductor matrix in steps, taking a picture at each position. The final image is formed as a composite picture.

The semiconductor is a special photodiode matrix with small sensor cells relative to the distance between the cells (Fig. 3). The size of the cells is 1 μm by 1 μm and the inter-cell distance is 8 μm. By moving the device in 1 μm steps between each picture, a high resolution image can be formed from the $8 \times 8 = 64$ sub-pictures. The resolution of the image can be adjusted by using matrices of different sizes.

CCD cameras do not require electron guns, deflection or focussing coils or evacuated glass envelopes. They do not need the cumbersome high voltage electronics associated with the photoconductive cameras and are therefore far more rugged and portable. CCD cameras are also less susceptible to damage from sources of bright light.

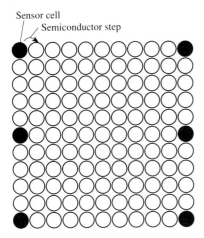

Fig. 3. Interpixel gaps in a photodiode matrix.

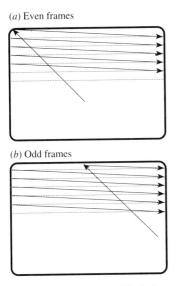

Fig. 4. Interlaced scanning. Each frame is composed of an even and an odd field.

Raster scanning

All television (TV) broadcasts depend on raster scanning. In both the camera tube and the TV display tube, the beam of electrons is focussed at a single point on the image plane. The deflection coils along the sides of the tubes cause the beam to scan across the image. The scan begins at the top left position of the image and proceeds to the right. At the end of the line the beam returns rapidly to the left edge (horizontal flyback) and the scan continues with the next line. At the end of the image (or field) the beam returns to the top left again (vertical flyback) to start another scan (Fig. 4(a)).

An interlaced scan is one in which the image is scanned in two fields (Fig. 4(*b*)). Only half of the scan lines are carried out in the first (even) field, the remainder being completed in the second (odd) field. The frame rate is therefore half of the field scan rate. An interlaced scan provides greater image resolution for a given video bandwidth. Because only half of the total number of lines required to form the picture are transmitted during the frame refresh period, the bandwidth required is halved. Of course, the overall imaging rate, or temporal resolution, is also halved as well.

In image analysis work a good quality monitor which is capable of high frequency, non-interlaced scanning is preferable, because the pixel resolution is higher and because the monitor exhibits less flicker.

Television signals

Fig. 5 shows the analogue signal from a single scan line with a monochrome camera. The black parts of the image return 0.3 volts and the white parts 1.0 volts. The horizontal blanking period refers to the part of the signal that contains no valid data because the scan has finished one line and is doing a

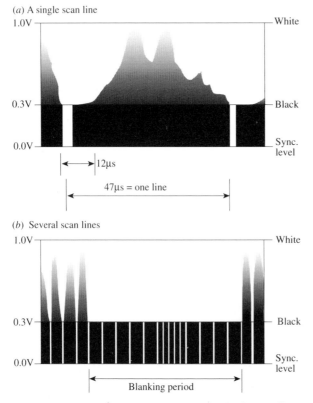

Fig. 5. Analogue signal resulting from a single scanline across an image with a monochrome camera.

Table 1. *RS-170 (USA) and CCIR (UK) video specifications*

Characteristic	RS-170	CCIR
Scan lines per frame	525	625
Active scan lines per frame	490	574
Frame rate (Hz)	30	25
Vertical frequency (Hz)	2×30	2×25
Horizontal frequency (kHz)	15.750	15.625
Horizontal blanking (μs)	11.23	11.82
Vertical blanking (ms)	1.27	1.28
Horizontal active scan (μs)	52.26	52.17
Aspect ratio	4:3	4:3

rapid flyback from right to left in preparation for scanning the next line. To identify the start of the scan a short synchronising pulse, called a sync pulse, is added to the signal. Similarly, a sequence of special short scan lines is used to indicate the vertical blanking period of the signal, i.e. the time necessary for the scan to recover from the bottom right of one image and start again from the top left (Fig. 5(*b*)). Some of the scan lines are lost in the frame synchronization period, reducing the number of active lines per frame.

The monochrome signal described above is common to the European (CCIR) and the American (RS-170) standards. Table 1 shows how their specifications differ in detail. The main differences lie in the number of scan lines per frame and the vertical frequencies, i.e. the frame rates.

When colour TV broadcasts began in the 1950s, it was considered essential to maintain compatibility with existing monochrome receivers. All current colour TV systems were established on that principle and three systems are widely employed at present. In the USA and Japan the NTSC (National Television Systems Commission) system is used, which transmits 525 line pictures at 30 frames/s, i.e. a field scan rate of 60 Hz. Two colour difference signals are transmitted 90° out of phase, which are combined in the receiver to form the chrominance signal. In a large part of Europe the PAL (phase alternating line) system is used, which transmits 625 line pictures at 25 frames/s, i.e. a field scan rate of 50 Hz. To overcome the critical phase relation of the colour signals in the NTSC system, their phase is reversed on alternate lines. Finally in France, the USSR (as was), Eastern Europe and the Middle East the SECAM (Séquential Couleur à Mémoire) system is used, also 625 lines at 25 frames/s. The two colour-difference signals are transmitted on alternate lines rather than being phase separated. As can be imagined, all systems are mutually incompatible.

Video signals from a colour camera may be in one of four forms:

1 A single composite signal, including sync pulses and colour modulations.
2 Three separate colour signals (red, green and blue) with the sync information encoded on the green channel.

3 Four signals, three being colour signals (red, green and blue) with a fourth, separate sync channel.

4 Two signals. One is the luminance signal which has the brightness and sync information, the other is the chrominance signal containing the colour information.

These are all analogue signals. Cameras have recently been developed which produce a digital output that can be accepted directly by a computer.

Gamma ratio

TV cameras tend to have a non-linear relation between the video signal produced and the light intensity reaching them. This is usually beneficial because it allows picture detail to be preserved at lower light levels. The ratio between the logarithm of the light and the logarithm of the signal produced is known as the gamma ratio. In a camera with a linear relation, gamma is unity. Vidicons have a gamma ratio of about 0.65 and TV displays are designed to have a gamma ratio of about 1.2 in order to correct this non-linearity.

Quantitative image processing work is much facilitated by a camera with a gamma ratio of unity. High quality CCD cameras can achieve this, with a deviation of less than 0.1% from linearity. This makes them ideal for image processing work.

Dark current and noise

Dark current refers to the background noise present in the camera. Even in the dark the pickup current is not zero, hence the name. On an image it will cause shading and noise (grain) in the darker parts of the image. Dark current noise is temperature dependent and in a vidicon camera the dark current approximately doubles for every rise in temperature of ten degrees celsius.

The noise in a well designed, high performance CCD camera is 100 to 1000 times lower than in a video CCD camera. High performance CCDs can also integrate the image to improve the SNRs. Since the CCD target comprises a semiconductor layer, the CCD camera suffers from the same dark current problems as the vidicon. CCD cameras used in the laboratory are therefore sometimes cooled to reduce the dark current, particularly in applications that require long exposure times in low light levels, such as fluoroscopy. In astronomy very long exposures are made using CCD cameras in which the semiconductor is cooled with liquid nitrogen.

Dynamic range

The dynamic range is the ratio of the largest signal that can be accurately recorded to the smallest resolvable difference in image intensity. A high performance CCD camera has a dynamic range of 100 000:1 (or 100 dB) compared to 200:1 (or 46 dB) for a video CCD camera. The effective resolution of the data stored in a computer is a function both of the dynamic range of the camera and the resolution of the associated electronics. Sometimes cameras have an improved dynamic range at the expense of their linearity (Lake, 1992).

Image lag

Image lag refers to the delay in following a moving or changing image. After a bright image is removed its pattern remains visible for a period. In most image acquisition applications this is not a problem, since the image is normally fixed. In image output devices, a long persistence phosphor in a monitor will reduce flicker.

Colour

Radiation with wavelengths between 400 nm and 700 nm is perceived as light by the human eye. As the wavelength increases from 400 to 700 nm, i.e. as the frequency decreases, the colour changes gradually through the visible spectrum from blue to red (Fig. 6). A narrow radiation band appears as a pure or saturated colour. A wider band makes the colour less pure (as in the way deep red changes to pink). The wider the band the whiter the colour appears (Gonzalez & Wintz, 1987).

RGB

The eye can be tricked into seeing non-existent colours. For instance, when two narrow frequencies, one of red and one of green, are added together they appear to be yellow. Similarly, when shining two different-coloured lights on a surface, the colours add together: the more colours are added, the closer to white the result becomes. Using this principle, colour TV can be made to work with the use of just three colours: red, green and blue. These are called the

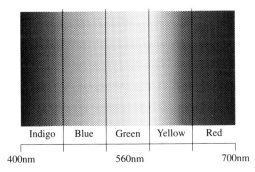

Fig. 6. The visible region of the electromagnetic spectrum.

Table 2. *Addition of primary colours*

Colours added	Result
Red + Green	Yellow
Red + Blue	Magenta
Green + Blue	Cyan
Red + Green + Blue	White

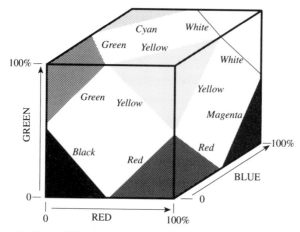

Fig. 7. The RGB colour cube.

primary or additive colours. Adding the primary colours together gives the results shown in Table 2. The RGB colour cube can be used to visualize the colour scheme in terms of the primary colours (Fig. 7).

CMY

When white light is passed through a coloured filter, colour is subtracted. The more colours are subtracted, the blacker the result becomes. The three subtractive or secondary colours are cyan, magenta and yellow. Subtracting the colours magenta and cyan from white leaves blue. Fig. 8 shows the CMY colour cube. To convert between RGB and CMY representations of colour, where the colour intensity is graded from 0 to 100, see the relationships in Table 3.

CMYK

Besides the two common systems described above, there are several other colour representations (Table 4). Colour printing involves the use of the secondary colours plus black, since it saves time and money to include black as

Table 3. *Conversion between RGB and CMY colour representations*

RGB to CMY[a]	CMY to RGB[a]
C = 100 − R	R = 100 − C
M = 100 − G	G = 100 − M
Y = 100 − B	B = 100 − Y

[a]Colour intensity is graded from 0 to 100.

Table 4. *Schema for representing colour*

Scheme	
RGB	Red, green and blue – primary colours
CMY	Cyan, magenta and yellow – secondary colours
CMYK	Cyan, magenta, yellow and black
HLS	Hue, light and saturation
HSV	Hue, saturation and value[a]
HSB	Hue, saturation and brightness[a]

[a]Synonyms.

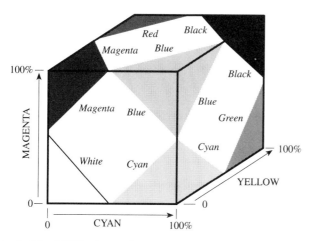

Fig. 8. The CMY colour cube.

an extra colour. This is the CMYK scheme, a variation of CMY which includes a value for black, K.

HLS

The HLS system is a format based on the hue, light and saturation of the colour. Hue describes the attribute of pure colour, for example, pure red or pure cyan. Hue therefore distinguishes between colours, for example between blue, red and green. In fact hue is represented as an angle on a circle with blue, magenta, red, and green at 0°, 60°, 120° and 240° respectively. For the light property, 0% represents black and 100% represents white. Saturation reflects how far the colour is from a pure colour, i.e. how far from a narrow frequency band of radiation. A pure colour has maximum saturation ($S = 1$), while grey has minimum saturation ($S = 0$). Adding white reduces the saturation, so that red is highly saturated and pink is relatively unsaturated. In Fig. 9 the HLS cone can be used to visualize the colour attributes (Foley *et al.*, 1990).

HSV

The HSV system is a format based on hue, saturation and value (also called HSB, where B stands for brightness). The hue has the same meaning as above. However, the saturation parameter is different from the HLS scheme. The saturation component characterizes the shade of the colour or how much white is added to the pure colour, a fully saturated colour having a low white component. A pure colour in both systems has a maximum value for S ($S = 1$). Adding white in the HLS scheme leaves $S = 1$, while L increases. Adding white in the HSV scheme decreases S while maintaining V. The value or intensity decribes the overall brightness of the colour and ranges from the darkest at 0% to the brightest at 100%. Fig. 10 can be used to visualize the scheme. Not all the values on the cone base have the same brightness.

The HSV system is, in certain respects, superior to the traditional RGB colour space. One advantage of this representation is that image processing times can be reduced. This is because in many applications it is not necessary to examine all three components of the image as is the case for RGB images. With the HSV system the examination of a single component, for example the intensity, may be adequate. The intensity component of an image corresponds to the greyscale version of an image and may therefore be employed by applications that only perform greyscale operations.

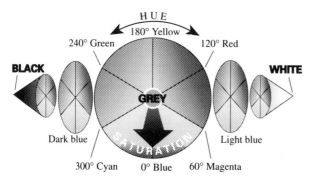

Fig. 9. The HLS colour cones.

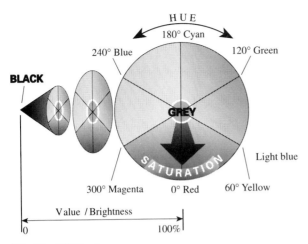

Fig. 10. The HSV colour cone.

Conversion between formats

The RGB and CMYK formats are suitable for hardware use, but the HLS and HSV versions are easier to manipulate in software. Conversion between formats is relatively straightforward.

Colour cameras

Cameras employ one of several methods for capturing colour images. In one system a high efficiency, dichroic light splitter (or prism) is used to divide the image into its red, green and blue components. Three pickups are required, one for each colour. This sort of camera is costly because it requires three pickups and precision optics. The colours need to be accurately registered and the low light bias levels must be coordinated. The second method uses a system of semi-reflective mirrors and dichroic filters to split the colours. This prism method is preferable because it is easier to align and it passes more light through to the pickups.

A cheaper alternative, which is employed in domestic camcorders, is to use a single pickup with colour striping either on the glass faceplate or on the semiconductor itself. The translucent colour wax is laid out in strips of colours, as shown in Fig. 11. The first strip allows only green light through. The next strip allows through both blue and green colours. In the electronics of the camera the value of the blue component of the image can be calculated by subtracting the green part. The next strip allows all three colours through, and the red component is calculated electronically by subtracting the green and blue components. The pitch of the stripes is about 40 μm and an optical filter is added to eliminate the banding effects that would otherwise be visible on the image. The presence of this filter is the reason why high quality lenses would be wasted on this type of camera.

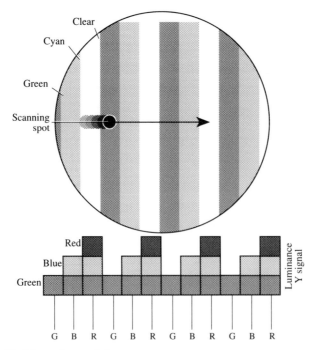

Fig. 11. The colour striping mask in a domestic camcorder.

Paradoxically, the best method of capturing colour images is to use a monochrome camera. Using a CCD camera, three or four separate pictures of the same image are taken with different filters to separate the colour components. This method has the advantages that there is no registration error, the colours can be carefully selected, and the cost is reduced because only a single pickup is required in the camera.

CCDs have a bias toward the infra-red part of the spectrum. In order to preserve a well-balanced picture, an infra-red-blocking filter is normally included in the light path.

Image display

For image processing work, monitors containing cathode ray tubes (CRTs) are used to display images. In comparison with TV displays for domestic use, monitors, for both workstations and PCs, have a higher video bandwidth and higher refresh rate.

Monitors

The important parameters in classifying a display are its resolution, refresh rate and the persistence of the phosphor. A CRT is of similar construction to a vidicon camera in using an evacuated glass envelope, deflection coils, accelerating grids and an electron gun. The layer of phosphor on the glass faceplate is stimulated by the stream of electrons from the gun. The electron beam is directed by the deflection coils in a raster scan across the faceplate in a similar manner to a vidicon. The electron beam is deflected by 45° either side of the centreline of the tube to reach the edges of the screen (Fig. 12). To make a more compact TV, the angle of deflection can be increased to about 70°, but this leads to significant geometrical distortion at the edges of the image.

Colour raster displays use three separate electron guns, one to generate each colour. On the inside of the glass faceplate there are groups of closely spaced phosphor dots, each triplet containing a red, green and blue dot. About 1 cm before the faceplate there is a shadow mask, which is a metal shield with finely spaced holes. The three electron beams are focussed at the same point on the mask, which is positioned carefully so that a given gun can illuminate only one colour of phosphor dots (Fig. 13).

The addressability of a screen is the number of pixels it can display. High quality CRTs currently have resolutions of 2048 × 2048 pixels. Resolution is only one of the parameters that define image quality. The other parameters are the pitch of the shadow mask, and the focus quality, which is defined in terms of the line width, spot size, bandwidth or number of raster lines.

The spot size is the smallest measurable detail which can be displayed. Because the spot is made up from several phosphor dots, the spot size is always larger than the pitch. Physically it is very difficult to make high resolution masks and matching phosphor trios, especially for larger monitors. Also a high proportion of the electrons hit the mask, heating it up and causing it to expand and move relative to the phosphor on the faceplate. Monochrome monitors have better resolution because they do not require shadow masks or phosphor trios.

The persistence of a phosphor is defined as the time from the removal of the excitation to the time when phosphorescence has decayed to 10% of the initial output. For most displays used in graphics equipment the persistence is 10–60 ms (Table 5).

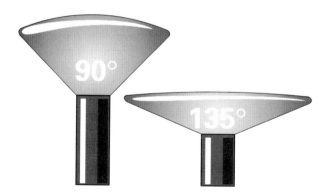

Fig. 12. Plan view of CRT tubes.

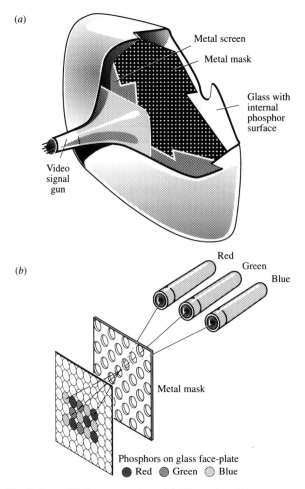

Fig. 13. Colour CRT construction. (*a*) The tube, (*b*) shadow shield mask and phosphor trios. In a precision in-line CRT, the three electron guns are in line with one another.

In comparison with monitors, TV and high definition television (HDTV) displays suffer from poor spot size, pitch and geometric resolution (caused by wide deflection angles). They are also designed to be much brighter and should be viewed from a distance of four metres or so, rather than the 450 to 900 mm usually used for a monitor. The limitation of the TV broadcast bandwidth means that TVs use a slow field refresh rate: 50 Hz in the UK and 60 Hz in the USA. At 50 Hz, most people notice perceptible screen flicker. At 72 Hz, as in a typical monitor, such flicker is not perceptible (Wyatt, 1991; Eccles & Romans, 1992).

Non-CRT displays

The advantages of liquid crystal displays (LCDs) are their low cost, low weight, small size and low power consumption. In the past their major disadvantage

Table 5. *Typical CRT monitor parameters*

Parameter	Television monitor	Normal monitor[a]	High resolution monitor
Horizontal pixels	430	1280	2048
Vertical pixels	574	1024	2048
Video bandwidth (MHz)	6	110	357
Horizontal scan frequency (kHz)	15	30–64	127
Vertical scan frequency (Hz)	60	60–90	60
Pitch (mm)	0.80	0.31	0.31
Spot size (mm)	2.00	0.65	0.60
Geometrical distortion (%)[b]	> 5	< 1	< 1

[a]For example, an SVGA standard PC monitor.
[b]Geometrical distortion is defined as the worst case positional error expressed as a percentage of the diagonal distance across the screen.

was that they were passive, reflecting only incident light, and therefore difficult to read in certain light conditions. Recently use of active panels has overcome this problem, although the displays are still not as bright and crisp as a CRT. LCDs are now becoming more common in personal computers, particularly in the laptop and notebook types. However, LCD displays are not yet capable of displaying images with the resolution or brightness of a CRT.

Colour printers

There are several types of colour printers and they vary greatly in output quality. Inkjet printers and impact printers with coloured ribbons compose the individual pixels from a number of adjacent coloured dots that, clustered together, appear like a new colour. The printers have four colours (CMYK) and the print head is traversed from side to side across the paper. Each colour component is added on a separate pass of the head. After completing a row of four passes, the paper is stepped down to the next row. These printers produce rather poor quality results because slight misalignments between the paper and printing head give rise to colour banding effects.

Dithering is a randomization of the cluster arrangement to mimimize cluster pattern effects. Dithering is necessary because many types of printers are incapable of adjusting the intensity of a given dot: it is either printed or not printed. Laser printers, for example, can print only black dots. Grey areas are simulated by clustering black dots to produce a single pixel. If a cluster of four dots is used to produce any single pixel, then different shades of grey can be

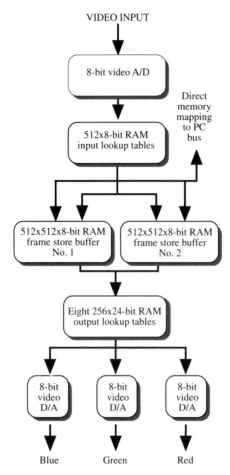

Fig. 14. Framegrabber.

produced. The patterns of any given greylevel are randomized, to prevent the formation of regular patterns. Colours are similarly dithered with CMYK combinations in each cluster.

A thermal wax printer has superior resolution and colour rendition, but also uses the dithering principle. The paper and wax are also relatively expensive.

In dye-sublimation printing the dye is heated, changing it from a solid to a gas. It returns to a solid when applied to the paper. This method creates subtle shades of colour without dithering. The results are of photographic quality for colour images, but monochrome pictures tend to be rather dull.

The highest quality results can be produced on film, rather than paper. Film recorders are capable of producing high quality slides or photographs. The recorder is connected either to the video output or to the computer bus directly.

Framegrabbers

The output from a camera will conform to some video standard, usually RGB or PAL in Europe, or CCIR in the USA. The image processing system is fitted with a device called a framegrabber which takes the analogue signal from the camera and digitizes it. The resultant data are stored in random access memory (RAM) (Fig. 14). The framegrabber has enough RAM to hold at least one digitized image. Frame sizes are usually between 512×512 and 2048×2048 pixels.

An image processing system may have more than one input device, so the framegrabber is normally fitted with a multiplexor or switch to select an input. The framegrabber may also be capable of accepting video signals in more than one format, so that it may be equipped with connectors for a variety of video types, e.g. RGB and PAL. The signal is then separated into three components, RGB or HSV, and then each part is passed through an analogue-to-digital convertor (ADC). The digital values are stored in three separate memory buffers. Fig. 15 shows how an analogue signal is digitized. If the ADC output is set at 12 quantization bits, then the number of possible values or quantization levels is 2^{12} or 4096. The total number of memory bits (m) required to store an image is:

$$m = n_p \times n_c \times n_q$$

where n_p is the number of pixels,
   n_c is the number of colours and
   n_q is the number of quantization bits per colour.
Thus to store a 2048×2048 colour image at 12 bits/pixel requires a total of 50 Mbits (or 6.3 MBytes) of memory.

The image in the buffer is output to a monitor by moving the data through digital-to-analogue convertors (DACs) to provide the RGB analogue signals. Between the frame buffer and the ADCs, the data are passed through lookup tables (LUTs), one for each colour component. Each LUT is a RAM buffer of the same size as the number of quantization levels. The LUT can be set up with any mapping of input to output data, the simplest being a straight line relationship. Data representing each pixel in turn are sent from the frame

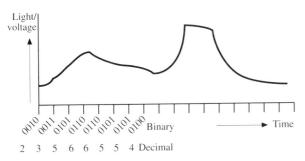

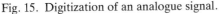

Fig. 15. Digitization of an analogue signal.

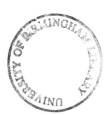

buffer to the LUT, and used to find a new value from the table (see Chapter 5). The image can be inverted simply by changing the LUT to a decreasing ramp. The simplicity and power of the LUT makes it a standard feature on framegrabber boards.

The computer interface to the framegrabber card gives it access to the image in the frame buffer and to the values in the LUTs. It also sends control signals to the card, for instance, to freeze an image or to switch from one input to another with the multiplexor.

Obviously the stored picture quality will depend on the number of pixels and the number of quantization levels used. An increase in either will require additional computer memory and probably a more expensive camera and framegrabber. The prices for computers, memory devices and framegrabbers have been falling steadily for some years and their performance has been improving. Currently it is thought that a realistic representation of a colour image can be obtained for most purposes at 2048×2048 pixels with 1024 quantization levels per colour (Atkin, 1992).

Frame processors

Frame processors are specialized versions of the standard framegrabber that incorporate additional computing power for high speed manipulation of images. The frame processor generally has two frame buffers and an arithmetic and logic unit (ALU) (Fig. 16). The ALU is a pipeline parallel processor which can perform rapid operations, such as convolution, between two datasets. Often the data can be processed in real time, so that the result of filtering the signal from a camera can be observed directly on a monitor.

Storage media

For ease of access, digitized images are usually stored on disk based, as opposed to tape based, media. Two forms of disk based systems are available using either conventional magnetic or optical technology.

Magnetic disk drives are often known as Winchester disks, after their place of origin. They are sealed units in which the disks rotate at high speeds, with low tolerances between the read/write head and the disk surface. The rotational speed is fixed, which leads to a low latency time, typically 10 ms, for accessing data on the disk. The largest disk drives use the Small Computer System Interface (SCSI) standard for interfacing to the computer. Currently SCSI drives of up to 2.3 GBytes unformatted capacity are available, although it is expected this limit may soon increase to 5 GBytes.

Optical disks use a laser to read the information from the platter. Normally these are write once, read many devices (WORM), although more recent drives now allow multiple writes, and so permit the erasing of data and the recovery of the disk space. WORM disk capacities of up to 2 GBytes are

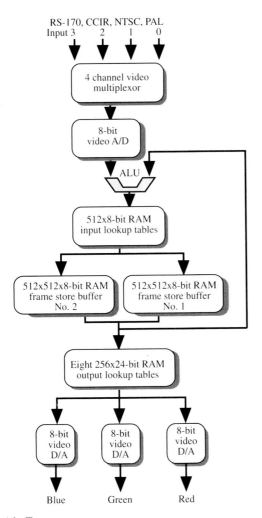

Fig. 16. Frame processor.

common and they can be used in multiplatter stacks of, say, 12 disks or in jukebox arrangements of 100–200 disks. Use of the latter does not permit multiuser access, since the retrieval of a particular disk for use in the jukebox is a relatively lengthy process, taking several seconds. Jukeboxes are particularly suited to large archives that are infrequently accessed, rather than on-line databases and image stores.

A form of optical disk using the compact disk standard is now becoming common, known as the compact disk, read only memory (CD-ROM). As the name implies this is solely a read only device. The CD-ROM holds 660 MBytes of data and this is unlikely to increase in the immediate future. Again multiplatter and jukebox drives are available for CD-ROMs. Disk access from optical drives is slow, typically 330 ms. This is due in part to the fact that the data are written to disk at an even density, which requires the rotational speed of the disk to vary in order to produce a constant linear velocity of the read head over the disk surface (i.e. the disk must rotate more slowly when accessing data on the outer tracks of the disk than when accessing data at the centre).

Computer architectures

Apart from the large data throughput required for image processing, computers must also carry out many types of specialized processing such as filtering, image registration, feature extraction and surface rendering. Most computers are still based on the simple 'von Neumann' architecture, in which a single processing unit handles all the computation with both program instructions and data held in the memory of the machine. Recent developments in integrated circuit technology, including the introduction of reduced instruction set chips (RISC) and more recently the pipelined and superscalar processors have increased the performance of individual CPUs markedly (Chapter 2). However, with the enormous processing power required for image processing, particularly in 3-D imaging work, it is not possible to imagine efficient image processing systems based solely on conventional computer architectures. High performance systems, therefore, invariably have additional graphics chips or specialist boards designed to relieve the computer CPU of some of the processing load. In the near future it is possible to foresee the combination of these and computers with many hundreds of processors operating in parallel to provide sufficient power to perform complex image processing tasks in real time.

References

Atkin, P. (1992). Better boards by design. *Image Processing*, **4**, 31–45.

Eccles, D. & Romans, G. (1992). High definition versus high resolution displays. *What sort of image quality? Advanced Imaging*, **7**, 16–20.

Fink, D. & Christiansen, D. (1989). *Electronic Engineers' Handbook*. New York: McGraw-Hill.

Foley, J. D., van Dam, A., Feiner, S. K. & Hughes, J. F. (1990). *Computer Graphics Principles and Practice* (2nd edition) Reading, MA: Addison-Wesley.

Gonzalez, R. C. & Wintz, P. (1987). *Digital Image Processing*. Reading, MA: Addison-Wesley.

Lake, D. (1992). Beyond camera specsmanship. Real sensitivity and dynamic range. *Advanced Imaging*, **7**, 54–6.

Prettyjohns, K. & Schumacher, J. (1992). High performance CCD cameras and applications that demand them. *Advanced Imaging*, **7**, 28–32.

Wyatt, P. (1991). Standards and the monitor market. *Image Processing*, **3**, 21–6.

4

Image file formats in biological image analysis

D-C. ABRAMS

Introduction

Graphical file formats currently available for bitmapped image storage are numerous, sometimes complicated and have yet to be standardized. However, there are two well-defined types of graphics file in common use, both of which have numerous aliases. The first of these is known as the bitmapped image file, also known as the raster, pixel or paint file. A bitmapped image consists of individual points or picture elements which collectively compose the image (Fig. 1). The second type of image file is the vector file, also known as the plotter, scalable or draw file. A vector file is similar to a computer program, which when executed creates the image at the output device. Vector images are scale independent and are therefore reproduced at the highest resolution of which the output device being used to display them is capable.

When viewed on a computer screen a vector image is often indistinguishable from its bitmapped equivalent. However, when displayed using a high resolution laser printer, a vector image often has a smoother appearance than its bitmapped equivalent. Although bitmapped images have a fixed resolution which is significantly degraded when the size of the image is enlarged, they are the commonest image type currently used in biological image analysis systems. For this reason only bitmapped image types will be discussed in this chapter.

Bitmapped images

Bitmapped images are the simplest form of image file format. Unlike a vector image file, which stores instructions to re-create the image, the bitmapped image file merely records the colour attributes of each element within the image. The theoretical image size may be as large as required, although the display is obviously restricted by the characteristics of the output device. In biological image analysis and image processing, images are usually generated by one of two methods. The first of these methods involves scanning the specimen with, for example, a narrow beam of light as in the case of confocal laser scanning microscopy (see Chapter 10). The scattered and emitted light

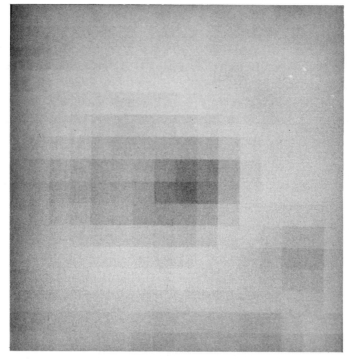

Fig. 1. A portion of a 512 × 512 image of respiratory mucosa which has been enlarged so that the individual pixels are visible. Each pixel represents approximately 0.35 μm^2 of the original section.

from the specimen is guided to light-sensitive detectors and converted to an electrical signal. The second method of image capture involves the use of a television camera (see Chapter 12). Computers can easily convert the electrical signals produced by these digitization devices to pixel values and hence produce bitmapped images.

A digital image is a graphical representation of an array of values which are stored sequentially, left to right and top to bottom, in the image file. These values, which are usually integers in the range 0 to 255, are used to represent the intensities of the pixels or to describe the colour components of the pixels in the image. A pixel is the smallest dot or picture element that comprises the image. The number of pixels that constitutes a row within the image is known as the image width. Similarly, the number of pixels in an image column is termed the image height. The depth of an image refers to the number of computer bits (binary digits) that are used to represent a pixel.

Binary images

The minimum number of bits that can be used to represent a pixel is one, and an image that consists of single-bit data is called a binary image. Such an image contains pixels which are either black (switched off) or white (switched on) and are represented by the pixel values 0 and 1 respectively. Binary images require less storage space than other types of images, although the information that can be stored in these binary image files is greatly reduced. Such images often result from operations performed on images of greater depth. For example eight-bit greyscale images can be segmented to produce a binary image (see Chapter 5). This process is often used for measuring the areas of objects by boundary delineation.

Greyscale images

If each pixel in a monochrome image can take more than two values, a greyscale image results. Four-bit data allows each pixel to have one of 16 (i.e. 2^4) greylevels. This range of greylevels is known as a greyscale, ranging from pure black at one extreme to pure white at the other; pixel intensities between zero and 15 are various shades of grey. The depth of a four-bit image is four times greater than that of a binary image. This means that four-bit image files are four times larger than binary files, but are capable of representing more information.

Eight bits is the most popular image depth currently used in biology. Each pixel can represent one of 256 greyscale values and therefore the amount of information that can be stored by these images is greater than can be stored by four-bit images. Although the computer is capable of distinguishing between the 256 greyscale levels, the human eye can distinguish only approximately 30 greyscale values. This means that it would be very difficult to distinguish by eye a five-bit image from an eight-bit image (Fig. 2). The more depth information required in an image, the greater the size of the image file. A binary image consisting of 512 rows and 512 columns, often referred to as a 512 × 512 image, would occupy 32 kBytes of storage space (Fig. 3). The 16-bit equivalent image would require 512 kBytes of storage space. In biology, eight-bit data are usually sufficient for storing the images obtained from microscopy.

Image depth

Image depth refers to the amplitude quantization, or greylevel quantization of the pixels. The number of possible greylevels (G) is given by:

$$G = 2^m$$

where m represents the number of bits used to represent each pixel. This is generally between 1 and 16, but may reach 64 for certain specialist applications. The depth of an image and the spatial resolution determine the overall quality of an image.

The depth to which an image will be digitized may be chosen according to its nature as well as its particular use. For example, digital images that will be subtracted are normally digitized to greater depth in order to retain sufficient quantization resolution in the resulting image.

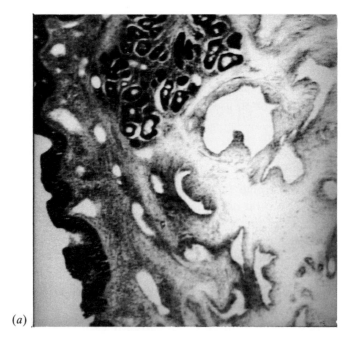

(a)

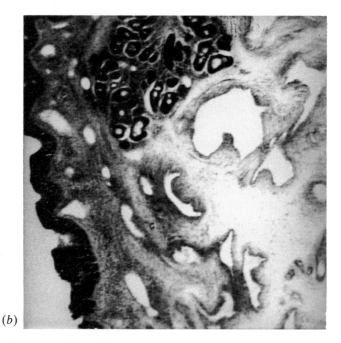

(b)

Fig. 2. These two 512 × 512 pixel, eight-bit images appear to be identical. (a) A five-bit image; this requires 160 kBytes of storage space. (b) An eight-bit image; this requires 256 kBytes of storage space. The reduction in image depth reduces the amount of image storage space required without significantly reducing the image resolution when viewed with the naked eye.

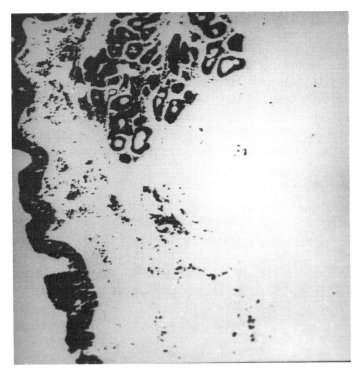

Fig. 3. A 512 × 512 pixel, binary image (i.e. 1 bit deep) of the haematoxylin and eosin stained respiratory mucosa shown in Fig. 1. The image was segmented by thresholding with a pixel value of 127.

Eight-bit images can be composed of either signed or unsigned integers. Unsigned images consist of positive pixel values that are in the range 0 to 255. The pixel values for signed images can take values from -127 to $+127$. Signed pixel values allow for negative information to be stored within the image. However, for image display the signed values are re-mapped to positive integers. The use of signed images in biology is somewhat limited, since the majority of biological images almost certainly consist of unsigned Bytes. Images may also consist of pixels of other numeric types, such as floating point and complex numbers. The depth of floating point images depends on the central processing unit (CPU) of the storing device. For example, the Fourier transform of an image may be stored as a complex image. In this case the real and imaginary parts of the image can be considered as distinct images of floating point type.

Colour images

A colour image can be constructed by combining various intensities of the three additive primary colours, red, green and blue. Although there are many ways to encode colour information, the majority of colour image file formats use the RGB (red, green and blue) system. Unlike greyscale images, where the intensity of a pixel is coded using a single value, the RGB system employs three values for each pixel. Each component of the RGB system is encoded using a particular number of bits. In the case of 24-bit colour images, each colour is coded with eight bits and it is the combination of these values that describe the final colour of the pixel.

Many of the colour image file formats use a two-stage mechanism for displaying colours. The displayed colour, which is encoded in the pixel values, is determined using a lookup table, also known as a colour palette or colour

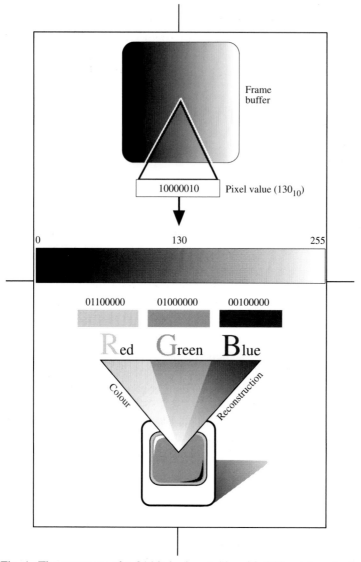

Fig. 4. The structure of a 24-bit lookup table with 256 entries. A pixel value of 130 is re-mapped to the colour brown. The pixel is displayed with a red intensity of 60/255, a green intensity of 40/255 and a blue intensity of 20/255.

table (Fig. 4). The colours that can be used to display the image are restricted by the lookup table, which in turn is governed by the output device. The output device may be capable of displaying thousands of colours, but an eight-bit lookup table can encode only 256 colours. Single-bit colour images can be represented only by eight different colours, while 24-bit colour images can be displayed using all 256 colours stored in the lookup table. In both cases the different images could use the same colour lookup table, but the number of available colours would be limited by the number of bits per pixel. This encoding scheme requires that the colour lookup table is stored with the image for authentic image rendition.

Colour images often convey more information to the observer (see Plate 1). This can be particularly important when analysing images obtained from histologically stained tissues. Technological advances in computing have already led to a proliferation of colour input and output devices.

Image file structure

An image file is usually composed of an image header, the image data or body, and sometimes an image trailer or terminator.

The image header

The image header contains information relating to the image size, the image type, pixel size, scaling parameters and other relevant characteristics of the image. The header may be coded in binary, or in standard ASCII characters. The image header information can be stored in a separate file, or may be incorporated into the image file prior to the image body.

The image body

The body part of the image file contains the pixel values. These are usually binary coded. The position of individual pixel values within the image file is critical because this positional information ensures that the correct pixel value is placed at the appropriate location in the reconstructed image. Pixel values are written sequentially from left to right for each row, and from top to bottom. In multiple-image files the individual images may be preceded by additional information specific for each image.

The image trailer

The footer, when present, may contain user-definable information describing the image. In MRC image format the footer is used to store information related to the acquisition of the image, for example, the zoom factor and the type of filter used during data acquisition. In an image file containing multiple images, the footer appears at the end of the file and not at the end of every image. A special termination sequence may be used to indicate, to the application program reading the image, that the end of the image file has been reached.

Types of images

TIFF format

The tag image file format (TIFF) was developed jointly by the Aldus Corporation and the Microsoft Corporation (Aldus, 1988), for the storage and interchange of scanned images in desktop publishing. A file format is defined by the image structure as well as the content of the image file. The TIFF image structure is complicated and contains an immense amount of information. A TIFF image file begins with an eight-Byte image file header, which points to one or more image file directories. These directories contain information about the characteristics of the image as well as pointers to the actual image data.

The most efficient file format for storing images is positional formatting. In this method the position of the values in the file describes the function of those values. For example, in one particular file format, the specification may state that Byte numbers 36 and 38 (counting from the beginning) describe the width and height of the image respectively. This positional formatting method is simple and easy to implement. The problem arises when it becomes necessary to modify the file format, to include additional information regarding the characteristics of the image, whilst maintaining compatibility with existing application software and image files. The developers of TIFF attempted to overcome this problem by defining fields in the image format. Each field is associated with a unique tag and contains specific information about the image. For example, tag code 256 describes the image width in pixels. An application program can access the information that it requires by selecting the appropriate fields and ignoring others. This strategy allows additional information to be added to later versions of the TIFF in the form of new fields.

There are currently five versions of TIFF: TIFF-B, TIFF-G, TIFF-R, TIFF-P and TIFF-F. TIFF-B is the simplest and is used primarily by bi-level scanners. Greyscale images are stored using the most widely used TIFF-G format. TIFF-R is a popular format for applications that employ full colour RGB images. TIFF-P is an alternative image file format for full colour images and uses multiple-bit planes. TIFF-P colours are produced with the aid of a colour lookup table. Finally, TIFF-F was designed as an image file format for facsimile machines, but is very rarely used.

The flexibility and strength of TIFF format is reflected in its use by a wide range of application software. However, simplicity has been sacrificed for robustness and this makes TIFF the most complicated file format commonly used. Due to the vast amount of data stored in a TIFF file, data compression is an integral component of the file format.

GIF format

The graphics interchange format (GIF) was developed by CompuServe (Compuserve, 1990; 1988) to exchange and display colour raster images, rapidly and efficiently, over the CompuServe network. The file format, which is completely hardware independent, includes a GIF signature, a screen descriptor, a global colour table, the data and a GIF terminator. A GIF file is able to store multiple images in a single file. These images may be displayed sequentially or simultaneously depending on the hardware and software controlling the image display. In a multiple image file there is a single copy of the header (signature, screen descriptor and global colour table), followed by the data blocks. Each data block consists of the data for a single image and an optional local colour table. The number of data blocks depends on the number of individual images within the file. Finally, the termination character appears at the end of the file and not at the end of each data block.

The signature, or 'magic number', identifies the image as a GIF file. Many other file formats also use a magic number, which is usually found in the image header. The screen descriptor describes image dimension, colour maps and other parameters relating to the characteristics of the image. A GIF image may contain two colour tables, a global colour table and a local colour table, both of which are optional. Which colour table is used is determined by the encoding and decoding software as well as the specifications of the output device. The GIF image data are encoded in the conventional manner, i.e. left to right and top to bottom. However, the decoding software can display the image using an interlace technique if desired. In this process the order in which the rows are revealed is altered so that the image is not displayed row by row. The GIF interlacing process renders the image in four passes. The first pass displays every eighth row starting from row zero. The remaining passes complete the image by displaying additional rows starting at other positions in the image. This allows image display to be terminated prematurely, should the image be unacceptable to the user. The GIF terminator instructs the decoder that the end of the image file has been reached and that there are no images remaining to be displayed.

Like Aldus and Microsoft, CompuServe also included mechanisms to allow for future enhancements to their image file format. GIF files are equipped with extension blocks for future use and all GIF decoders are designed to recognize these blocks and ignore them if they cannot be processed. This procedure enables earlier decoders to cope with updated GIF image files by neglecting the additional features. The incorporation of a sophisticated data compression algorithm allows GIF images to be decompressed and displayed simultaneously.

MRC format

The MRC image format was designed by the Medical Research Council for storing images acquired using the Bio-Rad Confocal Image System. The format is simple and consists of a 76-Byte header followed by the raster data and a footer. Like GIF, MRC format files are capable of containing multiple images. The MRC format, however, is a simple greyscale image format and therefore does not contain colour tables or any other formatting structures. All data are stored using positional encoding.

TGA format

The Targa image format is a popular format for personal computers. It is used by the Targa and Vista framegrabber boards to store images internally. The format consists of a short, simple image header followed by the image body which contains a colour table and the raster data. The Targa technical manual explains this format in more detail (Truevision, 1991).

VFF format

The visualization file format (VFF) is employed in the SunVision software suite which was developed by Sun Microsystems. The file format consists of an ASCII header followed by the binary data. The data are separated from the header with a standard ASCII formfeed character. This allows the header to be created or modified easily using a standard text editor.

Sun rasterfiles

Workstations are becoming commonplace in the laboratory. Sun Microsystems was the first manufacturer to produce a workstation with a bitmapped screen. The Sun rasterfile is a simple file format with provision for greyscale as well as colour images. The file starts with a 32-Byte header followed by an optional colour table and then the image pixels. The format of this file is described in the Pixrect Reference Manual (Sun, 1990).

Image formats in microscopy

Although there is no standard image format for biological image analysis systems, it is clear that few common formats include the necessary information for the processing and analysis of images obtained by microscopy. In microscopy it is important to preserve information relating to magnification, modality and sample identification. Some of the common file formats that may be encountered during biological image analysis are listed in Table 1.

Table 1. *Image file formats*

Format	Developer	Type	Note
CDR	Coreldraw	Vector	
CGM	ANSI	Vector and raster (in the same file)	Defined by ANSI/BSI/ISO
EPS	Adobe Systems	Vector	Encapsulated postscript
GEM	Digital Research	Bitmap	Four versions
GIF	CompuServe	Bitmap	
HPGL	Hewlett Packard	Vector	Hewlett Packard Graphics Language
IMF	Context Vision	Bitmap	
IMG	Digital Research	Bitmap	Ventura Publisher
IMG	Kontron Elektronik	Bitmap	VIDAS and IBAS format (128-Byte header)
IMG	Mayo Clinic	Bitmap	Analyze
TRS	Olympus	Bitmap	Olympus confocal microscope (256-Byte header)
PCX	ZSoft	Bitmap	PC paintbrush format
PIC	Lotus	Vector	Similar to HPGL
PIC	MRC	Bitmap	Bio-Rad confocal microscope format (76-Byte header)
PS	Adobe Systems	Vector	Postscript
RS	Sun Microsystems	Bitmap	Sun raster file
TGA	Truevision	Bitmap	Used by Targa framegrabbers
TIF	Aldus/Microsoft	Bitmap	Five versions
VFF	Sun Microsystems	Bitmap	Visualization file format – SunVision
WMF	Microsoft Corp	Vector	Windows metafile
WPG	Sintinel	Vector or bitmap (not both)	WordPerfect graphics file

Both SunVision and Analyze are very powerful packages for processing and analysing images obtained from a variety of modalities, including microscopy. Converting images between common formats can be achieved with the use of an image converter. However, converting images to a proprietary format such as VFF, MRC or IMG (Analyze) can be achieved by conversion of the existing image to a raw image file and then creating the required header. This usually involves writing a special computer program or using a utility such as the Unix 'dd' command to remove from the original image all file structures that are not required. An image header may be constructed to complement the raw image file, especially if the header can be written in standard ASCII characters. The new file is simply created by concatenating the header and the raw image file. The transfer of pixel dimensions, where possible, allows subsequent computerized measurements to be obtained in the correct dimensions and scale.

Colour images are more informative than their monochrome counterparts. This is especially true of images obtained from histologically stained tissues. The image file formats should therefore allow accurate image rendition and should be capable of storing text and graphics for image overlays. In microscopy the use of colour images rather than greyscale images can be advantageous. There are many methods available for describing colour spaces and in biology the most useful is the HSV system (see Chapter 3).

Image compression

One inherent disadvantage of storing high resolution images is that the image files can be extremely large and hence can occupy large amounts of disk space. For example, a confocal dataset consisting of 75 consecutive images, each 768×512 pixels, would occupy approximately 30 MBytes of storage space. There are two problems associated with large image files. The first is due to the amount of disk space that these large image files require for storage. The second problem is encountered when manipulating the files and relates to the file transfer speed. Images are often transmitted over networks for display or manipulation. Image transfer speeds are roughly proportional to the size of the images being transmitted. Large image files can take several seconds or even minutes to be transferred across a network.

To overcome these problems image files are usually compressed. Image compression involves coding the data in such a way that a sequence of image bits is replaced with an encoded version occupying less storage space. Algorithms used for data compression fall into two classes, image-preserving and lossy compression. Image-preserving, or reversible, algorithms maintain all of the image information so that an image recovered after compression is identical with the pre-compressed original. In lossy compression a certain amount of image degradation is permitted.

The degree of compression is expressed as the ratio of the size of the image prior to compression to the size after compression. Thus a compression ratio of 10:1 indicates that the compressed image occupies only 10% of the storage space of the original. The Unix compress command uses adaptive Lempel-Ziv coding, a method which is image-preserving. The compression ratios achieved in practice depend on the number of bits per pixel and the complexity of the image. In general, compression ratios of images from histochemically stained tissues are small, perhaps only 2:1, because of their complexity. Confocal microscope datasets can usually be compressed more. Binary images, obtained as the result of segmentation operations for example, can often be highly compressed. Depending on the total number of selected pixels in the binary image, compression ratios of up to 100:1 can be obtained.

Run-length encoding (RLE) is a common and simple encoding technique for image compression. The basic idea behind RLE is that pixel intensities are examined sequentially and translated into a sequence of number pairs. Each number pair consists of a pixel intensity and its frequency of occurrence. Consider the following pixel intensities:

189 189 189 189 189 190 190 190 190 190 190 190 191 191 191 190 190 190 190 101 101 101 50 50 50 50 50

Run-length encoding would reduce this sequence to:

189 5 190 7 191 3 190 4 101 3 50 5

This reversible method of encoding clearly reduces the amount of information required to store a sequence of pixel intensities. However, if a sequence of pixel intensities was obtained from a noisy image it might be less smooth. For example:

189 190 189 189 190 190 190 191 190 190 191 190 191 192 191 190 191 190 190 102 101 101 51 50 50 51 50

The encoded sequence would then be:

189 1 190 1 189 2 190 3 191 1 190 2 191 1 190 1 191 1 192 1 191 1 190 1 191 1 190 2 102 1 101 2 51 1 50 2 51 1 50 1

This actually requires more storage space than the original sequence. Pre-processing an image prior to compression, for example to smooth out noise spikes, can often be useful to increase the compression ratio.

A number of RLE-based compression methods have been developed to address various compression problems similar to the one discussed. Other methods of encoding include Huffman encoding (Huffman, 1952), LZW compression (Welch, 1984), arithmetic compression (Abrahamson, 1989) and lossy compression (Wallace, 1991).

Conclusion

There are many file formats available for storing graphics (Table 1). Many of these formats are continually being modified to contend with rapidly changing requirements. In this chapter I have attempted to introduce the concept of image file formats without exploring the technicalities. For a more detailed discussion of file formats, Kay & Levine (1992) provide simplified documentation on common file formats, many of which have not been mentioned here.

The portable bitmap utilities (PBM), primarily written by Poskanzer (1991), are a noteworthy set of tools for converting between various file formats and transforming image data. These tools and other useful utilities are publicly accessible via the Internet: consult the file PBMPLUS obtainable by anonymous FTP from ftp.ee.lbl.gov (128.3.112.20). A basic understanding of graphics file formats allows the biologist to convert between image files and hence permit images to be analysed or processed by third-party systems. An example of where this would be beneficial is in the field of confocal microscopy and 3-D visualization (see Chapters 10 and 18). It is often necessary to transfer confocal data from the original acquisition system to other 3-D visualization platforms.

References

Abrahamson, D.M. (1989). An adaptive dependency source model for data compression. *Communications of the ACM*, **32**, 77–83.
Aldus (1988). *Aldus/Microsoft Technical Memorandum*.
Compuserve (1990). *Graphics Interchange Format (Version 89)*. Columbus: Compuserve Incorporated.
Compuserve (1988). *Graphics Interchange Format. A Standard Defining a Mechanism for the Storage and Transmission of Raster-based Graphics Information*. Columbus: Compuserve Incorporated.
Huffman, D. A. (1952). A method for the construction of minimum-redundancy codes. *Proceedings of the Institute of Electronic and Radio Engineers*, **40**, 1098–00.
Kay, D. C. & Levine, J. R. (1992). *Graphics File Formats*. New York: Windcrest/McGraw-Hill.
Poskanzer, J. (1991). PBMPLUS: Extended Portable Bitmap Toolkit. Public network distribution.
Sun Microsystems (1990). *4.1 Pixrect Reference Manual*. Sun Microsystems.
Truevision (1991). *Targa File Format Specification Version 2.0. Technical Manual Version 2.2*. Indianapolis: Truevision, Inc.
Wallace, G. K. (1991). The JPEG still picture compression standard. *Communications of the ACM*, **34**, 30–44.
Welch, T. A. (1984). A technique for high performance data compression. *IEEE Computer*, **17**, 8–19.

5

Basic image processing operations on the digitized image

S. BRADBURY

Introduction

A recent survey has shown that many scientific papers are written in language so complex and rich in jargon that they are intelligible only to scientists who are already expert in that particular field. The field of image processing is no exception and many newcomers to this area of work find that the basic concepts are often explained in a mass of technical language, derived partly from computer studies and partly generated by the subject itself. In this chapter I will try to explain some of the basic operations performed during computer analysis of a digitized image in simple terms and at a very basic level.

We carry out image analysis every time we look at a scene; our eyes provide the input and the neuronal networks in the retina and in our brains are very good at sorting and classifying the large amounts of information presented to them in a complex image. The arrangement of features in a face or a landscape, for example, which form intricate patterns, can be processed very quickly, so allowing us to recognize individuals or places almost instantly, even when the data are incomplete. This type of operation is often very difficult for an automated image analysis system unless there is considerable preprocessing of the image. However, our eyes and brains are rather bad at counting and measuring features in an image. By contrast, given suitable images, these are operations at which image analysis systems excel.

Once a digitized image is stored in an image analysis system there are several reasons why it may need processing before measurement starts. Very often the original image is 'noisy', with occasional small white spots due to sudden surges that may originate in the power supplies. Contrast, although often introduced optically, may be low and needs to be enhanced, and often the complexity of the image is such that the amount of detail must be reduced before the extraction of the relevant features for measurement (the process known as segmentation). In practice, several processing operations will often be needed in sequence to transform an image into a form in which segmentation and measurement may be performed with certainty. Until quite recently, when high powered desktop digital computers with extensive RAM memory became available at affordable prices, all image processing was done by purpose-built hardware. A typical example of such an instrument was the Quantimet 720, then made by Cambridge Instruments. Even in the sophisticated processors available today, some image processing operations may still be carried out by hardware for reasons of speed, whilst the majority of image amendments demand actual arithmetical computations to be performed on the digital image.

In a modern image analysis system the sequence of events would be:

1 Obtain the best quality image on which to operate.
2 Capture, digitize and store the image in the computer memory.
3 Carry out image processing to improve or transform the image in some way.
4 Segment the image (i.e. indicate the relevant parts for measurement).
5 Measure the required parameters.
6 Process, present and store the measured data.

The necessity for obtaining a high quality image in the first place before attempting any form of analysis or measurement should be obvious, but is often overlooked and image analysis is attempted on images which are of poor quality. In many cases attention to elementary rules of microscope operation, for example (see Chapter 9), may well simplify the subsequent processes dramatically. Image capture and digitization form the subject of other chapters and will not be considered further here. The result of digitization is a series of numbers which, for a monochrome image, usually represent the brightness or greylevel measured at each of a large number of points in a sequential scan of the picture. Such a scan conventionally begins at the top left corner of the picture which is denoted by the x, y coordinates of 0, 0; the x coordinate increases with motion from left to right along a given line, whilst the y coordinate increases from the top to the bottom of the image.

In many systems the digitization is carried out at an eight-bit level, i.e. the range of brightness at each sampling point (often termed a pixel) is represented by a number ranging from 0 (black) to 255 (absolute white), which is the largest number that can be represented in a single Byte of computer storage. Such a digitized image would be said to have 256 greylevels. The number of pixels per image largely depends upon the amount of computer memory available as well as upon the detail required in any subsequent representation. It is clear that the larger the number of pixels, the higher will be the resolution of the image. An appreciation of this may be obtained by comparing the sharpness of photographs reproduced in a newspaper using a coarse screen (say 65 dots per inch) with those in a journal where the reproduction has been achieved with a screen having many more dots per inch. In image analysis a common practice has been the use of 512 × 512 pixels (a total of 262 144) per frame, but nowadays images of 1024 × 1024 pixels are not uncommon. If, on the one hand, the pixel number for a given image size is reduced (i.e. if the actual size of the pixel itself is increased) but the 256 greylevels are maintained, then resolution and quality soon deteriorate. Images of 256×256 pixels are acceptable, but those of 128×128 or 64×64 pixels show a marked chequer board effect which destroys the resolution. If, on the other hand, the number of pixels in an image is kept constant at, say 512×512, but the number of greylevels is reduced from 256 to 128 or even 64, then the perceived image quality does not suffer too much. Any further reduction has a marked effect on the quality.

If only one bit of information is stored per pixel (so allowing the information about eight pixels to be stored in each Byte of computer storage) then only the presence or absence of some quality at that point can be recorded, for example whether the pixel is bright or dark. Such an image is termed a binary image. It is economical of image storage space and easy to print. Binary images are often used to create what are termed masks, which are used for other operations and also for the logical manipulation of two images.

If the image is in colour then not only the brightness but also the colour of a particular pixel must be coded. In practice it is usual to sample the brightness of the red, green and blue components of a pixel either by using a special camera or by sampling through narrow-cut primary colour filters. It is obvious that such an approach will require three times as much image storage as a monochrome image. A valuable discussion of the features of a digital image will be found in Lewis (1990) as well as in Gonzalez & Wintz (1987).

Once an image is digitized and (usually) held in an area of computer memory designated as a frame store, processing to change its component pixels may then begin. The new values for pixel brightness are either substituted back into the original image, so destroying it, or into the corresponding locations of a transformed image. Although such processing is usually carried out in its entirety using programs loaded into the software as needed, an exception is the use of lookup tables, which are permanently stored in the computer memory. These speed up the processing dramatically, since with a lookup table a new value for a given pixel may be substituted very rapidly. For example, a lookup table may be constructed so that all pixels that have numerical values between 0 and 5 have their values replaced by the value 5, all with a value between 6 and 10 be altered to 25, those between 11 and 15 to 50 and so on (Fig. 1). In this example the value of an input pixel from the original image is assumed to be 12, so that the output for the corresponding pixel in the new image would be 50. Lookup tables are much used in certain areas of image processing to alter the contrast, to alter the number of greylevels in an image or to introduce false colour. This latter often simplifies the visual interpretation of an image when presented on the monitor or colour printer.

Image processing operations may be grouped for convenience into three main types, termed point processing, group processing and frame processing operations. In each category there are several possible available options, the implementation of which is often controlled by whether the maker of the image analyzer has provided the relevant software.

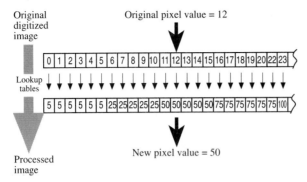

Fig. 1. A diagram to show the operation of a lookup table stored in the computer memory. A pixel in the original image with a brightness level of 12 will have a value of 50 substituted for it in the target or output image.

Point processing operations

An image is stored in memory as a matrix, in which the number in each location represents the brightness at that particular point in the image. In a point processing operation, an arithmetical operation is carried out on each pixel in turn and the new value either substituted for the old or, preferably, written into a new frame store so that the original image is always available for reference. Among some of the more common point processing operations on single images are:

> inversion
> pseudocolouring
> shading correction
> production of greylevel histograms
> greylevel traces
> contrast enhancement by histogram stretching
> image scaling and formation of binary images
> Boolean operations
> erosion, dilation and their sequential use, opening and closing
> skeletonization.

One of the simplest of such point processing operations is inversion; this is most commonly used with a lookup table in which a pixel value is changed so that the output provides a negative of the input image. Such a lookup table can be represented graphically (Fig. 2) which shows the mapping of the input to output. An inverting lookup table is convenient for use when the input is from, say, a photographic negative; it helps the operator visualize the successive operations more clearly when a positive image is displayed on a monitor.

The generation of pseudocolour images, already mentioned, where the colour of the output pixel generated depends on the numerical value of the input pixel, is another example of a simple point processing function which has

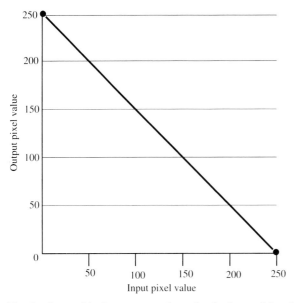

Fig. 2. A graphical representation of a lookup table; the ordinate represents the input pixel brightness values whilst those in the target image are given along the abscissa. This lookup table would serve for inversion or complementation; an input of 255 gives an output of 0 and vice versa.

considerable value for making the operator aware of small greylevel differences across the image. Pseudocolour images are especially helpful when setting what is known as the shading correction.

In any microscope or other imaging system an absolutely even illumination across a field is almost impossible to achieve, because of optical imperfections, misalignments of components or light source inhomogeneities. Such differences of image brightness are very difficult to perceive by eye but, if present, would make it very difficult to segment an image using greylevels alone (perhaps the most common method of segmentation). If a digitized image of a blank field is stored then it is possible to use this to correct any other image on a pixel by pixel basis either by subtracting the background image, pixel by pixel, from the new image or by dividing one image by another, sometimes called the ratio method. The subtraction technique may well result in some pixel values becoming negative, so it is usual to divide the difference value by 2 and then add 128, a rescaling which provides values within the acceptable range. Alternatively, a number representing the difference between the mean brightness of the reference background and the acquired image may be added to the pixel value obtained after subtraction. If the ratio method is used then the values are real numbers, but in order to avoid division by zero it is usual to replace all pixel values of zero with a value of 1 before the division is done. If the input television camera gives a linear output in response to brightness then the division method is preferable, whilst for cameras with a logarithmic response to brightness changes the subtraction method of shading correction is better.

Another point processing operation is the production of greylevel histograms. Here a count is performed of the frequency of each pixel value and the result expressed graphically (Fig. 3). From such histograms the contrast range of the image may be deduced. An image of low contrast will have a very peaked histogram extending over a short range of pixel values, whereas an image of good contrast range will extend over a much larger range of histogram values. It is a simple operation, again often carried out with the aid of lookup tables for speed, to expand or stretch a histogram or portion of a histogram so that the pixel values in the resulting image occupy the full range from 0 to 255. This is represented graphically in Fig. 4, where input pixels between 50 and 140 would be scaled to give an output that covers the full range from 0 to 255; Fig. 5 shows two actual histograms as they are reproduced by the printer of an image analyser to illustrate this operation. A variant on this procedure is not to accumulate the frequency of occurrence pixel values, but to plot as a line trace the value of the individual pixels along a single line (chosen by the operator) in the original image. This is the so-called greylevel trace (Fig. 6) which is often of great value in deciding where, for example, to set a thresholding level and to see whether the shading correction is adequate.

Pixels that have values outside a given range may be set to a common

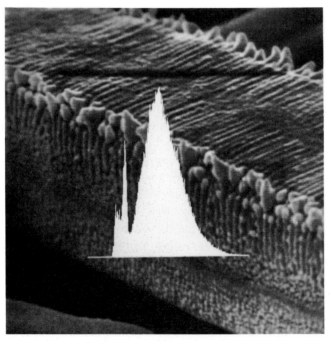

Fig. 3. A scanning electron micrograph of a diatom frustule, photographed from the screen of an image analyzer, with the bi-modal greylevel histogram superimposed.

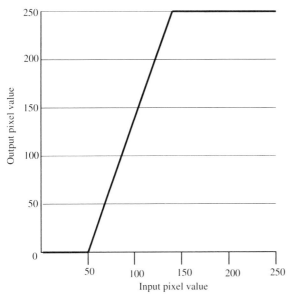

Fig. 4. A diagram of a lookup table for contrast expansion; input brightness values between 50 and 140 are expanded to occupy the full dynamic range from 0 to 255.

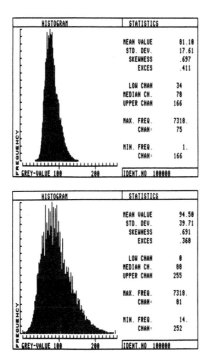

Fig. 5. Examples of the actual printer output from an image analyzer of an original greylevel histogram and that from the same image after the dynamic range has been expanded. Note that this particular manufacturer's image analyzer prints certain basic statistics related to the histogram at the same time.

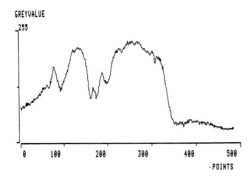

Fig. 6. A greylevel trace of a single line along the whole length (512 pixels) of an image.

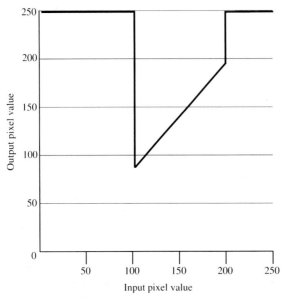

Fig. 7. A diagram of a lookup table which would effect background cleaning; input brightness values below 100 and above 201 are set to 255 (i.e. white) whilst those in between retain their original values.

predetermined value, so allowing the image to be cleaned up. Backgrounds, for example, may be eliminated both above and below pre-set values for the input pixels. Fig. 7 shows graphically a lookup table for a simple case in which all pixels below 100 and above 201 are to be set to a final value of 255 (i.e. to white). The pixels that make up the desired image lie between 101 and 200 and remain at their original value in the derived image. If only two levels of output value are chosen for this type of operation then a binary image results; in most such cases the final values of the pixels are chosen to be 0 and 255 giving an image in black and white only (the lookup table for this is shown diagramatic- ally in Fig. 8). Binary images may be stored economically in computer memory

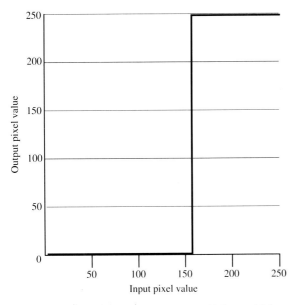

Fig. 8. A diagram of a lookup table which would form a binary image; input brightness values below 160 are set to black, those at or above 160 are set to white.

and single binary images are often the subject of further pixel-by-pixel operations (which may be called image amendments).

Operations carried out on binary images according to clearly defined logical rules are often called Boolean operations. The inversion of a single binary image may be thought of as a logical ⟨NOT⟩ operation; if a pixel is black in the input (represented by 0) then it becomes white (represented by 1) in the output and vice versa. Although this section is devoted to operations on a single image, it should be noted that, in practice, most Boolean operations combine two binary images derived from separate originals (Fig. 9, top row). Two commonly used logical operations on two images are the ⟨AND⟩ and the ⟨OR⟩. In the former, only those pixels that have the same value of 1 in *both* binary images will be represented by a 1 in the output image (Fig. 9 bottom row, left). The ⟨OR⟩ operation gives information in the output image (a pixel value of 1) if there is information in either of the original binary images (Fig 9, bottom row, right). The exclusive or operation, ⟨XOR⟩, yields an output image in which a pixel has a value of 1 only if its value in the first image is 1 and 0 in the other. The ⟨XOR⟩ operation is useful for giving an image of the difference between two images, so allowing the distinction between those parts of image 1 which are not in image 2 and conversely, i.e. those parts of image 2 which are not represented in image 1. It is clear that for this type of operation to be successful there must be very accurate registration of the two images. In practice this may require either image dilation or erosion (see below) before carrying out the Boolean operation. It is also possible to use the various

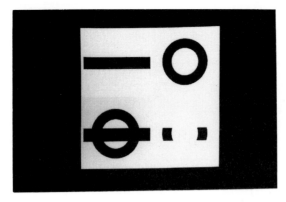

Fig. 9. Boolean operations on two binary images; the upper row shows the two original images – a bar and a circle; the lower row (left) shows the result of an ⟨AND⟩ operation – the black components of both images are present in the output. At the right on the lower row is the result of an ⟨OR⟩ operation – the resultant image shows black only in locations common to both images.

Boolean functions in sequence, e.g. the ⟨NOT⟩ followed by an ⟨AND⟩. Details of the possible applications of these operations will be found in Russ (1990) and in the Joyce-Loebl Handbook (1985).

It is easy when working with a binary image, to add or remove one or more pixels all around the border between the two states (Fig. 10). If a pixel is removed the operation is called erosion, and the converse, where one or more pixels are added to the edge, is dilation. It is clear that removal of pixels will eventually cause an irregularly shaped object (say a figure of eight) to break up into smaller objects (two roughly circular shapes in this case). Adding pixels to several close features will eventually join them all together. At the same time, however, if there are small holes or cracks in the image of any object these holes will be filled in by dilation, whilst erosion will remove surface whiskers. When these operations are used for the amendment of binary images, it is more usual for the erosion and dilation to be used in sequence; erosion followed by dilation is called opening. For example, if an image is eroded and then dilated by the same number of pixels, the erosion removes surface projections from large objects (thus smoothing their outlines) and at the same time causes very small objects to disappear completely. The subsequent dilation returns the large objects to their approximate original shape and size and they can then be measured.

The converse amendment operation is called closing and is a dilation followed by an erosion. The result of the dilation part of the closing will fill in cracks or holes in images of objects, whilst the subsequent erosion restores these final images to something close to their original size. It is clear that if there are several objects in close proximity to each other, the dilation of a

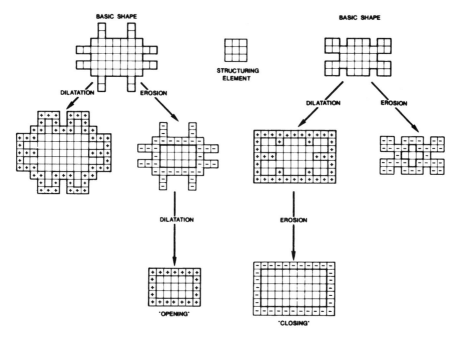

Fig. 10. Diagrams to show the effects of dilation and erosion and opening and closing. In this example the structuring element is considered to be a square pixel, although in practice other shapes may be used. At the top left a basic shape with protrusions is shown, whilst a shape with surface indentations is at the top right. In the second line the added or eroded pixels are indicated, so that the resultant shape may be seen. The bottom row shows the effects of opening (erosion followed by dilation) with the converse or closing operation on the right.

closing operation may cause the objects to coalesce irreversibly so that care is needed in the use of dilation (or closing) on an image. If all irregularities such as surface projections and holes and/or cracks are to be removed, it is preferable to do an opening followed by a closing rather than vice versa, since the opening will remove the surface projections, which might touch and cause the objects to coalesce if they were present during a closing operation. Skeletonization is a process whereby pixels are progressively eroded from the outside of a binary object until the resulting line between opposite edges is only a single pixel thick. It is clear that if this operation is performed on a circular or square feature then the result will be a single pixel; if the object has a triangular shape then a tripartite skeleton will be the result, whilst a circular object with an internal hole (e.g. the outline of a washer) will give a circular outline but only one pixel thick. The skeletons produced by more complex objects are often unpredictable: Fig. 11 shows the skeleton of the image of a complex logo. This process is not often used alone but may form part of an image amendment sequence.

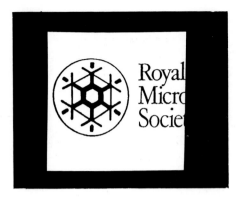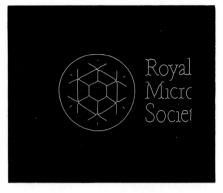

Fig. 11. The effect of skeletonization. The original image (the logo of the Royal Microscopical Society) is on the left and its skeleton on the right.

Group processing operations

In this category of image processing operations, the brightness of an individual pixel in a modified image depends on the brightness values of the group of pixels surrounding it and, for some operations, also by arbitrary values programmed into a one-dimensional (1-D) linear vector or into two-dimensional (2-D) square or rectangular matrices stored in the software. These matrices are used arithmetically to modify one of the group of pixels in the original image to produce a new value which is stored in a second, modified image before the whole operation is repeated on the next pixel. Such modifiers are often called convolution masks (often shortened simply to masks) or filters. This represents a spatial approach; other group processing operations which depend not on spatial relationships but on frequency are also possible. These Fourier transforms, as they are called, will not be discussed here; further details will be found in James (1987) and Lewis (1990), whilst a detailed theoretical treatment is given in Gonzalez & Wintz (1987).

One of the most common group processing operations – the median filter – simply involves ordering the values of the target pixel and the surrounding group in ascending order of magnitude. Let us suppose that a small area of the original image had pixel values as follows and that the central high value was the target value in this case:

    10   20   5
    15   210   20
    15   10   20

These pixels can easily be sorted by the computer into numerical order. In the example above this would be:

    5   10   10   15   15   20   20   20   210

The median value of these pixels (in this case 15) is then used as the output for the derived image. The high value (210) for the central or target pixel in the original image is most probably due to electronic noise originating in the camera, or the analogue to digital convertor, or the computer itself. As a result of the median filtering this is removed and a much lower value, more in keeping with the surrounding pixel values, is placed in the new image. The ordering operation is then repeated on the next adjacent pixel and so on until the whole image in store has been treated. The median filter is commonly used to remove noise without causing significant blurring of the image, which occurs with some other noise suppression filters.

The action of a filtering operation that involves not only the matrix of pixels in the original image but also the use of a convolution mask is illustrated diagrammatically in Fig. 12. Here the original values of nine pixels in the source image are illustrated together with a 3 × 3 mask containing a central

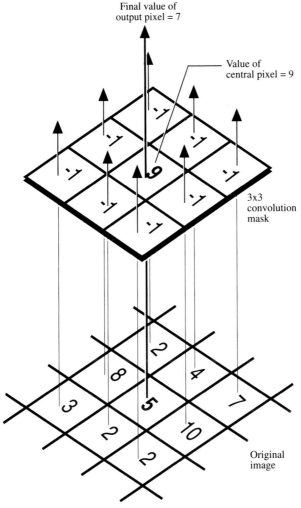

Fig. 12. A diagram to show the principle of a convolution filter or mask. This latter is a 3 × 3 high-pass matrix being applied to the central pixel in part of the original image. The output pixel in this case would have a value of 7.

value of 9 whilst all other values are -1. Its method of operation may be illustrated with reference to the target pixel in the original image which in our example has a value of 5. Its new or output value is computed from the sum of the result obtained by multiplying the value of the pixels in the matrix immediately surrounding the target by the corresponding value in the mask, as indicated by the arrows in Fig. 12. The result is thus given by:

$$[(2 \times -1) + (4 \times -1) + (7 \times -1) + (8 \times -1) + (5 \times 9) + (10 \times -1)$$
$$+ (3 \times -1) + (2 \times -1) + (2 \times -1)] = 7$$

The pixel that had a value of 5 in the original image would thus be replaced in the corresponding position in the output or derived image by a value of 7. The operation would then be repeated by performing the same calculation for the adjacent original pixel with a value of 10 and so on until the entire image has been covered. There are nine multiplications and eight additions involved when using a 3×3 mask in order to compute the value of each new pixel and, as there are 262 144 pixels in a 512×512 image, the total number of arithmetical operations required to modify an image is of the order of 4.5 million. For this reason, mask sizes are generally kept small (e.g. limited to say 9×9) although they may be increased for specialized purposes. It will be noted that the mask used in the example of Fig. 12 has values that sum arithmetically to 1 and is an example of a generalized high pass mask. Such high pass masks are used to enhance detail and sharpen up edges by allowing high frequencies to pass unchanged whilst attenuating low frequencies. Fig. 13 shows the effect of such a mask when applied to an X-ray of the pituitary fossa of the skull. Any noise present in the image will, however, also be enhanced.

The high pass filter is a variant of what is known as the inverse Laplacian filter, which has the form:

$$\begin{array}{ccc} -1 & -1 & -1 \\ -1 & 8 & -1 \\ -1 & -1 & -1 \end{array}$$

It will be noted that the central weight is 8 not 9 and thus the sum of the components of this 3×3 matrix is 0. When this is used alone the image would be set to black where the brightness is constant or changes only very slowly. It thus enhances the edges in the image. Such filters may be constructed to be directional and enhance edges that have a particular orientation.

Another category of filter is the low pass averaging filter which again may be used in moderation to suppress noise but at the expense of introducing blurring into the original image. A typical low pass 3×3 matrix would have the form:

$$\begin{array}{ccc} 1/9 & 1/9 & 1/9 \\ 1/9 & 1/9 & 1/9 \\ 1/9 & 1/9 & 1/9 \end{array}$$

It will be seen that the application of this filter averages the information in the

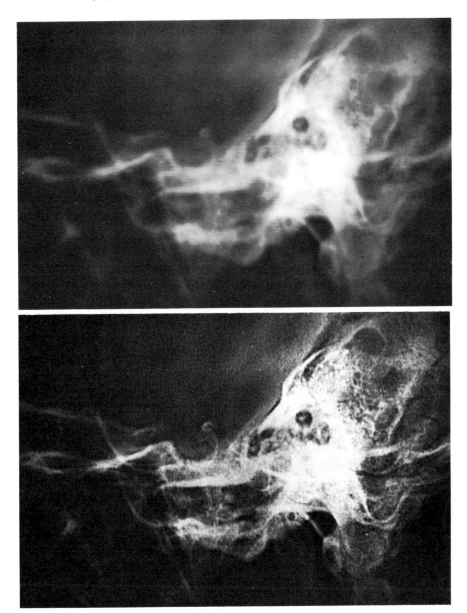

Fig. 13. The effect of a high pass convolution filter on an X-ray of the pituitary fossa in the base of the skull. These images, photographed from the screen of an image analyser show a marked apparent sharpening or enhancement of the edges in the processed image (lower panel) as compared with those in the image that has not been altered (top panel).

eight neighbouring pixels by replacing the value of each pixel by the average of it and its neighbours. This is expressed well by the notation used by Russ (1990) where the central or target pixel (P_0) and its neighbours are numbered as shown below:

$$
\begin{array}{ccc}
1 & 2 & 3 \\
8 & P_0 & 4 \\
7 & 6 & 5
\end{array}
$$

The simple low pass or smoothing filter may then be represented mathematically as:

$$ P_0' = \frac{1}{9}\sum_{i=0}^{8} P_i $$

There are many other types of filters: the Sobel and the Roberts filters are variants of gradient filters, related to the Laplacian operator mentioned above, as is the Kirsch operator. All of these may be altered in their effects by weighting them by altering the values in one or more of the locations in the 3×3 matrix. Filters may, of course, be used in sequence. Some of these filters are much larger than the simple 3×3 examples which have been considered here as examples. These will take more computational time to process an image but, with the speed of modern digital processors, this is of much less consequence than it was in the early 1980s. When using filtering, or indeed any operation on the image, the user must be aware of the danger of modifying the image too much. This could have the effect that the relevant information is transformed without the operator realizing the fact.

Frame processing operations

Frame processing operations are basically geometrical or spatial re-arrangements of the whole image and as such are of rather less importance in image analysis than the procedures discussed in the previous sections. Among frame processing techniques are:

1 x, y translations of the image.
2 Distortion correction.
3 Enlargement (zooming) or reduction.
4 Angular rotations of the image.
5 Rubber sheet transformations.

x, y transformations, angular rotations and enlargement or reduction are often used when a pair of images are to be aligned in order to measure similarities or differences between them. Rubber sheet transformations (sometimes referred to as image warping) are often required when images from curved surfaces or of plane surfaces viewed at an angle are to be dealt with. An example of the former would be an image of a sphere seen from a point (e.g. a planet seen from an orbiting satellite), whilst the latter situation is often encountered in scanning electron micrography where the object is tilted in order to improve the quality of the picture. In either case the object of image processing is to stretch the image so that it appears as a plan view of a flat object. In most cases if the position of the observation point is known or the shape of the surface is known then a set of equations may be determined that, when applied to the digitized image, will allow its correction. These equations may be relatively simple in mathematical terms, one of the commonest being to relate the address in the output image in terms of two functions of the input image address. Again using the notation of Russ (1990):

$$T(x, y) = \{U[S(x, y), V[S(x, y)]\}$$

where $T(x, y)$ represent the locations in the output image and $S(x, y)$ the locations in the input or source image. These latter are written as two functions U and V which are often quite simple polynomials, such as the bi-cubic form in which all possible cubic terms involving x and y and their products are present. The end result of this extensive calculation process is to produce coordinates that may not be integers and thus, in effect lie between pixels in the original image. The brightness value of the new pixel is often obtained by using the brightness of the pixel in the original image that is nearest to the new coordinates of the pixel. Alternatively, the new brightness value may be found by interpolating from the surrounding pixels in the original image. More details of image warping will be found in the works already cited.

Image editing

All the above techniques, whether applied to pixels, groups of pixels, or the whole image, will often effect dramatic improvements to the image. In favourable circumstances they may on their own allow the computing and measurement of the required parameters. All too often, however, ambiguities will be found in the output image and the measurements or segmentation remain unsatisfactory. For this reason almost all image analyzers provide some means (usually a light pen or linked optical cursor working on a digitizer tablet) to allow the operator to interact with and edit the image. It is of course a slow process and one in which subjective errors may well be introduced. Two of the more common editing operations on binary images are called Accept and Reject. They indicate whether an object should be measured or ignored by the computer. They may be invoked on individual objects or on all objects in an area which is delineated by the operator. In many cases an object is detected only around its circumference leaving a hole in the centre; by the use of another useful editing function (called Fill in many systems) the pixels forming any included areas may be set to 1 and so the object will appear as if it had been completely detected. Other image editing operations may be provided according to the practice of the maker of the instrument. It should be remembered, however, that extensive image editing slows down the measurement procedures substantially and if extensive editing is needed on an image then perhaps ways should be sought to improve the quality of that image.

References

Anon. (1985). *Image Analysis: Principles and Practice*. Gateshead: Joyce-Loebl.
Gonzalez, R. C. & Wintz, P. (1987). *Digital Image Processing*, 2nd edn. Reading, Mass:
    Addison-Wesley.
James, M. (1987). *Pattern Recognition*. Oxford: BSP Professional Books.
Lewis, R. (1990). *Practical Digital Image Processing*. London: Ellis Horwood.
Russ, J. C. (1990). *Computer-Assisted Microscopy: the Measurement and Analysis of
    Images*. New York: Plenum Press.

6

Study design

P. K. CLARK

Introduction

Good study design is very important in all fields of medical and scientific research. In this chapter, I deal with the statistical aspects of study design for medical research in general, and give examples relating to image processing. The main focus is on using image processing to examine some aspect of a clinical problem, e.g. comparison of the blood vessels in nasal mucosa between healthy people and patients with rhinitis. This assumes that a viable and reliable method of image processing has been found for the problem in question. A later section deals briefly with some aspects of developing image processing applications.

Study design is a fundamental aspect of statistics. It is possibly the most important topic – more important in many ways than analysis. For example, if the analysis is wrong it can be repeated, but if the design is wrong the results could be meaningless and a lot of time, effort, money and resources will have been wasted – not to mention the possible risk to the subjects or unnecessary use of animals.

Good study design always starts with the writing of a protocol – a blueprint for the study. This is discussed in the next section. In the subsequent sections, I examine the many types of study that can be performed in the medical field and discuss several aspects of the organization and structure of studies with the aims of improving their effectiveness and ensuring that the results are meaningful and can be interpreted with ease. Finally I describe two statistical aspects that are related to the development of image processing applications – accuracy and repeatability.

In general it is recommended that a statistician is consulted before designing any study and especially if more than one factor is likely to be studied. The books by Altman (1991) and Bland (1987) both include good chapters on study design.

Protocol

A protocol is a blueprint for your investigation. One will be needed when applying for a research grant, and is often necessary when obtaining ethical permission. In addition it will help when writing up your investigation, since the report may not be written until months, or even years, after the start of the study.

The protocol should be a full description of who would do what and to whom, including when, where, why and in what order it would be done. It should be detailed enough so that if the investigators changed, the new people would be able to become familiar with the study procedures without difficulty. It should also be detailed enough for a statistician to be able to understand the essential features of the study, and to prepare the most appropriate analysis.

As well as listing the details, the reasons for choosing between competing options should be given so that a proper interpretation of the results can be made. You should say which variables will be measured, what their values would tell you about the problem, and what you would expect to find. If you think of the paper you are going to write in terms of the major headings of Introduction, Methods, Results and Discussion, then a good protocol would effectively consist of the first two of them. Pocock (1983) explains protocols in more detail in the context of clinical trials.

Types of study

In the medical world there are two broad types of study:

1 Observational studies.
2 Planned experiments.

In observational studies the researchers choose the factors to observe or measure, but do not attempt to influence events. One example is the case-control study, where cases (people with a particular disease or condition) are compared with controls (other people without the disease or condition), e.g. patients with rhinitis and healthy people. Another type of observational study is one where the grouping of interest cannot be determined at the start, e.g. when studying bone density in female athletes taking part in different sports, the menstrual states of the subjects (amenorrhoeic or eumenorrhoeic) cannot be controlled by the researcher. Not all aspects of design apply to observational studies, for example randomization, but most do.

Planned experiments are based on deliberate interference with the subjects: the investigator deliberately controls or varies the experimental environment. These studies include laboratory and animal experiments and clinical trials.

There are two broad types of planned investigation – parallel-group studies and within-subject studies. For parallel-group studies there are two or more independent groups of subjects, each group being measured under different combinations of experimental conditions and/or treatments. A simple example is a clinical trial where individuals are assigned to one of two arms, or parallel groups, the subjects in each arm receiving a different treatment. In the rhinitis study, for example, the effect of a new treatment could be assessed by one group using a nasal spray containing this new treatment, the other group using a placebo spray.

In a within-subject study, each subject is usually measured under all combinations of experimental conditions and/or treatments. One example of this is the two-treatment, two-period crossover study. Each subject receives both treatments, but in a random order. This type of within-subject design usually requires fewer subjects than a study using independent groups of subjects. However, this type of investigation can be used only on a medical condition or disease which is essentially incurable – if the treatment in the first period has a permanent effect on a subject, then the effect of the treatment in the second period would be compromised and the comparison would be biased. It is also important to leave a 'wash out' period between the two treatment periods to avoid any carryover effect. Again using rhinitis as an example, if the new treatment produced only short term relief, rather than a cure, then each subject could receive both the active treatment spray and the placebo spray.

There are differences between the inferences that can be drawn from the results of observational studies and planned experiments. In observational studies any relationships found between variables can be considered to be only associations between those factors. It is unwise to infer any causality. That is, association (i.e. correlation) does not prove cause and effect. The results from planned experiments can often be treated differently: if there is a relationship between an outcome variable and a factor controlled by the experimenter, and the effects of the other factors have been taken into account, then causality may usually be inferred. However, if there is a relationship with an uncontrolled factor then the inference is the same as for an observational study.

In the context of the rhinitis study, rhinitis (or its absence) would be an observational factor because the experimenter cannot choose who gets rhinitis and who does not. However, the treatment (active or placebo) can be chosen by the experimenter, and can be regarded as a controlled variable.

Organisation and structure of a study

Selection of subjects

The most important feature of subject selection is ensuring that the subjects are representative of the population under study. This may not be very easy since often there is little choice: studies of disease rely on patients turning up at hospitals, and studies of 'normal' people require volunteers, often the researchers themselves. It can be difficult to decide whether these groups of people are truly representative of a more general population.

Another aspect of selection is homogeneity of subjects. If the population is heterogeneous, then the subjects need to be equally diverse. If there are any differences in background factors, such as age and sex, that are likely to affect the outcome variable, then these can be controlled for via stratification (see below) and designed into the experiment. Even in animal experiments, the animals do not need to be all alike. If different strains are thought to produce different results, then the strains could be used as a factor in the study. This would also avoid the risk of the results being valid for one strain only.

Controls

A control group is a set of subjects who are measured as far as possible under the same conditions as the experimental group, except for the condition or treatment under investigation. The difference in outcome between the two groups then gives a fairer estimate of the true effect of the treatment or condition being evaluated. Not all studies require controls; an example would be a study where the comparisons are of active treatments only. Similarly, in descriptive studies of a single group, experiments where each subject is measured under several different conditions (such as a crossover study), each subject acts as its own control.

Where controls are required, such as in case-control studies and studies comparing subjects under active treatments with untreated subjects, care has to be taken when selecting the controls. For case-control studies the controls should preferably be matched individually to each case by variables such as age, sex and any other factors which could be relevant such as social class, smoking or drinking habits. In other controlled experiments the subjects should be randomized to the control group or to the active treatment(s).

Where controls are used, it is recommended that the control group is assessed concurrently with the treatment group. This is to ensure that they are measured under the same conditions and that any temporal changes do not affect the results. Using a group of people assessed in the past, so called 'historical controls', is not encouraged. It is not possible to be sure that they were treated in the same way, or the response measured or assessed in the same way, as the treatment group. Also in the intervening period society could have changed and the control group may not now be representative of a currently selected control group. A further problem is that selection criteria may change over time; there is no guarantee that a group of subjects deemed suitable for a study in the past will all be suitable in the present.

Subjects can be used as their own controls. If the study measures each subject under all the different experimental conditions, then one of the conditions could be used as a control, as in a crossover study where one treatment is a placebo rather than an active drug.

Allocation bias – randomization

One source of bias that can arise is in the allocation of experimental conditions or treatments to subjects. This can occur in two ways:

1 The treatment and control groups may be different in respect of some background factor or factors that could cause a difference in the response variable.
2 Inappropriate allocation: experimenters can cheat by applying the experimental conditions to the subjects they think could best confirm their prejudices about the conditions. Also misunderstanding can arise as to the purpose of the study e.g. in a clinical trial it might be thought that the intention is treatment rather than investigation and a supposedly better treatment given to the more 'deserving' subjects.'

These problems can be avoided almost entirely by randomization, i.e. by allocating the treatments to the subjects on a random basis.

In image processing, bias can also occur in the selection of areas or cells within an image. Investigators sometimes choose areas or cells because they appear 'typical' of the type they are looking for. This is poor practice since this really means that the results will reflect what the investigator thinks is typical, rather than what is actually there. If selection of cells and/or areas of an image has to be made then this selection should be randomized to ensure there will be no selection bias. Methods for performing randomization are explained in Gore & Altman (1982).

Assessment bias – blinding

Where the image processing involves subjective assessment, which it often does, there is scope for the observer to introduce bias into the results, albeit unconsciously. This can occur when setting greylevels, marking out cell boundaries, or classifying cells into two or more groups. If the researcher does not know which treatments any subject has received, or which group they belong to, then the problem is much reduced. The practice of hiding the experimental conditions from the assessors is known as 'blinding'.

It can also be useful to hide the differences between the experimental conditions from the subjects so that their expectations have less effect on the outcome. For instance a placebo spray administered to a subject should appear identical with the active spray. The placebo effect should not be underestimated. Bland (1987) shows the results of a study of the relationship between the tablet colour and the efficacy of analgesics. The red placebo tablet appeared to be almost as effective as the best of the 'real' analgesics.

If only one of the two parties, investigator or subject, is blinded in this way then the study is said to be single blind. If both are blinded then the investigation is a double blind study.

Confounding

Confounding is the term used to describe the situation when the effects of two factors are indistinguishable. A simple example will illustrate the problem.

Suppose that in the rhinitis study two assessors (say A and B) were to be used to determine the blood vessel volume in each subject. Then if assessor A always looked at the subjects given the active treatment and assessor B always looked at the placebo treatment (or control) group, any differences between the treatments might simply be a reflection of the difference between the assessors. We say that the effect of the treatments is confounded with the effect of the assessors.

This problem can be avoided by treating the assessors as a factor in the experiment, using randomization of assessors as well as conditions, or by having both assessors examine each image.

Study size and power

When planning an experiment it is important to make some estimate of the number of subjects required, since without this information it could be impossible to tell if the study has a good chance of producing worthwhile results. You also need to know if you can recruit enough subjects in a short enough time. Estimating the study size also entails considering the size of an effect or difference expected. This is worthwhile in its own right.

From a statistical point of view the most important aspect is the power of the study. In general the larger the study the greater the power. Also the smaller the size of the effect which is to be detected, the larger the study size needed, so that looking for subtle differences needs a large number of subjects.

If no significant difference is found after completing the study then it could be the result of two possibilities:

1 That there really is no difference.
2 That there is a difference, but the study had insufficient power (i.e. it was too small) to detect it.

Without a power based assessment of the number of subjects needed it could be very difficult to avoid the second situation. Many studies have been ruined because they had insufficient power to detect a real difference, and the time, effort and money were wasted.

Altman (1991) gives an easy graphical method for calculating study sizes, and Lachin (1981) gives more information and some relevant formulae.

Stratification

Stratification can be used to reduce the amount of uncontrolled variation in a study, thus allowing smaller effects to become more apparent and fewer subjects to be used. The procedure is to divide the subjects according to a background factor which could affect the outcome variable, and then take this factor into account in the randomization and analysis. For instance in an investigation comparing the effects of two different diets on weight loss in human beings, it might be considered that the two sexes would react differently. Men and women should therefore be randomized to the diets separately, and the sex of the subjects taken into account in the analysis. Using a background factor like this is also known as 'blocking'.

It is strongly recommended that the same number of subjects is allocated to each possible combination of conditions and/or treatments. This ensures that the design is 'balanced' and makes it much easier to analyse and interpret than an unbalanced design with unequal group numbers.

Simplicity

A very important aspect of study design is simplicity. When designing a study the golden rule is to aim for simplicity rather than complexity. Choose the simplest design that will answer your questions and do not try to answer too many questions at once.

A complex design may not stand up to the rigours of the actual study. Simple studies have fewer things to go wrong and any mishaps will be less likely to cause serious problems. There is always a danger that the subjects will not comply with complicated procedures. It can prove very difficult to organize the collection of many different specimens and perform many different types of measurement and assessment, and holes in the data can arise very quickly. Having a simple study allows you to concentrate on the quality of the data rather than the quantity.

A simple experiment is also easier to analyse. A complex design which produces many missing data can be very difficult to analyse. For example, multiple regression requires every subject to have a valid value for each variable in the regression equation. If you have a lot of variables, all of them with some missing data, you could end up with no, or at best very few, subjects with a complete set of data. This causes very serious problems with the analysis, and with the interpretation of results based on only a few of the subjects in the study.

Simple studies with simple analyses are usually much easier to interpret. Do not design a study leading to an analysis you do not understand. If you cannot understand the analysis, how can you explain the results to anyone else?

Developing new image processing applications

When a new application of image processing is being investigated two areas of statistical concern can arise:

1 Accuracy – are the image processing measurements close enough to the 'real' ones?

2 Repeatability – are these measurements repeatable, i.e. is there only small variation between different measurements of the same parameter.

In this section I give a brief outline of these two aspects.

Accuracy

The only way to be sure of the accuracy of an image processing procedure is to use objects of known size and/or shape. It is also very useful to use objects of differing sizes to see if the accuracy is the same for most objects. If objects of known size are not available (and even if they are) it is very useful to compare the results of a new procedure with those from other, proven methods. See Bland & Altman (1986) for details on comparing two methods of making the same measurement.

Repeatability

Repeatability can be assessed by measuring each object several times. You should also use more than one person to do the measuring as there can be great between-observer variation (Jagoe *et al.* 1991).

Another aspect of repeatability is the relationship between the various sources of variability in the measurements, i.e. the relative sizes of the variability between subjects, within subjects, between areas within subjects, between sections within areas, between cells within areas etc. Fleiss (1986) gives a good introduction to repeatability (he calls it reliability), but the subject of sources of variation, often called variance component analysis, is a large and complex field; Healy (1989) gives further information.

Repeatability can be difficult to measure, but is a lot easier if the study design is balanced, i.e. there is the same number of areas for each subject, the same number of sections per area, and the same number of cells per section. If this is the case then the repeatability can often be calculated with relatively simple statistical software such as Minitab, but if the data are unbalanced then specialist variance component software really has to be used.

References

Altman, D. G. (1991). *Practical Statistics for Medical Research*. London: Chapman and Hall.

Armitage, P. & Berry, G. (1987). *Statistical Methods in Medical Research* (2nd edition). Oxford: Blackwell Scientific.

Bland, J. M. (1987). *An Introduction to Medical Statistics*. Oxford: University Press.

Bland, J. M. & Altman, D. G. (1986). Statistical methods for assessing agreement between two methods of clinical measurement. *Lancet*, **1**, 307–10.

Fleiss, J. L. (1986). *The Design and Analysis of Clinical Experiments*. New York: John Wiley & Sons.

Gore, S. M. & Altman, D. G. (1982). *Statistics in Practice*. London: BMA.

Healy, M. J. R. (1989). Measuring measuring errors. *Statistics in Medicine*, **8**, 893–906.

Jagoe, R., Steel, J. H., Vucicevic, V, Alexander, N., van Noorden, S., Wootton, R. & Polak, J. M. (1991). Observer variation in quantification of immunocytochemistry by image analysis. *Histochemical Journal*, **23**, 541–7.

Lachin, J. M. (1981). Introduction to sample size determination and power analysis for clinical trials. *Controlled Clinical Trials*, **2**, 93–113.

Pocock, S. (1983). *Clinical Trials: a Practical Approach*. New York: Wiley.

7

Principles of stereology

M. A. BROWNE, C. V. HOWARD and
G. D. JOLLEYS

Introduction

Stereology comprises a set of simple and efficient rules for quantifying 3-D microscopic or macroscopic structures. These rules have been designed to obtain information from sections visualized with a microscope, but are also suitable for other forms of image data such as MRI, ultrasound or CT scans. The results obtained from stereological estimators are based on geometrical statistics. To ensure that the estimates are unbiased, the sections must be obtained in an appropriate manner. The most important condition is that the sampling should be random. For all stereological measurements, the object to be investigated must be sampled randomly in 3-D space. For some measurements the object must be randomly orientated in 3-D space as well.

Systematic bias and precision

Bias is a measure of the accuracy of an estimate, i.e. how closely it approaches the true value. After an infinite number of trials an unbiased estimator will converge on the correct result. A biased estimator, on the other hand, will converge on a value that is incorrect. Bias cannot be detected in a single experiment.

In Fig. 1 the centre of the target represents the true value. For an estimator with zero bias, the mean of a series of estimates will tend towards the true value, as shown in Fig. 1(a) and 1(b). In contrast, the biased estimators shown in Fig. 1(c) and 1(d), will tend towards some other value.

Precision is a measure of the scatter of the estimates. Precision and variance are inversely related: a high precision estimate is said to have low variance. Precision and bias are essentially independent, so that it is possible to have a high precision, biased estimator as shown in Fig. 1(c). A high precision, unbiased estimator, as shown in Fig. 1(a), is the type to be preferred.

The results obtained with an estimator depend on a number of factors. The most important condition is that the estimates are unbiased. The stereological

96

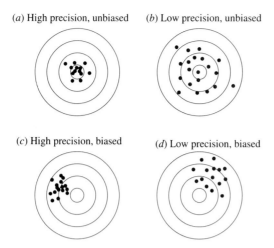

(a) High precision, unbiased   (b) Low precision, unbiased

(c) High precision, biased   (d) Low precision, biased

Fig. 1. Precision and bias in estimation procedures.

estimators in the Digital Stereology System (Confocal Technologies, 1992), when used with appropriate sampling, are unbiased.

Sectioning

Sectioning a 3-D object reduces the dimensions of its features. For example, a volumetric feature will appear in the section as an area; a linear feature such as a tubule will be seen as a number of profiles per unit area. In general, geometrical features of dimension D will appear with dimensions $D-1$ in the resulting sections (Table 1). As an example, consider the object shown in Fig. 2. Sections taken from the object exhibit 3-D features in 2-D.

The histological section or polished plane surface is a 2-D geometric probe. Features are cut in proportion to their L_1 dimension. Volumetric probes may be created by taking stacks or pairs of sections.

The grid shown in Fig. 3 contains points (L_0), lines (L_1) and areas (L_2). To translate this grid randomly, it is only necessary to move it such that one corner

Table 1. *Reduction in feature dimension by sectioning*

Dimension of feature		Dimension of section	Note
L_3	$\Rightarrow$	L_2	Volume is reduced to area
L_2	$\Rightarrow$	L_1	Area is reduced to length
L_1	$\Rightarrow$	L_0	Length is reduced to points
			Points have zero dimensions and cannot be sectioned

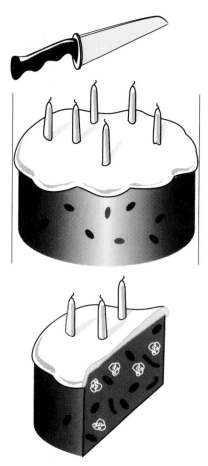

Fig. 2. Random sectioning of a complex body. For a uniform random section to be taken from this object, the knife must have an equal chance of falling anywhere between the two vertical lines.

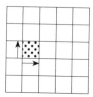

Fig. 3. Grid containing points, lines and surfaces.

of a grid square can appear with equal chance anywhere within the area of one grid square. Because the grid is a repeating pattern, all elements of the grid will be randomized at the same time. The grid allows uniform random sampling. In general, uniform random sampling is employed at all levels in stereology since it gives rise to estimates with lower variance than purely random sampling.

Ratios and densities

Stereological estimators are ratio estimators. Measurements are made in a sample from the complete specimen, known as the reference volume. Thus the numerical density of particular objects in the reference volume (ρ_N) is:

$$\rho_N = N/V_R$$

where N is the number of objects of interest and

V_R is the reference volume.

Similarly, the length density (ρ_L) is:

$$\rho_L = L/V_R$$

where L is the length of interest.
The surface density (ρ_S) is:

$$\rho_S = S/V_R$$

where S is the surface area of interest.
The volume density (ρ_V) is:

$$\rho_V = V/V_R$$

where V is the volume of interest.

The above quantities all refer to the reference volume, i.e. the volume of the sample which has been measured. In order to obtain results relating to the whole specimen, it is necessary to know the specimen volume. Thus the total number of objects of interest (N) in the specimen is:

$$N = \rho_N V_S/V_R$$

where V_S is the volume of the specimen.

In biological systems, the measurement that is usually the most relevant is the total quantity. Ratios, although unbiased, have a number of potential pitfalls and are often too insensitive to identify differences between experimental groups. In a ratio, either the numerator or the denominator or both quantities may change. This is known as the reference trap and is particularly dangerous when working with histological sections, which may undergo shrinkage during sample preparation. For these reasons total quantities should be estimated whenever possible.

Model based and design based solutions

There are basically two ways of formulating stereology: design based and model based. In the design based approach, the structure of interest is fixed and the test system is randomly positioned and/or oriented by experimental design. In the model based approach, the structure of interest is randomly positioned and/or oriented; the test system is, or may as well be, fixed. For example, a model based approach is used in the Fullman method of metallurgical grain sizing (Fullman, 1953). In this protocol an arbitrary section is taken and linear probes (lines) of known length are overlaid on the image, usually via the microscope eyepiece. The number of intersections between the linear probes and grain boundaries is counted and a mean grain diameter is computed from the ratio. This assumes that the grains are isotropic and spherical, i.e. that mean diameter is a meaningful measure. Section and probe orientation can be arbitrary. In contrast, a design based approach makes no assumptions about the isotropy or spatial characteristics of the sample. Instead the structure of the sampling at all levels is designed to be isotropic and uniform random in space. Such a sampling structure then forms a uniform sample taken from the whole population or material and is guaranteed unbiased.

From the point of view of the underlying mathematical theory it does not matter which formulation is adopted, as long as the relative positions between the structure and the test system are random. Estimates in each approach refer to different populations.

Nested analysis of variance

Stereological experiments are usually nested in their design because of a hierarchical sampling scheme (see the description of the fractionator below). This means that experiments usually begin with complete organs or batches and conclude with measurements. At the end of the experiment, the observed variance between organs or batches is greater than the real variance between them. This is because at each level of an experiment, the variance is increased.

In a typical experiment, the variance between batches or individuals may be 70%, the variance between blocks from individuals may be 20% and the variance between sections 8%. At the measurement level, the contribution to the total variance may be only 2%, so that more precise measurements can improve the precision of the overall experiment only by 1% or 2%. Note that the observed variance consists of both the true variance and a measurement error arising from the inability to study all components of an entity (that is the whole population, organ or section).

In a stereological experiment, it is not usually necessary to measure more than 100 events (points, intersections or profiles) in an individual field, if the sampling regime is optimum (Gundersen & Jensen, 1987). The measurement from one field is usually a single ratio. Although the variance of the measurement is usually high in absolute terms, in relative terms it is normally very low. Higher experimental effects are obtained by examining more individuals and more blocks per individual.

To improve the precision of an experiment a good working rule is to 'do more less well', i.e. add another individual or batch to the experiment, rather than measuring more features (Gundersen & Osterby, 1981).

Unbiased sampling strategies

The general rule in stereology is to ensure uniform random sampling, i.e. every part of the specimen should have the same chance of being included in the sample. This means that the sample will be representative of the entire specimen and will allow the results obtained to be related to the whole specimen. The 'fractionator' illustrates an approach to uniform random sampling and, in general, this approach should be adopted prior to the sectioning stage in most stereological experiments.

The fractionator

The fractionator (Gundersen, 1986) is the simplest of all sampling schemes in stereology and for that reason the most powerful. When estimating the total number of particles in a specimen, it is usually impractical to count them all. Instead the particle number is estimated in a known fraction of the reference space. The fractionator principle involves sampling particles uniformly at random with a known and predetermined probability, and then deriving the total number in the reference space from the number in the sample and the sampling probability. The principle is illustrated in Fig. 4. The fractionator avoids the reference trap.

The fraction of the object or sample of interest selected for measurement will obviously depend on the scale of the features and the object itself. Clearly even 1/10 000th part of an object such as a kidney will represent a very large quantity of material for microscopic analysis, so the scaling must be done to suit the experimental conditions.

Unbiased counting systems

The unbiased 2-D counting frame is shown in Fig. 5. Profiles of features that fall within the frame are counted, provided they do not touch the exclusion edge or its extensions (Gundersen, 1977). The guard area ensures that only complete features are sampled. Features that intersect the boundary are rejected, since they would inevitably bias the estimate.

The unbiased 2-D counting frame can be extended into three dimensions, forming a parallelepiped, as illustrated in Fig. 6 (Howard *et al.*, 1985). Particles intersecting the brick are sampled provided that they do not intersect the fully drawn surfaces.

Cavalieri's principle

The total volume of an object can be measured using Cavalieri's principle. There are three stages:

1 The object is sliced into sections. The slices need not necessarily be of equal thickness, although they almost always are. The starting position of the first slice in the object must be random. Subsequent slices will then be uniform random.

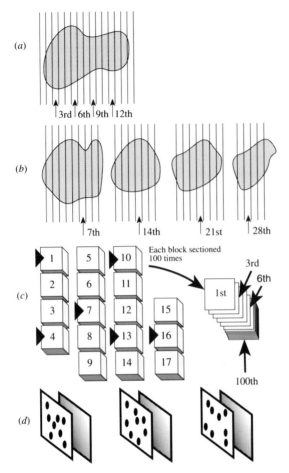

Fig. 4. The fractionator. (a) The first stage is to take one third of the material with uniform random probability. (b) The second stage is to cut the sampled sections into strips and take uniform random strips, e.g. every seventh strip starting with strip 7. (c) The third stage is to cut the sampled strips into blocks and select every third block, for example, in a uniform random manner. (d) The fourth stage is to section each sampled block exhaustively and then take a pair of sections e.g. every hundredth section, thus applying uniform random sampling. The fifth stage is to use the dissector principle on the section pairs selected in the previous stage to count all features appearing in one section but not in the next.

2 The total area of each section is estimated using the point counting method. Corresponding profiles should be counted with each subsequent section.

3 If the distance between the sections is equal then the volume of the object may be estimated by multiplying the distance between the sections by the total surface area (Fig. 7).

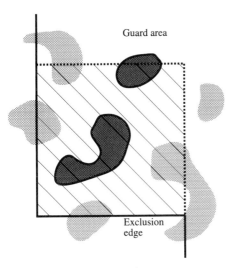

Fig. 5. The unbiased counting frame. Profiles of features that intersect the frame but do not intersect the exclusion edge (solid line) are sampled. The guard area ensures that only complete feature profiles are sampled.

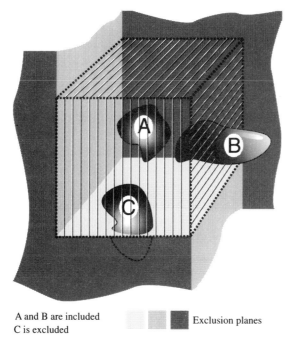

Fig. 6. The unbiased sampling brick for use in 3-D sampling of specimens, especially useful in confocal microscopy.

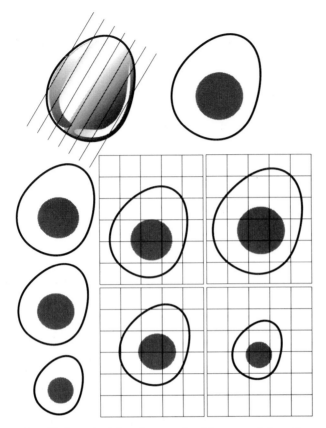

Fig. 7. Cavalieri's principle. A set of arbitrary serial sections is created from the specimen and the Cavalieri estimator is then used to calculate the total volume using point counting in a uniform random grid. The volume fraction of yolk to egg can be estimated by similar methods (see below). Needless to say this is a destructive technique. In the above example, the domain of each point is 100 mm^2 and the slice thickness is 5 mm. Therefore an unbiased estimate of the volume of the yolk is $24 \times 100 \times 5 = 12000$ mm^3 and of the volume of the egg is $62 \times 100 \times 5 = 31000$ mm^3.

Volume density

If points are randomly dispersed in space, the number of points appearing in any 3-D object will be proportional to its volume. Volume density may be obtained by counting the number of points falling within the object of interest and dividing it by the number of points falling within the reference space. To do this, a random section is taken through the object and a 2-D grid is placed randomly on the resulting plane. In 3-D, this grid has been randomly positioned within the object. The estimator is unbiased but will have a high variance associated with it. The variance can be reduced by counting a number of sections. It is important to make this measurement on thin sections to avoid the problems of over-projection (an artefact due to finite section thickness).

The dissector

The dissector (Sterio, 1984) is a geometric probe that samples isolated objects in 3-D space with uniform probability. Two serial sections are compared. They can be either physical or optical sections and it is essential that accurate registration is maintained between them. First, particle profiles are selected with a 2-D unbiased sampling frame (USF) on the so called 'reference section'. Then, the other, 'lookup' section is checked for profiles of the same particles. Only if the profiles are not present in the lookup section will they be counted in 3-D, for their tops will appear in the volume bounded by the 2-D frames and the distance between sections. Knowing the 2-D frame area and the distance between the sections the numerical density of the particles can be estimated. The most effective height between the sections is 25–30% of the average particle height.

It is essential to know whether two profiles from the same non-convex particle lie within the same frame. This problem can be overcome with optical sections by using the unbiased brick method, in which a guard volume around the brick is examined, or by having prior knowledge about the objects.

A histological section is a biased, non-representative sample of the cell population and is biased in the height-weighted distribution. A cell that is twice as high as another, in the direction normal to the section, has twice the chance of being in the sample. By counting only those particles that appear in one section of the dissector pair and not the other, the method provides a uniform sampling regime for cell counting in 3-D. Techniques based on profile counting on 2-D sections will inevitably be height-weighted and therefore biased. The orientation of the particles can also lead to large biases with 2-D measures. The dissector is unaffected by orientational anisotropy, capping and truncation effects.

The optical dissector

The dissector procedure is based on the use of physical dissection, where sections are physically cut. In contrast, the optical dissector obtains thin sections by exploiting the optical sectioning abilities of confocal and conventional microscopes. The plane of the section can be moved through a thick specimen to achieve the desired effect. Conventional and confocal microscopes require a microcator fitted to the stage in order to measure movement in the z-plane accurately.

High numerical aperture oil immersion lenses, with similarly matched condenser lenses, give the smallest focal depth. If the oil used has a refractive index equivalent to the embedding material, then the movement in the z-plane will be equal to the focal plane movement.

The method is carried out by focusing down a random distance into a thick physical section. Any profile appearing in focus in this section will not be counted in 3-D. The criterion for a profile to be considered present in any section may be that of maximum clarity of the nuclear membrane. The optical section is racked down through the specimen and any new profile is counted as a particle in 3-D if it appears within the acceptance region of the 2-D sampling frame (see Fig. 3). In practice, the height of the dissector is decided in advance. The focus is used on each particle in turn to obtain maximum clarity of the nuclear membrane and then the microcator is checked to establish if the particle was in the dissector volume. It is not usually recommended to have more than about ten events per dissector because of the practical difficulties of keeping track of them.

There are numerous advantages to using the optical dissector: the major advantage is that the sections are, by definition, perfectly registered.

Generation of isotropic directions

The dissector, and the techniques described above for volume estimation, can all be used with sections of arbitrary orientation. However, most of the other estimators used in design based stereology require the use of isotropic geometric probes, i.e. a probe that has the same properties in all directions. Techniques of sampling have been developed by stereologists to ensure that isotropic probes can be implemented in practice.

To generate isotropic directions in space, two random angles are required, selected from planes at right angles. The first angle, ϕ, is uniform randomly generated (as occurs by spinning a bottle). The second angle, θ, needs to be sine-weighted, otherwise the directions obtained will be biased towards the pole of the sphere. The relationship between ϕ and θ is shown in Fig. 8. An isotropic section is a plane perpendicular to the isotropic direction. To perform uniform sampling the sections must be uniform random.

In practice, for specimens where there is no obvious axis of anisotropy, isotropic, uniform random (IUR) sections may be obtained by cutting the block of material and randomizing the orientation before embedding. For material that has an appreciable degree of anisotropy, this will not suffice and a more formal protocol is necessary. The orientator, described below, has been developed by Mattfeldt *et al.* (1985) to create IUR sections.

The orientator and IUR sections

As mentioned previously, isotropic sections are necessary for many stereological techniques. Fig. 9 shows an example of the creation of IUR sections from a highly anisotropic body, a carrot. The sectioning procedure is as follows. The specimen, which will normally be a block selected in a uniform random manner from the material of interest, is placed approximately in the centre of the first circle. A random number is selected using a random number generator (e.g. 7 in Fig. 9). The specimen is cut perpendicularly to the plane of the circle along the selected direction. The cut must go through the centre of

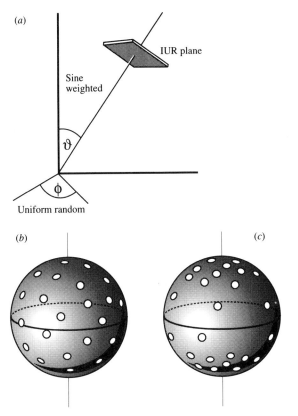

Fig. 8. Generation of isotropic directions. (*a*) Two angles ϕ and θ are shown with their relationship to a Cartesian coordinate system. An IUR plane is one that is normal to the anisotropic direction chosen by the generation of ϕ in a uniform random fashion and θ in a sine-weighted manner. (*b*) The effect of sampling in IUR directions and (*c*) the effect of sampling with a uniform random orientation in both ϕ and θ.

the circle. The cut surface creates a new edge, which is placed on the second circle with the new edge aligned along the 0–0 direction. The divisions of the second circle yield cosine-weighted sections that are therefore normal to sine-weighted directions (see below). A random number is selected and the specimen is cut, normal to the plane of the clock, in this direction (e.g. 9 in Fig. 9). The resultant section is isotropic uniform in the specimen, i.e. its orientation is one chosen from all possible orientations with uniform probability.

Vertical sections

In many circumstances it is desirable to section a sample in a preferred direction, e.g. a skin biopsy, so that a knowledge of the structures of interest can be applied to the interpretation of the results generated by the stereological study. Furthermore it may prove difficult to generate IUR sections in any case.

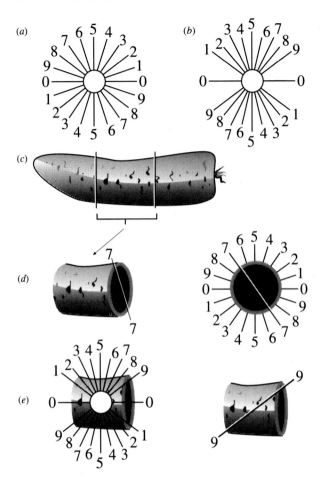

Fig. 9. The specimen and the apparatus with the two clocks, the left one (*a*) having uniform random directions and the right one (*b*) having cosine-weighted directions. (*c*) A part of the carrot is placed on the uniform-weighted clock and (*d*) a random number is chosen to select the first cutting angle, 7 in this instance. (*e*) The cut portion from the uniform clock is placed onto the cosine-weighted clock (so that the section is normal to the sine-weighted direction) with the original longitudinal axis of the carrot oriented along the 0 line and a second random number is taken, 9 in this example, and the IUR plane is cut. The carrot is reconstructed to show the position of the selected IUR section.

Vertical sections provide an alternative and, in many respects, a better way of enabling isotropic linear probing of a sample. To generate vertical sections, take any horizontal plane (arbitrary or of some physical significance, if preferred) and define a vertical direction perpendicular to this. Then cut sections in the vertical direction but with uniform random orientation about the vertical direction and uniform random translation, as shown in Fig. 10. The same vertical direction must be maintained for all sections from each specimen.

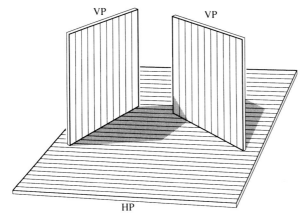

Fig. 10. Vertical sections are taken relative to an arbitrary but fixed plane in the specimen. The orientation about the vertical direction is chosen uniform random and then a random $x-y$ translation is applied. VP, vertical plane; HP, horizontal plane. Reproduced with permission from the Journal of Microscopy (Baddeley *et al.*, 1987).

Any isotropic direction in space can be obtained in a set of sections preferentially oriented around a defined normal (vertical) to a horizontal plane.

Surface density estimation

The estimation of surface area is an important technique in any study of structure or function. The surface density (surface area per unit volume) of micro- or macrostructures is an essential property in studying processes that take place either as a result of surface interaction or across surfaces, as is the case with transport and diffusion processes, for example.

The unbiased estimation of surface density involves probing the 3-D structure with isotropic linear probes and evaluating the intersection count per unit length of the probe. As discussed earlier, a linear probe (L_1) is used as a probe for a surface (L_2) feature and the sum of their order is three. The classical relationship that describes the surface density in terms of the intersection count and the total length of testing lines used to probe the sample (Weibel, 1979) can then be used to estimate surface density (ρ_S):

$$\rho_S = S/V = 2N_I/L,$$

where S is the surface area of interest,
V is the volume of the object,
N_I is the number of intersections and
L is the total length of line falling within the object.

The use of isotropic linear probes is essential if an unbiased estimate of surface density is to be obtained. This can be achieved in both IUR and vertical sections as described above. In IUR sections, probes with a uniform orientation distribution are applied, thus probing isotropically in 3-D. In vertical sections the orientation distribution of the probes must be sine θ-weighted and for this reason it has been normal practice in manual stereology to utilise cycloidal testing lines, which individually exhibit sine θ-weighting (Baddeley *et al.* 1987). However in digital stereology it is more efficient to utilize a multiplicity of linear probes which collectively exhibit the desired orientational distribution. These are often known as 'needles'.

It is interesting to note that because the intention is to count the number of intersections between isotropic linear probes and feature profile boundaries, there is no need to apply a 2-D unbiased sampling grid in this case. All feature profiles, complete or otherwise, contribute to the surface density within the field of view. So long as the total length of testing lines is known, an unbiased estimate of surface density is obtained.

Estimation of length density

The probability that a given structure is hit by a randomly positioned and randomly oriented section is proportional to its linear dimension or length. The number of times a linear structure is cut by or intersects a section will depend on the total length of the structure and the area of the probing section. To estimate the total length, the reference volume containing the object must be known. However, to estimate the length density or length per unit volume the reference volume is not required. It is important that the sampling sections or planes are IUR, not vertical, since the geometric probe in this case is 2-D (L_2) and the only way that a 2-D probe can be applied isotropically is at the sectioning stage. Furthermore, the intersections between the section and the structure must be counted without bias. Thus a 2-D USF is used for counting.

In practice, two rules are frequently used in this estimator, the 2-D unbiased counting rule and a point counting rule (for area determination). Thus the frame that is applied to successive fields of the sample may have a dual function. On the one hand it may be used to sample intersection points without bias and on the other it may have a low density raster of points (possibly one point per frame) associated with it for area fraction determination. As the USFs are moved through the successive fields of view, the number of points falling within the object of interest is recorded, as well as the number of intersections accepted. Thus the calculation of the length density estimate can be carried out for the total reference volume, by using the sum of all USF areas (as shown in the first equation below). Alternatively, the estimate can be computed with respect to the object of interest by using the fraction of the total USF area (from the fraction of points in the raster) falling within the object of interest. In the latter case all intersections within the object of interest must be counted, irrespective of whether the point in the USF intersects the object of interest. A typical situation is shown in Fig. 11, where the feature, the section and the counting frame are clearly visible.

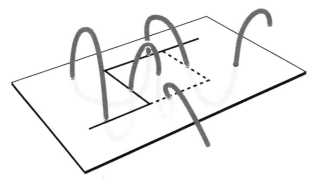

Fig. 11. The linear feature is shown intersecting the sampling section, with the 2-D unbiased counting frame overlaid to ensure appropriate counting of intersection points. Regions of the linear feature that are above the section are drawn as dark lines, while those below are drawn in pale lines. $N_I = 3$ for this section.

If the area associated with each counting frame is known, then the length density (ρ_L) or length per unit volume is:

$$\rho_L = L/V_R = 2\,N_I/\Sigma a_f,$$

where L is the total length of the feature,

V_R is the reference volume,

N_I is the number of intersections between the feature and the section, within each counting frame and

a_f is the area of each unbiased counting frame.

If the length density within a given object is required, and the USF has one point per frame as illustrated in Fig. 12, then the above expression can be modified as follows:

$$\rho_L = 2N_I/(N_P a_g)$$

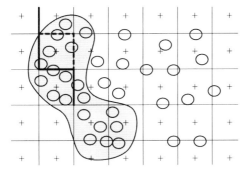

Fig. 12. The object of interest here is shown as a shaded area, while the surrounding material is unshaded. The dissector frame tessellates throughout the field and has associated with it a single point per frame. The intersection count of the linear features (shown as black elliptical outlines) is used to estimate N_I and the point count (points shown as +) to estimate the total area frame falling within the object of interest, N_P. In this example $L_V = 2 \times 18/5a_f$, where a_f is the area of the frame in real units at the magnification used for observation.

where N_P is the number of points falling in the object of interest and
a_g is the area of each dissector grid.

Note that in Fig. 12 the USF tessellates throughout the section, ensuring a uniform sampling scheme. It is not essential to provide complete coverage of the section, since it is usually more efficient to subsample. The power of the USF is readily apparent here because it ensures that each intersection between the structure of interest and the section will be counted only once. The number of testing points that are associated with the dissector area and fall within the object of interest may be used to evaluate the area fraction of that object and, from the description of the volume fraction estimator, it will be apparent that the area fraction is an unbiased estimate of the volume fraction. Hence the combined counting scheme gives length density in the object of interest, or alternatively in the total reference volume.

Particle sizing

The surface areas and volumes of particles can be estimated indirectly or by direct methods.

Indirect methods

Particle sizes can be estimated indirectly using a combination of number and stereological size estimators. For example, the mean particle volume (V_m) can be estimated from:

$$V_m = \rho_V/\rho_N,$$

where ρ_V is the volume density and
ρ_N is the number density.

Similarly the mean particle surface area (s_m) is:

$$s_m = \rho_S/\rho_N,$$

where ρ_S is the surface density, or surface area per unit volume.

Direct methods

Particle sizes can be measured directly by selecting them according to the dissector rule and measuring their volume using the Cavalieri principle. This approach requires a knowledge of shrinkage and of section thickness.

The point sampled intercept

Gundersen & Jensen (1983; 1985) developed a method for measuring the mean particle volume from single sections. The first step is to sample particles in proportion to their volume. This is done by projecting points into 3-D space and measuring the volume of any particles that are selected by the points. The second step is to measure the length of a number of isotropic lines passing through the point within the selected particle.

In practice IUR sections are used and a grid of points is placed onto a micrograph. The direction of the lines must be uniform random over 180°, to complete the process of creating IUR lines in 3-D space. Vertical sections may also be used for particle sizing but the grid must consist of sine-weighted lines. An unbiased estimator of the volume-weighted mean volume (V_m) is:

$$V_m = (l_1 + l_2 + l_3)^3\, \pi/3,$$

where l_i is the length of the i-th intercept.

Because these measurements can be made on single sections, the technique is very useful in electron microscopy. The method is very efficient, usually requiring only between 50 and 100 intercepts for a stable estimate.

The nucleator and the selector

The nucleator and the selector are methods that require pairs of sections, or a series of sections, taken by a uniform random technique from a block. Two of the sections are used to make a dissector. The nucleator (Gundersen, 1988) is best suited to cells containing only one nucleus or nucleolus. The cell is sampled only if the nucleus or nucleolus is captured by the dissector. The dissector thickness does not need to be known. If the cells of interest do not exhibit any unique features, then the selector (Cruz-Orive, 1987) may be used instead.

Having obtained a sample of particles, then the volume of each particle must be estimated. Since each particle was sampled with equal probability, then the arithmetic mean of the volume estimates is an unbiased estimate of the mean cell volume in the number-weighted distribution. The volume of each particle is estimated using a few point sampled intercepts that must be isotropic in 3-D space. The orientation of the serial sections must therefore be either IUR or vertical.

The nucleator demands that only the profiles containing the cell nucleus, or other identifiable feature, are measured, while the selector requires that complete particles are scanned through successive sections, thereby providing profiles for a Cavalieri-type volume estimation.

Measurements with the nucleator proceed by drawing lines through a random point within the nucleus or nucleolus, whose orientation properties are chosen depending on the section characteristics, i.e. IUR or vertical. The length of a number (typically four) of intercepts from the point to the cell boundary is measured (Fig. 13). The mean cell volume (V_m) is given by:

$$V_m = 4\pi\, (l_1 + l_2 \ldots l_n)^3/3n,$$

where l_i is the length of the i-th intercept and
n is the total number of intercepts measured.

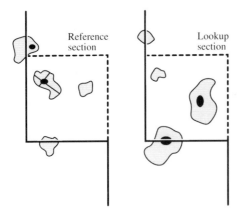

Fig. 13. The dissector pair used to select particles or cells for the nucleator. A particle in the acceptance region of the dissector is selected for measurement in the reference section as shown. Isotropic intercepts are generated radially from the random point within the nucleolus. The intercept lengths from the point to the edge of the cell l_1, l_2 and so on are then used in the estimation formula.

The star volume estimator

The star volume estimator is the analogue of the point sampled intercept estimator for non-discrete features. It has been used successfully in the study of voids and the continuous phases of samples where transport and diffusion are important. For example, the permeability and porosity of water and oil-bearing rocks appear to be related to both the mean free, line-of-sight path length of voids and the void volume fraction. The star volume estimator is related to both these parameters.

The estimator measures isotropic intercept lengths in three directions. The star volume (V^*) is given by:

$$V^* = \pi \, (l_1 + l_2 + l_3)^3/3,$$

where l is the intercept length.

An example of void characterization is shown in Fig. 14. The regions of interest are sampled using the familiar point sampling grid and the linear probes must be applied isotropically. This requires that the sample sections are IUR or vertical in nature. In fact sampling is identical to that for point sampled intercept. However, there are potential problems with the estimator, whose properties are not fully understood. For example, it seems best to use the estimator at the lowest possible magnification so that extensive voids or continuous-phase features can be measured to their furthest extent to minimize the danger of bias introduced by edge effects.

The spatial grid

The spatial grid technique can be employed to measure the surface of a single object, given a stack of perfectly registered sections through it (Sandau, 1987).

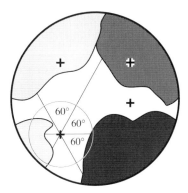

Fig. 14. A void (unshaded) in a multiphase structure. The star volume is computed from the mean of the cubes of the isotropic intercepts. In this example only one set of intercepts is shown, another would be generated in this field for the other point falling within the void to the right.

The only constraint is that the stack must be IUR. A probe that is a 3-D grid of lines in space is used. The probe is mapped out by sweeping a 2-D grid with lines in the x and y axes through space in the z direction. The intersections of the x and y lines on the 2-D grid then trace lines in the z direction.

On a 2-D rectilinear grid of lines, a single point has two adjacent sides of a grid element associated with it. A 3-D grid of points has three adjacent grid line elements associated with each single point, as shown in Fig. 15. Sets of these elements in a 3-D grid form right prisms, and the length of line associated with each point in the lattice is equal to the sum of the three sides of the prism.

In the spatial grid, these 3-D grids are thrown into space and the number of intersections between the test grid and the object of interest are measured (N_I). The total length of test line per unit volume (L/V), associated with the grid, enables the total surface area of an object to be calculated. This technique gives an efficient, low variance estimate. The grid must be perfectly registered between sections and so the technique lends itself to confocal microscopy.

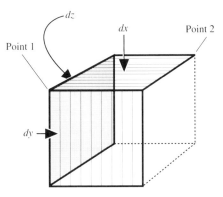

Fig. 15. The basic prism in a 3-D spatial grid consists of a point and three associated sides, of dimensions dx, dy, dz. The interlocking prisms form right parallelepipeds. In the special case where $dx = dy = dz$, the lattice is made up of cubes.

To estimate the total surface of an object it is necessary to know the total number of intersections of the grid with the object and the linear dimensions of the basic prism of the grid.

The position of the grid with respect to the object must be uniform random and the orientation isotropic – that is IUR. In a design based approach it is therefore important to make sure that the orientation of the object is properly randomized. The estimator has a low variance associated with it because of the antithetic effect of using three orthogonal sections as a single sample. Note that this estimator cannot be used with vertical sections.

To derive the basic relationship between the 3-D lattice parameters and the estimate, the classical result for surface density is used:

$$S/V = 2N_I/L,$$

so that:

$$S = 2N_I V/L.$$

In a spatial grid, each element or prism of the grid has one point, three sides and a volume associated with it, as shown in Fig. 15. Each prism can be described by its elemental dimensions, dx, dy, dz and the volume to length ratio (V/L) for each prism is then:

$$V/L = ((dx.dy.dz)/(dx + dy + dz)).$$

The estimate of S is calculated by substitution into the original equation:

$$S_{est} = 2((dx.dy.dz)/(dx + dy + dz))\Sigma I,$$

where ΣI is the sum of all intersections in x, y and z.

This formulation works well when the spatial grid is cubic, i.e. when $dx = dy = dz$, but in most practical applications it is not possible to achieve the same resolution in x, y and z, usually for physical reasons. In such cases the basic prism will normally have a larger dz than dx or dy. Another formulation of the estimator handles the intersection counts for x, y and z independently and provides more reliable estimates when using the anisotropic spatial grid. It will be noticed that it degenerates to the form above in the case of a cubic grid:

$$S_{est} = 2\{(dx.dy.dz) \cdot [(\Sigma I_x/dx) + (\Sigma I_y/dy) + (\Sigma I_z/dz)]/3\},$$

(see Fig. 16).

Practical considerations

The spatial grid is designed to be used with technologies that allow the non-destructive sectioning of macroscopic and microscopical specimens. Examples include magnetic resonance imaging, X-ray computerised tomography and confocal microscopy. In confocal microscopy an optical section can be moved up and down through the specimen.

On the optical section a 2-D rectangular grid is superimposed. An empty micrograph is included above and below the stack of sections through the

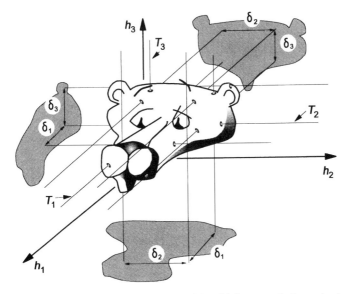

Fig. 16. A means of visualizing how the spatial grid is passed through the object of interest and the surface is intersected by the grid lines as shown. The lines marked T_1, T_2 and T_3 will all intersect at one point on the grid, within the object of interest. h_1, h_2 and h_3 represent the Cartesian coordinates of the system and δ_1, δ_2 and δ_3 the dimensions of the grid, corresponding to *dx, dy* and *dz* in the formulae above. Figure reproduced with permission of Ute Hahn, University of Stuttgart, Germany.

feature of interest. The section is repeatedly stepped down a known distance through the specimen. In each section the number of intersections of the grid with the boundary of the object in x and y are recorded. This task can often be performed automatically.

Intersections of the spatial grid in z are recorded by comparing adjacent sections. Points on the grid that fall outside the profile boundary of the feature on one section but fall inside on the next represent a line of the grid in z that has entered the object in 3-D. Conversely, a point that lies within the profile of the object on one section but outside on the next represents a grid line in z that has left the object in 3-D. Therefore it is possible to keep a tally of the entrances and exits of the grid lines in z with the object, as illustrated in the examples, provided that the sections are perfectly registered. The empty sections above and below the stack are necessary to commence and terminate the z intersection count correctly.

The volume of the object can be estimated by Cavalieri's Principle when the spatial grid is used. The result may be nonsensical if the object of interest consists of muralia (e.g. membranes within a cell).

Total length from total vertical projections

Length density can only be estimated from single sections if they are IUR. Gokhale (1990) has shown that length density can be estimated on projections of slabs with vertical orientation properties, provided the thickness of the slab is known. A new estimation of the total length of a space curve has been proposed by Cruz-Orive & Howard (1991) where the thickness of the vertical slab need not be known provided the whole curve is present in the slab. This may be the case, for example when attempting to evaluate the length of the dendrite tree for an individual neurone. A space curve can be projected onto a vertical plane. If it is projected onto a cycloid or similar set of sine-weighted testing lines, these can be imagined to be drawn up through the 3-D projection to form a set of sine-weighted surfaces, which in vertical slabs are isotropic in 3-D. The intersections of linear features with these isotropic surfaces are a measure of the total length and can be quantified simply by counting the number of intersections of the feature with the testing lines in the projections. The total count is scaled to deliver an unbiased estimate of the total length of the curve.

$$L_{\text{est}} = 2(a/l).(1/m).(1/n).\Sigma I_j,$$

where L is the length of the curve,

a/l is the area to length ratio of the testing lines,

m is the linear magnification,

n is the number of projections and

ΣI_j is the total number of intersections over all projections.

There is a potential source of bias in this estimator, in the masking of one linear feature by another that occupies the same position in the 2-D projec-

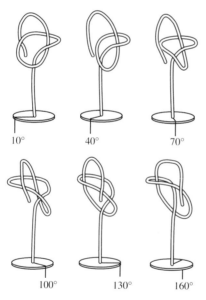

Fig. 17. The total length estimation procedure with six uniform random projection angles to produce the vertical projections. In this case the angles selected are 10°, 40°, 70°, 100°, 130°, 160°. The cycloid test grid is shown for this manual operation of the estimator. Figure used with permission from the Journal of Microscopy.

tions. The net effect of this is to cause an underestimate of the total length. It is an especially serious problem in dense tree-like structures.

Fig. 17 shows an example. Here a cycloid testing system is used, but sine-weighted linear probes may be preferable. In this case the total length of the piece of bent wire will be estimated. Each projection is overlaid onto the testing grid and the number of intersections between the two is counted. This is repeated for a number of uniform random projections (in this case six) and the above formula is used to estimate the total length. For relatively simple curves the estimator delivers a very low variance, unbiased estimate. Recently, for example, it has been shown to be useful for the measurement of dendritic tree length in neurones (Howard *et al.*, 1985).

References

Baddeley, A. J., Gundersen, H. J. G. & Cruz-Orive, L. M. (1987). Estimation of surface area from vertical sections. *Journal of Microscopy*, **142**, 259–76.

Confocal Technologies. (1992). *Digital Stereology Users Manual*. Liverpool: Confocal Technologies Ltd.

Cruz-Orive, L. M. (1987). Particle number can be estimated using a disector of unknown thickness: the selector. *Journal of Microscopy*, **145**, 121–42.

Cruz-Orive, L. M. & Howard, C. V. (1991). Estimating the length of a bounded curve in three dimensions using total vertical projections. *Journal of Microscopy*, **163**, 101–13.

Fullman, R. L. (1953). Measurement of particle size in opaque bodies. *Journal of Metals*, 447–52.

Gokhale, A. (1990). Unbiased estimation of curve length in 3-D using vertical slices. *Journal of Microscopy*, **159**, 133–41.

Gundersen, H. J. G. (1977). Notes on the estimation of numerical density of arbitrary profiles: the edge effect. *Journal of Microscopy*, **111**, 219–23.

Gundersen, H. J. G. (1986). Stereology of arbitrary particles. *Journal of Microscopy*, **143**, 3–45.

Gundersen, H. J. G. (1988). The nucleator. *Journal of Microscopy*, **151**, 3–21.

Gundersen, H. J. G. & Jensen, E. B. (1983). Particle sizes and their distributions estimated from line and point-sampled intercepts. Including graphical unfolding. *Journal of Microscopy*, **131**, 291–310.

Gundersen, H. J. G. & Jensen, E. B. (1985). Stereological estimation of the volume-weighted mean volume of arbitrary particles observed on random sections. *Journal of Microscopy*, **138**, 127–42.

Gundersen, H. J. G. & Jensen, E. B. (1987). The efficiency of systematic sampling in stereology and its prediction. *Journal of Microscopy*, **147**, 229–63.

Gundersen, H. J. G. & Osterby, R. (1981). Optimising sampling efficiency of stereological studies in biology: or do more less well! *Journal of Microscopy*, **121**, 65–73.

Howard, C. V., Reid, S., Baddeley, A. J. & Boyd, A. (1985). Unbiased estimation of particle density in the tandem scanning reflected light microscope. *Journal of Microscopy*, **138**, 203–12.

Mattfeldt, T., Mobius, H. J. & Mall, G. (1985). Orthogonal triplet probes: an efficient method for unbiased estimation of length and surface of objects with unknown orientation in space. *Journal of Microscopy*, **139**, 279–89.

Sandau, K. (1987). How to estimate the area of surface using a spatial grid. *Acta Stereologica*, **6**, 31–6.

Sterio, D. C. (1984). The unbiased estimation of number and sizes of arbitrary particles using the disector. *Journal of Microscopy*, **134**, 127–36.

Weibel, E. R. (1979). *Stereological Methods*, vol. 1 *Practical Methods for Biological Morphometry*. London: Academic Press.

PART 2

Image acquisition

8

Samples and preparation methods

D. R. SPRINGALL and J. M. POLAK

Introduction

In the past few years, many new morphological techniques have become available to the investigators of biological systems. These techniques permit the visualization and precise localization at the tissue or cellular level of the mechanisms controlling cell function, in terms of the synthesis and storage of cell products and their precursors, and the sites of action of regulatory factors. To detect stored secretory products or constitutive molecules, immunocyto-chemistry may be used; the gene or mRNA directing the synthesis of a particular product can be detected and quantified using *in situ* hybridization. Specific binding sites that act as receptors for a regulatory molecule on a target cell may be localized and quantified by measuring the binding *in vitro* of labelled ligand. Radiolabels are usually used followed by autoradiography. These types of study have previously been carried out by biochemists and molecular biologists, using extracts of whole tissues. The microscopist can now add more detailed information at the cellular level. This has the advantage that changes in a group of cells that constitute a small proportion of a tissue, or changes in the tissue localization of a factor with no significant changes in the amount, can be readily detected. This valuable information would be lost if the tissue had to be homogenized and extracted before examination.

The availability of these techniques has required that methods be devised to produce quantitative data and to extend the classical morphometric techniques (Aherne & Dunnill, 1982). Such methods are described in greater detail in other chapters of this volume. However, the advent of these techniques has, in turn, demanded that the histological or cytological techniques should be optimized to yield the best possible preparations. There is no point in spending valuable time analysing preparations that are not the best that can be obtained because the resultant data will be of limited value and will not reflect accurately what is happening *in vivo*.

Quantitative data can be obtained from these various types of preparations in two main ways. One way is to measure the total area of labelled structures, and to express this as a proportion of the area of the section or a particular tissue within it. By using stereological techniques or confocal microscopy, volume rather than area measurements can be made. The other way is to measure the intensity or density of the labelling itself as an estimate of the concentration of the species detected by the labelling method employed. The two may also be combined to produce a measure of the overall load of a factor within a given tissue. Which of the methods is used will depend on the type of information required. It should also be noted that area/volume measurements will reflect to some extent the tissue concentrations of a species because the sensitivity of a method to detect that species will vary depending on how that method is carried out and on factors such as the concentration of probe used. Thus, low levels of the species may or may not be detected in a method-dependent way.

Preparations

The production of preparations such as tissue sections or cell smears for image analysis generally involves four main steps: obtaining the material, fixation, processing and staining.

Material

Material for image analysis can be tissues or cells, the latter either *ex vivo* or in culture. Unless the material is to be observed whilst alive, as in investigations of cell or organelle motility, the main essential is that it should be obtained as fresh as possible and processed rapidly, the better to reflect the situation *in vivo*. The type of processing will depend on the staining technique to be employed, but will generally involve some type of fixation and possibly also embedding. It is also important to consider the type of analysis to be undertaken; for example, if stereological techniques are to be used it is necessary to take the whole organ in order to permit the random selection of slices (see Chapter 7). Whatever method of analysis is employed, it is essential to obtain a representative sample of the tissue, i.e. several blocks from each case.

Fixation

For most techniques, fixation of the tissues will be necessary. The fixation and any subsequent processing steps will inevitably cause some distortion, usually shrinkage, of the tissue. This will vary with the type of tissue and may need to be accounted for by making measurements of the dimensions of blocks of the tissue before and after fixation and processing.

A host of fixation protocols and fixatives have been used, but it is possible to make some general rules. The main ones are that the fixation should be rapid and preserve the tissue as well as possible but not destroy the species to be detected. Within reasonable times of fixation this is largely a function of the type of fixative used. These fall into two main categories: precipitant and crosslinking (Springall, 1986).

The precipitant fixatives include organic liquids such as methanol, ethanol, acetone and chloroform. They act by dehydrating the tissue, removing lipid, and distorting the tertiary structure of proteins. Their main advantage is that they cause little damage to the antigenicity of proteins. Their disadvantages are that they are rather inefficient at anchoring small molecules in the tissues, thus allowing them to diffuse, and are less effective at preserving tissue structure and size. Precipitant fixatives are therefore useful for the immunocytochemical detection of some labile antigens, but not so good for small molecules. They are usually excellent for fixing cell preparations as they also permeabilize the plasma membrane by removing lipid, thereby allowing better penetration of the staining probes.

The crosslinking fixatives include the more reactive chemical species, such as formaldehyde and glutaraldehyde. These denature the proteins in tissue by a complex series of reactions that lead to links being formed between adjacent protein chains. They are therefore very effective at preserving tissue, but tend to cause more damage to antigenicity. However, they are excellent for many immunocytochemical and *in situ* hybridization schemes. Generally, formaldehyde-based fixatives are favoured by light microscopists whereas glutaraldehyde is preferred by electron microscopists because it is better at preserving tissue structure.

For some techniques it is essential that the tissues are not fixed. These include immunostaining of highly labile antigens and for receptor–ligand binding studies. In these cases, unfixed frozen sections are required.

The actual fixation procedure may be accomplished by immersing the tissue in fixative or by perfusing it via the vasculature, which yields better results as the fixation is more rapid. If immersion fixation is used the tissues should be sliced thinly so that one dimension does not exceed 3–4 mm; for electron microscopy the tissue should be cut, whilst immersed in the fixative, into 1 mm cubes. The fixation step may also be performed after frozen sectioning of the tissue or even after the staining. Post-fixation of frozen sections allows the variation of fixation conditions to be achieved simply and reduces dimensional changes induced by the fixative (although this may be offset by such changes caused during sectioning, which may be greater with unfixed tissue). However, it has the disadvantage that very soluble species may be lost or at least translocated. Fixation after staining is necessary for certain techniques such as in *in vitro* ligand binding, that require that the substance to be detected is undamaged. It should only be used where really necessary as the staining procedure is liable to cause severe damage to the structure and tinctorial properties of the tissue.

The same rules apply to fixation of isolated cells and cell cultures as to tissues (Springall, 1986). However, fixation times are usually much shorter because the fixatives do not have so far to penetrate, and the cells can be fixed either whilst still wet or after preparing a smear on a glass slide that is then allowed to dry to increase cell adhesion to the slide. The latter is not usually used for adherent cell cultures, and will cause considerable distortion of the cell structure, but is a very effective way of permeabilizing the membranes.

Processing

Subsequent processing steps are required only for tissues, since cell preparations may be taken straight to the staining procedure. In order to allow sections to be cut, the tissues are frozen or embedded in a solid matrix, usually paraffin wax or plastic.

Freezing is the least damaging of these processes in terms of degradation of tissue components and bioactive molecules, but can cause damage to the architecture. This is largely due to the formation of ice crystals and is minimized by washing the tissues after fixation in buffer containing a cryoprotectant such as solutions of 10–15% buffered sucrose, and by rapid freezing to reduce the size of crystals or to prevent their formation. A good method is to immerse the tissue in isopentane or dichlorodifluoromethane which has been cooled in liquid nitrogen.

The most common embedding medium for light microscopy is paraffin wax. The tissue is first dehydrated using alcohol and then cleared in a solvent that is miscible with the wax before being immersed in the molten wax. All of these steps can lead to distortion of the tissue and further damage to its constituents. Plastic embedding media are used for electron microscopy and for some applications in light microscopy. Hydrophobic epoxy resins such as Araldite, and hydrophilic crosslinked acrylics, such as methacrylate, are the main types of resin used. They offer the advantage that very thin sections can be prepared. This is essential for electron microscopy and is very useful for light microscopy because the same cell can appear in several sections, thus allowing different techniques to be used on serial sections to investigate colocalization of two or more antigens or mRNA or both.

Staining

The staining techniques that may be applied to gain quantitative information are outlined below. It is important to emphasize that while these are mostly standard laboratory methods, it is often necessary to adapt them for quantification, even if the results are then not as aesthetically pleasing or striking as they could be. For example, it may be necessary to reduce the intensity of immunostaining in order to measure optical density to quantify an antigen, or to reduce the exposure or the radioactive labelling when producing autoradiograms. This is needed, if the autoradiograms are to be quantified at the microscopical level using grain counting methods, in order to avoid artefacts caused by the high density of silver grains and grain clumping (Chapter 21).

Synthetic machinery

Application of hybridization techniques, based on those of classical molecular biology but performed at the microscopical level, permits the precise localization and thus characterization of the cells possessing the synthetic machinery for particular products (Polak & McGee, 1990). Demonstration of mRNAs is based on the mutual affinity of complementary nucleic acids and can be achieved either by Northern blotting, using gel-electrophoresed tissue extracts or, by *in situ* hybridization, applying the technique to histological sections of tissue and thereby permitting the precise localization of specific mRNA species at the cellular level (Fig. 1). The *in situ* hybridization technique involves the application to the tissue section or cell smear of labelled DNA or RNA probes complementary (cDNA or cRNA) to the species to be detected. Different types of probes are currently used, including double-stranded cDNAs, cRNAs (riboprobes) and synthetic oligonucleotides. For riboprobes, a cDNA sequence is subcloned adjacent to a promoter within a bacterial plasmid, which is then linearized and transcribed to produce a complementary RNA sequence (cRNA or antisense probe) to the mRNA of interest (Gibson & Polak, 1990). The RNA probe is labelled by incorporating a nucleotide marked with a radioisotopic or non-radioactive reporter molecule. Following hybridization, washes of

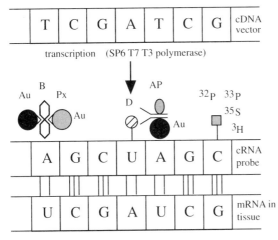

Fig. 1. Schematic illustration of hybridization using cRNA probes to detect mRNA. The cRNA probe is prepared from the cloned cDNA sequence inserted into a vector and transcribed using the appropriate polymerases to generate the 'antisense' cRNA sequence and the 'sense' mRNA sequence. These are labelled by including a base linked to a reporter molecule such as biotin (B), digoxigenin (D) or a radiolabel (^{32}P, ^{33}P, ^{35}S or ^{3}H) in the transcription mixture. The probes are then hybridized with separate tissue sections and the label revealed by an appropriate method (e.g. streptavidin or antibody labelled with gold (Au), peroxidase (Px) or alkaline phosphatase (AP), or autoradiography) to localize the mRNA (antisense probe) and non-specific binding (sense probe) as a specificity control.

appropriate stringency ensure that nonspecific probe-binding is minimized. Alternate control sections are hybridized with a non-complementary (sense) RNA probe as a method control. The labelled cRNA that has hybridized is detected by an appropriate technique to allow localization of the tissue mRNA. Labels currently used include:

1 Radioisotopes (^{35}S, ^{32}P, ^{33}P, ^{3}H), detected by autoradiography.
2 Biotin, detected either by gold- or peroxidase-labelled streptavidin, or else by antibody to biotin.
3 Digoxigenin, detected by gold- or alkaline phosphatase-labelled antibody (Giaid *et al.*, 1989: see Plate 2).

The autoradiographic method is often favoured due to its higher sensitivity. It also has advantages for quantification in that autoradiography is a thoroughly investigated and well-established technique for such purposes. Autoradiography is described in Chapter 21.

Stored products

Information regarding stored products can be obtained by radioimmunoassay of tissue extracts, which provides quantitative levels of the molecule as well as allowing its chemical characterization by procedures such as chromatography, and/or by immunocytochemistry using specific antibodies (Polak & Van Noorden, 1986). The reaction product can then be visualized at the microscopical level to provide precise information about the type of cell that is storing a particular antigen. Immunocytochemistry can be used to visualize the stored product at light and electron microscopical levels (Polak & Van Noorden, 1986; Polak & Varndell, 1984) and the basic technique has reached a very high degree of sophistication and sensitivity; proteins that are stored in low concentration in a particular cell type can now be analysed accurately and reliably (McBride *et al.*, 1990).

A variety of immunohistochemical staining techniques using various labels are available. The immunostaining may be performed by direct, indirect, or bridge techniques (such as the avidin–biotin or unlabelled-antibody bridge methods; see Fig. 2). The labels (Plate 3) may be a fluorescent dye, a variety of enzymes such as peroxidase, alkaline phosphatase and glucose oxidase that require a histochemical reaction to localize them, or colloidal gold, which is usually silver enhanced for light microscopy (Springall *et al.*, 1984). All of these methods and labels are applicable for image analysis (see also Chapters 19 and 20).

Receptor binding sites

Many techniques are available for investigating receptor binding sites. To obtain numerical assessment of binding sites, the classical method is to deter-

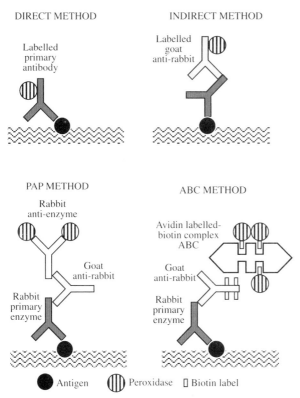

DIRECT METHOD

Labelled
primary
antibody

INDIRECT METHOD

Labelled
goat
anti-rabbit

PAP METHOD

Rabbit
anti-enzyme

Goat
anti-rabbit

Rabbit
primary
enzyme

ABC METHOD

Avidin labelled-
biotin complex
ABC

Goat
anti-rabbit

Rabbit
primary
enzyme

● Antigen   ⬚ Peroxidase   ▯ Biotin label

Fig. 2 Diagram of immunostaining methods showing direct, indirect and bridge methods such as the peroxidase–antiperoxidase (PAP) and avidin–biotin complex (ABC). A variety of different labels are used, including fluorescent dyes, enzymes and colloidal gold. In the multistep methods, antibodies are applied sequentially with washing steps between to remove the excess, unreacted reagent.

mine radiolabelled ligand binding to membranes isolated from tissue homogenates. For the analysis of the mRNA coding for a particular receptor, classical molecular biology techniques including *in situ* hybridization (q.v.) are used. However, for the precise localization of active binding sites, such as those for regulatory peptides, within any tissue, the technique of choice is *in vitro* receptor autoradiography with image analysis (Palacios & Dietl, 1989).

In vitro receptor autoradiography was first introduced in 1979 and its use has increased steadily. The same principles apply to both isolated membrane preparations and *in vitro* autoradiography; both use radioligands, but the latter employs tissue sections and the detection of bound radioactivity is carried out using autoradiography (Fig. 3). Serial tissue sections are incubated with radiolabelled ligand and the same concentration of radiolabelled ligand with an excess (usually 500–1000-fold) of unlabelled ligand. The latter is a competitive-inhibition control and is used to localize and measure the amount of non-specific binding of the ligand. After the incubation, the sections are washed to remove unreacted ligand, and autoradiograms are produced either by apposing

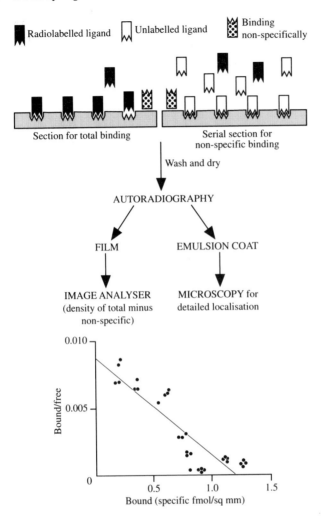

Fig. 3. The *in vitro* autoradiography technique to determine specific ligand binding sites. Radiolabelled ligand applied to tissue sections at appropriate concentration binds specifically with receptors or non-specifically. The specific binding is competitively inhibited by simultaneously applied unlabelled ligand or other antagonist/agonist. The labelled section is then subjected to autoradiography with film to generate quantitative data or by dipping in liquid emulsion to give preparations suitable for microscopic localization of the binding. The binding density is measured by determining the optical density of the image in the area of interest in a section, converted into radioactivity units from a standard curve prepared from simultaneously exposed radiostandards, subtracting the value for non-specific binding in the equivalent area. Knowing the specific activity of the ligand, the radioactivity units can be converted to the quantity of ligand bound and expressed per unit area of tissue.

the sections to autoradiography film or by dipping the slides in liquid photographic emulsion.

Film type autoradiograms (Fig. 4) can be used to obtain quantitative data on ligand binding of specific tissue structures and thus to derive binding character-

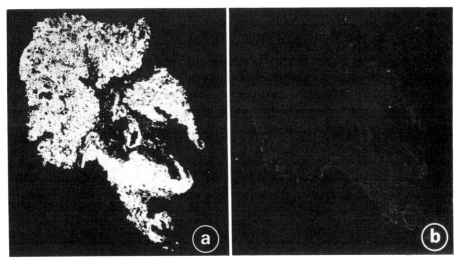

Fig. 4. Film autoradiograms showing the binding to human lung of the vasoconstrictor peptide endothelin-1 (ET-1) labelled with [125]I. Total binding is shown in (*a*) and non-specific binding, determined by incubating in the presence of an excess of un-labelled ET-1, in (*b*).

istics such as the dissociation constant (K_d) and maximum binding (B_{max}) of the ligand binding in a given tissue (Davenport, Hill & Hughes, 1989). Emulsion dipped preparations, whilst being excellent for precise microscopical localization of binding (Fig. 5), are not suitable for quantification because the immersion in hot aqueous emulsion can disturb the binding equilibrium and remove ligand. If microscopical quantification is necessary (e.g. to measure binding to small blood vessels or capillaries), it is possible to use emulsion dipped coverslips but the technique is difficult. Quantitative data can be obtained by using image analysis to compare the integrated optical density of specific areas of the autoradiograms with those of simultaneously exposed standard sections containing known quantities of radioactive material (Davenport *et al.*, 1989).

Conclusions

The application of image analysis has added greatly to the amount of information that can be obtained from morphological studies. When these include techniques such as immunocytochemistry, *in situ* hybridization and labelled-ligand binding, the possible yield of information is further increased. Although the use of such analysis is still in its infancy, it is nowadays feasible to study the synthesis and storage of any molecule for which the relevant probes are available. Such quantitative data may be either the overall load of the antigen in a tissue, thereby allowing comparisons of levels in a disease or following manipulation, or the actual intracellular level, which adds the previously unattained dimension of comparisons between cells. But the technique is still

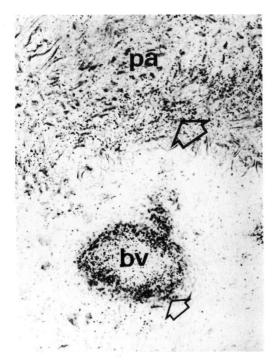

Fig. 5. Microscopic view of the total binding of ^{125}I-ET-1 in blood vessels in human lung, as in Fig. 4. The labelling appears as silver grains concentrated over the vascular smooth muscle.

developing; methods are being devised to add more sophisticated tools that will permit the quantitative analysis of tissue distribution of specific molecules as well as automation of many basic operations that are currently rather time consuming. Image analysis has become an essential part of the move towards a more functional morphology.

References

Aherne, W. A. & Dunnill, M. S. (1982). *Morphometry*. London: Edward Arnold.

Davenport, A. P., Hill, R. G. & Hughes, J. (1989). Quantitative analysis of autoradiograms. In *Regulatory Peptides*, ed. J. M. Polak, pp. 137–53. Basel: Birkhauser Verlag.

Giaid, A., Hamid, Q., Adams, C., Springall, D. R., Terenghi, G. & Polak, J.M. (1989). Non-isotopic RNA probes. Comparison between different labels and detection systems. *Histochemistry*, **93**, 191–6.

Gibson, S. J. & Polak, J. M. (1990). Principles and applications of complementary RNA probes. In *Modern Methods in Pathology: In Situ Hybridization*, ed. J. M. Polak & J. McGee. Oxford: Oxford University Press.

McBride, J. T., Springall, D. R., Winter, R. J. D. & Polak, J. M. (1990). Quantitative immunocytochemistry shows calcitonin gene-related peptide-like immunoreactivity in lung neuroendocrine cells is increased by chronic hypoxia in the rat. *American Journal of Respiratory Cell Molecular Biology* **3**, 587–93.

Palacios, J. M. & Dietl, M. M. (1989). Regulatory peptide receptors: visualisation by autoradiography. In *Regulatory Peptides*, ed. J. M. Polak, pp. 70–97. Basel: Birkhauser Verlag.

Polak, J. M. & McGee, J. O'D. (1990). *In Situ Hybridisation: Principles and Practice*. Oxford: Oxford University Press.

Polak, J. M. & Van Noorden, S. (1986). *Immunocytochemistry: Modern Methods and Applications* (2nd edition). Bristol: John Wright.

Polak, J. M. & Varndell, I. (1984). *Immunolabelling for Electron Microscopy*. Amsterdam: Elsevier Science Publishers.

Springall, D. R. (1986). Immunocytochemistry in diagnostic cytology. In *Immunocytochemistry: Modern Methods and Applications* (2nd edition), ed. J. M. Polak & S. Van Noorden, pp. 547–67. Bristol: John Wright.

Springall, D. R., Hacker, G. W., Grimelius, L. & Polak, J. M. (1984). The potential of the immunogold-silver staining method for paraffin sections. *Histochemistry*, **81**, 603–8.

9

Light microscopy

P. J. EVENNETT

Introduction

The light microscope is probably the most familiar and most important source of images in histology. But because the microscope uses light to produce its images, important differences from everyday naked eye vision are frequently not recognized; observation of features whose dimensions may be close to the wavelength of the imaging radiation brings special problems that do not exist when observing larger objects. Artefacts can be formed which are ignored by an experienced observer, but which have special significance when images are analysed by machine. Even though sophisticated image analysis software may be available, software that is capable of elaborate manipulation of an image, it is undeniably better to present the analysis system with a high quality image from the microscope.

The microscope

The function of a microscope is to provide information about fine detail in an object. Clearly magnification is a prime requirement, providing the sensing device (the eye, film or video camera) with an enlarged image of the object. Magnification is relatively easily achieved, and requires no finesse on the part of the microscope designer or user. Skill is, however, required to ensure that the magnified image contains information about the object in sufficient detail – resolution – and with sufficient variations in brightness and/or colour – contrast. Indeed it is a combination of these qualities of resolution and contrast that determines the usefulness of a microscopical image. In addition, it is important that microscope images be free from distortion of shape or thickening of outlines, and that the illumination be uniform across the field of view; deficiencies in these respects are likely to be misinterpreted by the analytical system and give rise to spurious results.

Correct operation of a microscope is a procedure which is easily followed when the optical design is understood in simple terms. A modern microscope consists essentially of an illuminating and an imaging system, each incorporating two lens systems, together with the lamp, the specimen, several diaphragms, a sensing device for the final image (eye, film or video camera), and mechanical parts for support and adjustment (the stand). In microscopy, the lenses that make up the illuminating and imaging systems are not normally single elements, but systems of multiple lens elements designed to provide optimal image quality.

The imaging system

In terms of simple geometrical optics, the objective lens acts like the lens of a projector. A projector lens forms an enlarged image of the transparency on a screen; the microscope objective forms a magnified image of the specimen, the primary image, towards the top of the eyepiece tube. (This image can be seen by removing the eyepiece and holding a piece of thin paper across the tube; it may be necessary to increase lamp brightness and refocus a little.) The eyepiece acts as a magnifying glass, examining the central part of the primary image and, in conjunction with the lens of the eye, transfers the image to the retina. An objective lens of short focal length will produce a primary image of higher magnification than one of longer focal length, since magnification depends on the ratio of lens-to-image and lens-to-specimen distances.

Because the specimen is imaged in the primary image plane and also on the retina, these three optically linked locations are known as conjugate planes; since this set of planes includes the field of view, it is known as the field set of conjugate planes.

The information gathering power of a microscope objective lens is limited by diffraction, and depends on the angle of the cone of rays which it can accept from the specimen; this is known as the aperture of the lens. Refraction of light at the coverglass–air interface causes the aperture angle outside the specimen to appear larger than the angle within the preparation, which is where it can be considered to be most important. To take account of this, the information gathering power of a microscope objective is expressed as a number, the numerical aperture (NA), which is the product of the refractive index of the medium through which the lens operates (air, or an immersion medium such as water, glycerine or oil) and the sine of half the aperture angle (Fig. 1). Because an immersion medium has a higher refractive index than air, immersion objectives may have larger NAs than dry objectives, collect more information about the specimen, and thereby provide superior resolving power. The smallest distance (d) that can be resolved by a microscope objective can be calculated from:

$$d = 0.6\lambda/NA$$

where λ is the wavelength of light, usually approximately 0.5 μm.

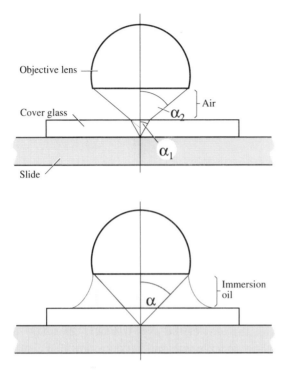

Fig. 1. Numerical aperture.

The illuminating system

It is necessary for the specimen to be illuminated uniformly over an area at least as large as that being observed. A simple way of providing uniform illumination is to throw on to the specimen an image of a uniformly illuminated surface – in the past this was provided by white clouds in the sky, for example. Almost all modern microscopes use artificial light and follow the system devised by August Köhler in 1893, which provides even illumination over a field of controllable area, with the illuminating angle adjustable to suit object-ives of different aperture. In Köhler illumination the lamp collector lens appears as a uniformly illuminated surface, which is imaged on to the specimen by means of the condenser lens, acting like a camera lens (Fig. 2). The system will operate as designed only when these two lenses are correctly adjusted.

For the lamp collector lens to provide a uniform field of illumination, the filament of the lamp must be positioned close to the first focal plane of this lens. In many microscopes this adjustment may be preset in manufacture, or rendered less critical by the inclusion of a diffuser. Where adjustment is available and any diffuser can be removed, correct setting is achieved when a centred and sharply focussed image of the lamp filament falls just beneath the condenser lens; adjustments may also be provided for the centralization of the

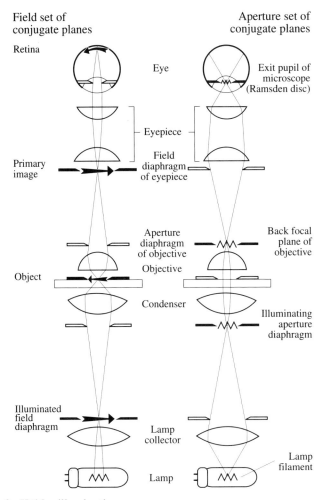

Fig. 2. Köhler illumination.

filament image on the condenser. Once it is correctly set, readjustment of the lamp and/or collector lens should not normally be necessary.

The position of the condenser lens requires frequent readjustment, principally because of variations in thickness of slides. Microscopes designed for Köhler illumination are fitted with an iris diaphragm, the illuminated field diaphragm (IFD), situated just after the lamp collector; it is so named because it controls the area of the field which is illuminated. The condenser must be adjusted to form a sharply focussed image of this diaphragm on the specimen, concentric with the field of view. The illuminated field diaphragm is thus another (and the first) member of the field set of conjugate planes. Focusing the illuminated field diaphragm on to the specimen not only fulfils the criterion by which the designer intended the condenser to be adjusted, but also provides a practical benefit important in image analysis: it enables the diameter of the area of specimen illuminated to be controlled by adjusting the IFD. This in turn enables the area of the primary image to be reduced to that which is under examination, and thus to reduce stray light reflecting from internal parts of the microscope. Such reflections frequently cause a so-called hotspot, a spurious bright patch, usually in the centre of the image, which the analysis system may wrongly interpret as a feature.

Köhler illumination also requires a second iris diaphragm, fitted just before the condenser lens; this is known as the illuminating aperture diaphragm because it is used to control the illuminating aperture, the obliquity of the angle of rays as they enter the specimen, and, in effect, the numerical aperture of the condenser. For optimum imaging of a well-stained specimen, the aperture of the condenser should be adjusted so that it is just a little smaller than the aperture of the objective lens in use.

Rays from any one point within the illuminating aperture pass through all parts of the specimen within the illuminated field parallel one to another and are brought to a focus in the back focal plane of the objective, where they form an image of the illuminating aperture diaphragm. (The back focal plane of the objective is the plane where parallel light entering the lens, as if from infinity, is brought to a focus; it is equivalent to the position of the film with respect to a camera lens.) A further image of this diaphragm is formed just above the eyepiece, in a position known as the exit pupil of the eyepiece or the Ramsden disc.

A second set of conjugate planes is now apparent, the aperture set, its members interleaved between those of the field set. The filament is imaged first on the illuminating aperture diaphragm, then in the back focal plane of the objective and finally in the exit pupil of the eyepiece.

Setting up a microscope for Köhler illumination

Adjustment of the imaging system of a microscope is almost entirely confined to focusing the image; most of the pitfalls in the setting up of a microscope lie in the adjustment of the illuminating system. A typical procedure is outlined below, together with the reasons which lie behind each important step. This procedure assumes the use of a modern upright (rather than inverted) microscope with built-in Köhler illumination system.

1. *Initial setup.* Open all diaphragms, raise the condenser to its highest position, put a well-stained specimen on the stage, move the ×10 (or similar magnification) objective into position, and switch on the lamp.
2. *Focus the objective lens* to obtain a sharp image of the specimen by using the coarse and fine focus controls. This first important step sets the correct relationship between specimen and objective lens.
3. *Focus the condenser.* Close the illuminated field diaphragm (IFD) and adjust the height of the condenser until a sharp image of the IFD is seen superimposed on the image of the specimen. This adjustment sets the correct relationship between the condenser lens and the specimen.

4. *Centre the condenser lens*. Make the image of the IFD concentric with the field of view using the condenser centring screws. This adjustment brings the condenser lens on to the optical axis of the microscope as defined by the positions of the IFD and objective lens.

5. *Adjust the area of field illuminated*. Open the IFD until its image is just outside the field of view; readjust the condenser centralization if necessary. This ensures that illumination falls only on the area of specimen within the field of view, and that the diameter of the primary image is only a little larger than the field-limiting diaphragm within the eyepiece; light does not fall on the internal walls of the microscope, to be scattered, to produce hot-spots and to reduce contrast in the final image.

6. *Adjust the illuminating aperture*. Remove an eyepiece, look into the microscope tube from about 100 mm above the tube, and observe the back focal plane of the objective, the disc of light at the base of the tube. Close the illuminating aperture diaphragm (IAD) until the image of the iris is just a little smaller than this disc of light (the aperture of the objective). Replace the eyepiece. The working aperture of the condenser is now slightly smaller than the aperture of the objective lens. This results in an increase in contrast due to reduction in stray light scattered from the extreme edges of components of the objective lens. Do not close the diaphragm too far: this will cause a serious deterioration in the quality of the image (see the section on contrast, below).

7. *Adjust the brightness* using the control on the lamp power supply, or by inserting grey filters as appropriate. Note that none of the microscope's optical adjustments or diaphragms can be used to control brightness without also adversely affecting the quality of the image.

8. *After changing to a higher power objective*, which will generally have a larger aperture and higher magnification:
   a. Reduce the opening of the IFD to match the smaller area of specimen which will fill the field of view because of the higher magnification of the new objective. The better view of the IFD may permit more precise adjustment of condenser focus, but a large readjustment should not be necessary since the relationship between condenser and specimen remains unaltered.
   b. Open the IAD to fill the larger aperture of the new objective, as described in step 6 above.

9. *After changing to a lower power objective*, which will generally have a lower magnification and smaller aperture:
   a. Increase the opening of the IFD to match the larger area of specimen now within the field of view.
   b. Reduce the opening of the IAD to match the smaller aperture of the new objective, as in step 6 above.

   With objectives of magnification less than about ×10, the field of view may not be illuminated to its edges even when the IFD is fully open. Some condensers have a top element which can be swung out, or other device to enable a larger field to be illuminated; special condensers are available for use with objectives of extreme low power. Resist the temptation to defocus the condenser to enlarge the illuminated area; uneven illumination will almost certainly result.

10. *To change slides.* Since the thickness of slides is variable, slight readjustment of objective and condenser focus may be necessary on changing slides; other adjustments should remain approximately correct.

Defects of the optical system

Because of diffraction, and aberrations and other defects of the optical system, a microscope image can never be identical with the object. Diffraction presents a fundamental limitation which cannot be circumvented, involving both wavelength and aperture, and provides the theoretical basis for calculating the minimum resolvable dimension (d), as described above.

A single lens suffers from chromatic and spherical aberrations, and may have a field of view which is not flat and which may be distorted; the effects of all these defects have been minimized in objectives of modern design.

Chromatic aberration is the inability of a lens to focus light of different colours in a single plane, with the result that features in the image are surrounded by coloured fringes. All currently available microscope objectives have a good degree of chromatic correction, and even the simplest, the Achromats, provide a good quality image. The highest degree of chromatic correction exists in Apochromatic objectives, while the less expensive Semi-Apochromatic or Fluorite objectives perform almost as well.

It is unlikely that inadequacy of the chromatic correction of objectives will cause serious problems in image analysis, but there is a serious risk from a related cause. In many optical systems, the correction for chromatic aberration is split between the objective lens and the eyepiece; the primary image still contains a chromatic error, which is later corrected by a compensating eyepiece. Objectives from different manufacturers, and even from different systems from one manufacturer, may require different degrees of compensation by the eyepiece. When fitting a video camera to a microscope it may sometimes be useful to omit the eyepiece, or perhaps to use one of more suitable magnification from another manufacturer. Whenever such an incomplete or unmatched optical system is used, chromatic correction in the final image should be checked by examination of a high contrast specimen such as an electron microscope grid mounted in balsam under a coverslip; search for colour fringes especially towards the edges of the field of view. Some modern objectives such as the Nikon CF and the Zeiss ICS systems produce a chromatically fully corrected primary image which is suitable for direct presentation to a video camera.

Spherical aberration is the defect that causes rays that pass through the centre of a lens to come to a focus in a different plane from those passing through the periphery. It is more serious for lenses of larger aperture, which in effect have more periphery, and results in a serious blurring and lack of contrast in the image. Microscope objectives are well corrected for this aberration too, but for this to be effective, attention must be paid to two factors. Objectives are corrected to operate at a particular tubelength – the distance between the objective and the eyepiece. Formerly, this distance was most often set at 160 mm, but many recent microscopes are designed for infinity-corrected objectives, corrected to produce their primary image in conjunction with a tube lens, with a parallel raypath in between. Objectives of different tubelength corrections are not normally interchangeable. Incorrect tubelength is unlikely to be a problem unless optical parts have been transferred from one instrument to another injudiciously. The related factor, however, which is a frequent cause of poor images due to spherical aberration, is that objectives are made to work with a specified thickness of coverglass and mounting medium above the specimen. Errors are most noticeable with dry objectives of larger aperture, about 0.65 and above; oil immersion objectives are relatively insensitive since there is no significant optical difference between a little more glass or mountant and a little less oil. Where the performance of an objective is sensitive to spherical aberration, the required coverglass thickness is engraved on the lens mount. The commonest value is 0.17 mm, the thickness of a Number $1\frac{1}{2}$ coverglass; objectives are also available corrected for the relatively thick walls of culture vessels, used particularly on inverted microscopes, and large aperture dry objectives are normally supplied with a correction collar to optimize spherical correction for a given specimen. In order to reduce image degradation from spherical aberration, the correct thickness of coverglass should be used, together with the bare minimum of mounting medium. Use of oil immersion objectives even for low magnification work (magnifications of ×40, ×25 or even lower are available), though inconvenient, will avoid any difficulty from this cause.

Flatness of field is an important attribute of an objective to be used for any form of image acquisition from the microscope. During direct observation, if the field of view is curved, we automatically compensate by refocusing our eyes and the microscope; however, a video image will not be sharp all over, being blurred either in the centre or at the edges. Objectives with a flat field of view are available from all manufacturers, usually designated by the syllable 'Plan' included in their name, and are strongly recommended for use in image analysis.

Distortion of the image is a defect that may pass unnoticed. Examination of a square grid may reveal pincushion or barrel distortions due to unequal magnification across the field of view. Since a similar defect could arise from the video system also, a check on the linearity of the image being analysed is strongly recommended. A simple test can be performed by measuring the area of a clearly defined unambiguous feature positioned in several different parts of the field.

142   P. J. Evennett

Contrast

Specimens used in histology are usually stained, and they present their information in the image in the form of variations in brightness or shades of colour. The procedure outlined above is designed to give an image of the highest resolution of which the microscope is capable, using such a specimen where contrast is due to differential absorption of light. Sometimes a specimen may be weakly stained or faded, or some features of interest may not be stained at all. The best solution would be to use a properly stained specimen, or to find a staining technique that provides contrast in all relevant features, but this may not be possible.

It is a common (and somewhat reprehensible) practice in such cases to increase contrast by reducing the illuminating aperture, most simply by closing the illuminating aperture diaphragm. This certainly does increase contrast, and its judicious use may be necessary as a last resort where sufficient contrast is not available by more acceptable methods, but it must be recognised that this practice leads to an image which is a less faithful rendering of the original object, and in which outlines of all features appear thickened – hence the increased contrast. Closely adjacent features are thus merged in the image, leading to a reduction in resolving power, and features appear to be surrounded by successive light and dark bands and thus to have an unnaturally large area. Moreover, decreasing the aperture of the condenser increases its depth of field, as with a camera lens, and can bring into focus any hairs, dust and contamination from normally invisible planes within the illuminating system. Furthermore, if the reduction in illuminating aperture has been achieved by a random maladjustment of the system, uneven illumination across the field of view may result, with the possible superimposition of an image of the lamp filament.

Strict adherence to the correct procedure for Köhler illumination is strongly recommended wherever possible.

Colour filters

Where a feature is weakly stained, but does show some colour differentiation from its surroundings, contrast can be increased by the use of colour filters. In essence, colour filters make it possible to alter the way in which the colours in an image are rendered in monochrome as shades of grey. Consider a section containing objects stained either red or blue-green (e.g. alcian blue) against a clear background. If a red filter is inserted, the background becomes red and any red objects will be seen in lower contrast against it. The blue-green objects, however, which appear to be blue-green simply because they absorb red light, will become darker and appear in higher contrast against the red background. For an illustration of this effect see Bradbury (1985). Hence the general rule is

Table 1 *Complementary colours*

Colour	Complementary colour
Red	Cyan (blue-green)
Green	Magenta
Blue	Yellow
Cyan	Red
Magenta	Green
Yellow	Blue

that filters of colour similar to the object of interest will lighten the tone of that object in a monochrome image, and filters of complementary colour will darken the object. Colours and their complements are shown in Table 1.

In addition to simply manipulating contrast to provide a good image, colour filters may be used, according to the principles outlined above, to select features of different colour as separate categories in analysis. For example, lysosomes might be coloured blue following a histochemical technique using an azo dye, while the cells might be counterstained in red. A strong red or yellow filter will allow selective measurement of the blue areas, while a blue or cyan filter will enable the total area of the cells to be established.

Phase contrast and differential interference contrast

Several methods of enhancing contrast which involve manipulating the illuminating and/or imaging rays are in common use in microscopy for direct observation, but they should be used only with great caution for image analysis since they introduce serious artefacts into the image, rendering it difficult to separate the relevant from the irrelevant by accurate segmentation.

A phase contrast image is characterized by the dark or bright halo which surrounds each contrasted feature. Differential interference contrast, while providing a superb high resolution image, provides asymmetrical, azimuthal contrast, giving the appearance of a 3-D object illuminated obliquely from one side. Because of the halo or shadow, in both these cases the true area of a feature is not represented in the image. These methods may be found useful for counting objects, where the enhanced contrast at, for example, cell boundaries might be helpful. However, where segmentation of the image into its components is based on greylevels, this process will be confused since a given feature may be represented by a wide range of values from bright to dark. Where necessary, skilled use of the image analyser might overcome this problem, but it could cause difficulty for the unwary beginner. These contrast methods will not be covered further here; for details the reader should refer to James & Tanke (1991) and Richardson (1991).

Dark ground

Like phase contrast and differential interference contrast, dark ground images may be of limited value in image analysis. A dark ground image is formed by illuminating with a hollow cone of light which is so arranged as not to enter the objective lens directly; the object is seen by virtue of the light that it scatters, appearing in high contrast, bright on a black background. Dark ground imaging is particularly suitable for isolated particles that scatter light strongly, though difficulties can arise with contaminant particles such as dust, which also fall into this category.

Special condensers are available for dark ground; these produce hollow cone illumination by a combination of refraction and reflection of light. Such condensers are essential when it is necessary to produce a dark ground image with a large aperture immersion objective. However, for objectives of aperture up to about 0.65, dark ground images can easily be improvised using standard equipment. If a phase contrast condenser is available, use of one of the larger annuli, designed for the largest aperture objectives, will be found to produce a good dark ground image.

A do-it-yourself dark ground method can also be used with condensers of traditional design and objectives with an aperture up to about 0.65. This requires a piece of transparent material, glass or plastic, of suitable size and shape to be fitted immediately below the lower lens of the condenser – ideally a disc to suit the filter tray, where this is fitted. An opaque circular stop attached centrally will obstruct the light that would otherwise pass directly into the objective, and provide the necessary hollow cone illumination. The size of this stop depends on the aperture of the objective, and may conveniently be determined by trial and error.

Fluorescence

Using modern techniques and equipment, fluorescence microscopy is capable of producing an image almost ideally suited to the requirements of analysis, since the image as presented to the video camera may already be segmented into its features of interest. A fluorescent substance absorbs energy from radiation of shorter wavelength (ultraviolet, blue or green), and emits part of this energy as radiation of a longer wavelength (such as green, yellow or red, respectively). Most tissue specimens used in histology will not themselves usefully fluoresce (or autofluoresce) but they may be rendered secondarily fluorescent by the specific attachment of a fluorescing substance or fluoro-chrome. Fluorescence microscopy may be used to enhance the results of some conventional techniques such as periodic acid–Schiff (PAS) or Feulgen or, more usually nowadays, to demonstrate sites of the highly specific antibody–antigen reaction, the antigen being labelled with a fluorescing marker such as fluorescein isothiocyanate (FITC). By this technique, high contrast in the image can be provided, extremely selectively, of features carrying a specific antigen, and of these features alone.

A modern fluorescence microscope will use the technique of epifluorescence, in which the specimen is illuminated from the same side as that from which it is observed (Fig. 3). Light containing energy in the required part of the spectrum, usually from a mercury arc lamp, is directed via a series of collector lenses into the microscope objective by a special partially reflecting mirror (a dichroic mirror) arranged at 45° behind the objective. The objective lens acts like the condenser in transmitted light Köhler illumination and projects an image of the illuminated field diaphragm on to the specimen. Light resulting from fluorescence of the specimen is collected by the objective lens, passes through the mirror and forms an image in the normal way. It should be noted that the objective lens acts as its own condenser, and is thus always in correct alignment with itself. Moreover, when the illuminated field diaphragm is correctly adjusted, the objective illuminates only the area under observation, and this area changes along with the different fields of view of objectives of different magnification. The important consequence of this for fluorescence microscopy is that whatever objective magnification is used, all the radiation that passes through the objective aperture falls on to the area being observed, and is thus available for exciting fluorescence.

The specific control of the ranges of wavelengths in the exciting radiation and in the image results from the special properties of the dichroic mirror and

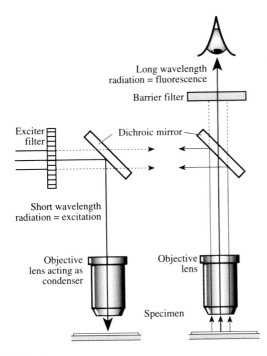

Fig. 3. Epifluorescence.

its associated exciter and barrier filters. The mirror is arranged to have the property of reflecting into the objective light of wavelengths shorter than a specified value (arranged to contain the waveband required for exciting fluorescence in a particular fluorochrome), while transmitting light of the longer wavelengths which result from the fluorescence. The mirror is usually mounted as a unit with the appropriate exciter and barrier filters specific for a particular application.

Several considerations are important in achieving good fluorescence microscopy, beyond the selection of a filter combination appropriate for the fluorochrome in use. Fluorescence images commonly lack intensity, and the fluorescence fades, sometimes with dramatic speed, on exposure to the energy in the exciting radiation. In order to maximize brightness in the image, objectives of large numerical aperture should be chosen, since the light-transmitting power of a lens depends on the square of its aperture. In fluorescence microscopy, light passes through the objective lens twice, once for excitation and once for imaging; improvements due to increased aperture will thus be proportional to the fourth power of the aperture, and will be highly significant. Brightness of an image is also inversely related to the square of the magnification, since light passing a given aperture may be required to cover a smaller or larger area. A bright image in fluorescence will thus result from using objectives of large aperture and low magnification, together with a viewing system using eyepieces and any magnification changer also of low magnification. Special immersion objectives are manufactured for fluorescence microscopy, using water, glycerol or oil as immersion medium; examples are ×16/0.65 water-immersion and ×40/1.4 oil. When attempting to collect a video image from a specimen that fluoresces particularly weakly, it will be found advantageous, where the equipment allows it, to direct all of the imaging light to the video camera and none to the binocular viewing tube. Where this cannot be done, it may be necessary to fit temporary caps over the eyepieces (empty 35 mm film containers are very suitable) to prevent entry, through the eyepieces, of room light, which can interfere with the image.

Apart from careful choice of fluorochrome and mounting medium, efforts should be made during observation to minimize fading by restricting irradiation of the specimen. The exciting radiation should be occluded whenever observations are not being made, and work should proceed as quickly as possible. Once an image has been acquired by the analysis system, irradiation of the specimen should be stopped. It is also most important to ensure that all components of the system are themselves free from fluorescence; this includes all relevant optical parts of the microscope, slides and coverslips, mounting media and, in particular, the immersion fluids.

Epifluorescence equipment may also be used in another way, not involving fluorescence, to provide contrast. Two common techniques result in the specimen being labelled by highly reflective metal particles: autoradiography, where sites of activity are marked by the presence of small grains of silver, and immunogold techniques, where the antibody is labelled with small particles of gold. Using a suitable filter block containing a partially reflecting mirror without the usual wavelength-selecting properties, the specimen will be illuminated and observed by light of the same colour; colour filters inserted into the illuminating path will cause the reflections to be coloured. The highly reflective metal particles appear bright against a dark background.

It is worth pointing out that when epi-illumination equipment is fitted to a microscope, the normal transmitted light pathway remains available for other imaging techniques. Thus observation and analysis of the fluorescence or reflection image, with its precise localization of specific substances, can be combined with or rapidly followed by a bright field, phase contrast or differential interference contrast image to show the sites of localization in their context within the tissue.

The microscope stand

Apart from the obviously desirable properties of being rigid, adaptable, and suitable for the optical system in use, it is particularly important that the microscope stand be fitted with a good quality mechanical stage, preferably rotatable and centrable, to facilitate precise positioning of the area to be analysed. In more complex systems, movements of the stage may be driven by stepper motors controlled from the analysis equipment, permitting systematic sampling of large areas of the specimen.

The drawing tube

Most analysis of images from the light microscope will probably make use of images acquired directly by means of a video camera, but in some cases it may be more appropriate to work from a permanently recorded image, a photomicrograph or drawing of the specimen, entered into the system by a video camera fitted with a suitable lens. The details of photomicrography are beyond the scope of this chapter (see Evennett, 1989; Thomson & Bradbury, 1987), but the equipment designed to facilitate drawing may have a special use in image analysis. A drawing tube is available as an attachment for many microscopes. It is inserted between the body of the microscope and the binocular head, and enables the user to see, usually through both eyepieces, an image of the drawing paper and pencil superimposed on the normal microscope image of the specimen. The outlines of features can thus be traced on the paper. Provided the geometry of the system has been set up correctly, in particular with the paper perpendicular to the direction of observation, it should provide a correctly proportioned drawing (this may be checked by drawing the markings of a stage micrometer lying in the vertical and horizontal axes, and measuring the distances in the drawing).

The drawing tube may also have another use in image analysis. If the system permits data to be entered from a digitizing tablet, this can be used in conjunction with the drawing tube to provide a simple method of image acquisition. The image of a small, coloured, light-emitting diode attached to the cursor of the digitizing tablet and placed beneath the drawing tube, can be clearly seen through the binocular and traced around features in the microscope image. This method may lack accuracy, depending on the skill of the user, but it is simple and cheap, and it permits direct editing of the image, separating features of interest from the irrelevant.

Attachment of the video camera

A microscope is designed principally to produce an image in a form appropriate to enter the human eye; several factors must be considered when adapting a microscope to present its image on to a surface, such as a video camera sensor or photographic film. These concern both image quality and the ability of the video system to extract and handle the information resolved by the objective lens of the microscope.

The video camera used for image analysis should preferably not have a built-in lens as home video cameras do. The simplest kind of camera will have the same standard screw lens mount as used on 16 mm film cameras, the so called C-mount, which is a female screw thread, one inch (25.4 mm) in diameter, with a pitch of 32 threads per inch (not SI units, but the standard was originally defined in inches). In the normal configuration, the image should be formed 0.69 inches (17.53 mm) behind the flange of the mount. More complex video cameras may have internal beamsplitters and separate sensors for the three primary colours, and will require the image to be presented deeper within the camera; these also are fitted with special mounts often peculiar to a particular manufacturer's instruments.

The easiest way to attach a video camera to a microscope, suitable for the simpler cameras with a single sensitive surface, is to arrange for this device to lie in the primary image plane of the microscope. This method is cheap, requires no optical parts, and is mechanically very stable: it simply needs a tube of appropriate length, made to fit in place of the normal camera tube of the microscope, and carrying a fitting for the video camera. A suitable adaptor can be made in most laboratory workshops. This method may perform satisfactorily with some equipment and for some applications, but it is subject to two criticisms: there may be a problem with the correction of chromatic aberration, and the relationship between the magnification of the primary image and the size of the video camera sensor is fixed.

As described above, many objective lenses, particularly those of older design, produce a primary image which is not fully corrected for chromatic aberration; correction is normally completed by the use of a compensating eyepiece. If the primary image from such an objective is picked up directly by a video camera, features will be subject to colour fringing, particularly towards the edges of the field of view. Whether this defect is considered important will depend on the type of objective lens, the fineness of resolution of the video camera, and the nature of the work being done. Objectives fitted to some recent microscopes are designed to produce a fully corrected, aberration-free primary image, and are not subject to this limitation.

The alternative method of presenting the microscope image to a video camera requires the use of a lens system, preferably provided by the microscope manufacturer or one of the firms that specialize in video microscopy, which is designed to match the optical system of the microscope. Such an optical interface makes it possible to alter the size of the image as it is presented to the camera, by choosing suitable components or even by using a zoom system.

The relationship between the fineness of detail contained in the primary image and the information handling ability of the video camera and subsequent analysis system is an important consideration when designing the video camera interface. This relationship, together with the absolute size of the camera's sensing device, will also have an implication for the proportion of the visual field of the microscope that can be included in the video image.

As described in earlier chapters, for analysis the microscope image must be divided into picture elements or pixels. These may correspond to the separate sensing elements of a CCD camera, or result from digitization of the image within the analysis equipment; the number of pixels comprising one image frame will be known for any particular system. Each resolved feature should be magnified to such a degree that it falls on several pixels at the camera and thus in the image presented for analysis.

The considerations involved are best illustrated using some real values as an example. Suppose an objective of magnification ×25 and NA 0.65 is in use, with light of wavelength 0.5 μm. Substituting in equation 1 gives a value for resolved detail of about 0.5 μm in the specimen. This detail will be magnified 25-fold by the objective, up to 12.5 μm in the primary image. The video camera may have a sensor of say 10 × 10 mm, from which an image of 512 × 512 pixels may be collected – each pixel thus being about 20 μm square. Clearly the 12.5 μm detail resolved by the microscope will require further magnification of at least twofold, and preferably a little more, in order for it to be sufficiently large to be handled by an analysis system using 20 μm pixels. This extra magnification might be provided by a magnification changer system before the primary image, or by an optical interface, with appropriate magnification factor, between the microscope and the video camera. In the above example, the objective lens quoted (a real one) has a relatively large aperture (high resolving power) for its magnification, and the assumption has been made that the work requires the system to be capable of handling the finest detail resolved by that lens. Conditions may not always be so stringent, and the advantages and simplicity of collecting the primary image directly may be considered overriding.

Where more complex equipment is available, adjustment of the relationship between the objective's magnification factor and the requirements of the video system is most conveniently done using a continuously variable or zoom system between the microscope and video camera. Failing this, a magnification changer with fixed magnification steps, such as the Zeiss 'Optovar' will be found useful.

Conclusion

The light microscope is a more complex piece of equipment than is appreciated by most of its casual users. It is unusual in that it is technologically almost perfect, its ultimate performance being limited principally by the laws of nature. Because it appears superficially to be simple, the majority of micro-scope users make no effort to understand it. In consequence most light microscopes are misused, and their versatility is underexploited. It should be remembered that with a microscope you do not see, or analyse, the specimen, but an *image* of the specimen, and the fidelity of the information in this image relative to the original specimen depends on the skill of the user.

References

Bradbury, S. (1985). Filters in microscopy. *Proceedings of the Royal Microscopical Society*, **20**, 83–91.

Evennett, P. J. (1989). Image recording. In *Light Microscopy in Biology: a Practical Approach*, ed. Alan J. Lacey, pp. 61–102. Oxford: IRL Press.

James, J. & Tanke, H. J. (1991). *Biomedical Light Microscopy*. Dordrecht: Kluwer Academic Publishers.

Richardson, J. H. (1991). *Handbook for the Light Microscope*. New Jersey: Noyes Publications.

Thomson, D. J. & Bradbury, S. (1987). *An Introduction to Photomicrography*. Oxford: Oxford University Press and Royal Microscopical Society.

10

Confocal optical microscopy

A . B O Y D E

Introduction

The basic physical principle of any scanning microscope is that the sample is scanned with a radiation probe which illuminates discrete points in the sample. The probe is scanned over the sample, usually in a pattern something like a television raster. The signal from the interaction of the radiation probe with the sample is collected and used to reconstruct an image. The pioneer scanning optical microscope used the image of a cathode ray tube as a spot source of illumination for a light microscope (Young & Roberts, 1951). The subsequent development of such unitary-beam scanning optical microscopes has been strongly dependent upon the advantages of lasers, which give a powerful source of monochromatic radiation which can be concentrated in one spot.

Most of the real specimens that are examined with light microscopes are either translucent or, if they are surface reflective, are not flat. In both cases, light interacts with the sample over a considerable vertical range. It is therefore reflected (or in the case of fluorescent light, emanates) from a thick layer. It helps if the specimen is illuminated very brightly at the focal plane of the objective lens, but light still interacts with the sample in depth and this unwanted reflected or fluorescent light can enter a conventional imaging system.

The principle of the confocal scanning microscope is that scattered, reflected, or fluorescent light from out-of-focus planes is eliminated. This can be done by combining the idea of illuminating discrete spots in the focal plane with that of detecting the required signal from the same spots (Fig. 1). A real or a virtual aperture in the illuminating channel is imaged in the plane being focussed on. In the usual case of reflection and epifluorescence illumination this is performed by the objective lens. In the detection channel, a conjugate aperture is placed so that the light from only the illuminated spot in the sample will pass. The second or confocal aperture then obstructs the scattered, reflected or fluorescent light from out-of-focus planes, greatly reducing the overall signal intensity. This increases the probability that the detected light signal comes from the single point being measured. The analogue signal can be converted to

152   *A. Boyde*

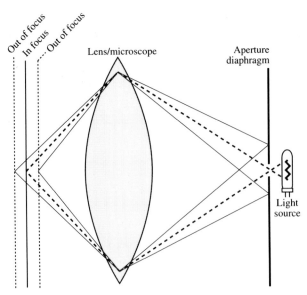

Fig. 1. The confocal principle. A real or virtual aperture is imaged by the objective lens into a plane of focus in or at the surface of the sample. Light reflected from, or fluorescence emanating from, this spot will return to the image at the same confocal aperture. Light reflected, scattered or fluorescing from out-of-focus planes is intercepted by the solid regions of the aperture diaphragm on the return path.

a digital value to assess the degree of reflection or fluorescence relating to that point at that time.

Historical development

It is a peculiar fact that the success of the early confocal microscopes was ignored by the biological microscopy community, yet biologists were closely associated with their invention and construction. The flying spot microscope was invented by Young & Roberts (1951). The improvement in imaging resulting from either illuminating a single microvolume in a specimen or collecting light only from that one spot was known to Mellors & Silver (1951). They used multiple beam, Nipkow disc scanning in illumination or detection for microscopic photometry. In confocal microscopy or spectroscopy, both are achieved simultaneously. Minsky (1961) created a single spot, on-axis, cathode ray tube (CRT) image with a 10 s frame speed in a transmission and reflection confocal light microscope which used mechanical scanning of the specimen with conventional incoherent illumination.

Weber (1970) described a transmission Nipkow-disc-based confocal configuration using two discs. Petran & Hadravsky (1968a; 1968b) described their 1964 invention of both transmission and reflection configurations for microscopes using a single two-sided disc (see also Egger & Petran (1967) and Petran *et al.* (1968)). They had first thought of, but rejected on grounds later detailed by Boyde & Petran (1990), the idea of using only one side of a disc for aperturing in both illumination and detection (Frosch & Korth, 1975; Xiao & Kino, 1987). The efficiency and utility of disc scanning were well known in the 1950s and 1960s, to the extent of understanding proper space-filling designs for the aperture array in the Nipkow disc (Nipkow, 1884; Reed, 1962).

Weber (1970) also described a transmission confocal light microscope with an x-scanned stage, fixed apertures, and the two-sided mirror scanning later adopted by Brakenhoff & Visscher (1990; 1992) in their precursor of the commercial Insight™ real time CSLM now manufactured by Meridian Inc.

An alternative method for deriving focal-plane-specific illumination which works well for certain classes of object is to illuminate the sample with a slit of light at right angles to the direction of observation. MacLachlan (1968) used this principle and showed how any method for reducing the instantaneous depth of field could also be used to increase it by through-focussing whilst recording, or observing, the image stack.

Lukosz (1966; 1967) provided a theory relating to the extension of the resolving power of the light microscopy beyond the classical limit, but both Minsky (1961) and independently, Petran & Hadravsky (1968a; 1968b), realized that they had achieved it through confocal (synonym tandem) scanning.

The term 'confocal' cannot strictly be applied to the use of microscopes with real or virtual slits as spatial filters. However, this is common practice and the great merits stemming from the ease of manufacture and alignment and the better signal available from slit confocals were seen by Egger *et al.* (1969), who described a slit disc scanning reflection confocal light microscope. Many relatively recent commercial instruments have gone back to these advantages (Newport Instruments, BioRad Viewscan DVC-200, Lasertec Corpn 1LM21, Meridian Insight).

Baer (1970) described novel microscopes with arrays of slit sources and slit detectors, appreciating the advantages for their use in fluorescence in biology. He also described a means of scanning with no moving parts utilizing lateral chromatic dispersion. Baer again realized that the depth of field could be increased by through-focussing whilst recording and that this could be done so quickly with a fast scanning system that a controlled increase in depth could be acquired for real time viewing. Furthermore, he saw how instant stereo could be obtained from the longitudinal chromatic dispersion of the objective, that the elevations of reflective features could be found by determining the focus level for peak brightness, and also that a range of heights could be determined from a single focus plane when using white light and an objective with an appropriate range of longitudinal chromatic dispersion. Baer's remarkable contributions also included the means for acquiring direct stereo images by oblique through-focussing.

The first laser scanning CSLM was described by Davidovits & Egger (1972), who employed lens scanning in a reflection (epi-illumination) configuration. Slomba *et al.* (1972) described a mirror beam scanning laser CSLM.

The first published biological observations with a confocal microscope were those of Egger & Petran (1967) and Petran *et al.* (1968) made with an early version of the multiple beam disc scanning CSLM, the tandem scanning microscope (TSM). This version was superseded by a more elegant design in 1970. Several papers in the Czech language describing applications appeared in 1972 under the authorship of Petran, his doctoral student Sallam al Sattar, and his colleague Hadravsky (Petran & Hadravsky, 1974; Petran & Sallam-Sattar, 1974; Sallam-Sattar & Petran, 1974).

Frosch & Korth (1975) described one-sided disc scanning CSLMs (1sTSM). They again saw that the depth of field in a CSLM could be increased by incrementing the focus at high speed with a high speed scanning system and showed that this could be visualized in a direct photograph, or with a video camera. Frosch & Korth also described *xyz* data storage for the first time, thus realizing one of the most important practical and theoretical advantages of confocal scanning.

Sheppard and colleagues in Oxford independently developed on-axis laser scanning for transmission and reflection confocal light microscopy. The advantages of using annular pupils for illumination and detection were shown by Sheppard & Wilson (1979). They also calculated the confocal depth discrimination advantage in the reflection mode, showing that the signal reduced to 50% at 0.71λ defocus, where λ is the wavelength of illumination (Sheppard & Wilson, 1978).

Brakenhoff and colleagues in Amsterdam independently developed very high precision, specimen scanning, on-axis laser confocal microscopes. They concentrated first on the transmission mode (Brakenhoff, 1979; Brakenhoff, Blom & Barends, 1979), and later published images of bacteria (Brakenhoff, Barends & Binnerts, 1981).

Several designs of slit confocals, with high speed, rotating polygonal mirror scanning, mainly conceived for work in clinical ophthalmology, were described by Koester (1979; 1980a; 1980b). Roberts (1982) described a slit confocal arrangement using opposite sides of the objective.

An early commercial CSLM offered by Oxford Opto-Electronics in 1979 failed to sell. Possibly the first commercial sale was in 1983: that of the Plzen TSM built for University College London and funded by a research grant obtained on the strength of successful documentation of through-focus image series recorded in Plzen in 1980 and 1981 (Boyde, Petran & Hadravsky, 1983).

Weber, now at Zeiss with colleagues Schmidt *et al.*, wrote another all-embracing patent which included the use of diode arrays in both illumination and/or detection; mirror scanning, infra-red, visible and ultraviolet wavelength ranges, fluorescence, phosphorescence, and Raman spectroscopy (Schmidt *et al.*, 1983).

Sheppard & Wilson (1981) produced their theory of the 'direct view' disc scanning CSLM utilizing, by way of illustration, a two disc arrangement as envisaged by Weber (1970). Other important contributions from the Oxford

group included that of Hamilton & Sheppard (1982) on the confocal interference mode; Cox, Sheppard & Wilson's (1982a) demonstration of the improvement in resolution with an offset detector aperture, and (1982b) of the
improvement in resolution in the fluorescence mode. Hamilton & Wilson
(1982a; 1982b) and Cox & Sheppard (1983) described digital scan control and
data storage, extended focus or range imaging and the production of stereo
images in reflection CSLM (preceded by both Baer, 1970 and Frosch & Korth,
1975).

Åslund *et al.* (1983) and Carlsson *et al.* (1985) described probably the first
mirror beam scanning laser CSLM using mirrors in a separate black box. This
paved the way for the commercial development of their own design as the
Sarastro, later Molecular Dynamics, CSLMs. They also claimed the invention
of *xyz* scanning and digital data recording (Carlsson, 1986). This was, however,
one of many re-inventions in the field.

Three-dimensional fluorescence images from digital *xyz* datasets from slow
speed, laser CSLMs were published by Wijnaendts van Resandt *et al.* (1985),
Carlsson *et al.* (1985), and Van der Voort *et al.* (1985). All these papers were
submitted after directly recorded, stereo, 3-D fluorescence images from real
time, disc scanning TSMs had been shown publicly in 1984 (see Boyde, 1985b).

Mendez (1982; 1985) considered speckle in laser CSLM, an important
problem since widely ignored.

The patent relating to the ultimately successful BioRad MRC500 series laser
CSLMs (White, 1987) was preceded by several others. These included Bille
(1986) and Webb (1988), describing instruments that worked at full television
(TV) rate (Schmidt *et al.*, 1983). In contrast, the BioRad instrument contained
a polygonal mirror scanning on the line axis and a galvanometer mirror
scanning on the slow frame axis.

Horikawa (1988) taught the importance of placing beam deflection mechanisms at conjugate pupils, described both a black box configuration with both
scan axes controlled by galvanometer mirrors (the industry norm in the period
1988–91) for work in reflection, fluorescence and transmission confocal light
microscopy and the use of acousto-optic deflection (AOD) to achieve a TV
rate reflection instrument. Houpt & Draaijer (1988) made a combined fully
confocal in reflection and slit confocal in fluorescence instrument using AOD,
the forerunner of Noran's Odyssey video rate CSLM (VRCSLM). Horikawa
(1990) described an AOD VRCSLM which was slit confocal in both reflection
and fluorescence.

Goldstein (1988) and Goldstein *et al.* (1990) described a working model of a
'no moving parts' instrument using a laser spot imaged on an image dissector
tube.

Webb & Wornson (1989) used a cylindrical lens to broaden the laser beam to
create a line scanned by a mirror, the detected signal (from the eye, since this
was conceived again for clinical ophthalmology) being directed to a linear array
of detectors.

Keldermann *et al.* (1989) described interesting inverse confocal configurations designed to give minimum brightness at focus.

Confocals were a long time in being recognized. Perhaps one reason was that Minsky did not publish a paper, but only a patent. The TSMs invented by Petran and Hadravsky (1968*a*; 1968*b*; 1970) to view the internal structure of living tissues were successful from their inception and used to examine eye, brain and muscle tissues. Whilst the intensity of the image forming light was sufficient to observe living and moving tissue with the unaided eye, the fact that such tissue was necessarily moving meant that, at that time, no image recording technique was available that could capture the information for transmission to third parties. For this reason, only those who had seen one of these TSMs working with live tissue were impressed. Very few people saw one, because there was only one instrument, and it was on the wrong side of the 'iron curtain'.

Types of CSLM

Real time, direct view, white light CSLMs: TSMs

The disc scanning CSLMs are multi-beam, real time, direct view systems with no inherent need for digital image storage or the use of computers in the image reconstruction process.

The tubelength of the standard Royal Microscopical Society (RMS) threaded objectives is 160 mm, i.e. an intermediate image plane lies 160 mm behind the objective lens. Take a reflection microscope configuration illuminated through the objective, place a small aperture in this intermediate image plane and the aperture will be imaged in the focal plane in the specimen. Now place an identical aperture 160 mm behind the objective and bring the returning imaging light from the focussed-on plane to a focus at the level of that aperture: it will normally be necessary to use a beam splitter to separate the illuminating and imaging apertures and rays. The arrangement described makes it possible to illuminate only a discrete spatial spot and to collect the rays from that spot separately from other reflected, scattered, or fluorescent rays into a detector aperture (Fig. 1).

To make a confocal scanning microscope that scans at great speed, an array of apertures could be used that could be moved physically at the level of the intermediate image plane (Figs. 2–4). If a large number of apertures are used (Fig. 4), the specimen may be illuminated with a large number, possibly a thousand or more, of scanning beams simultaneously, giving perhaps tens of thousands of scanning lines. This gives a major advantage in speed. Obviously, the illuminating and detecting apertures have to be scanned in tandem, hence the original name of TSM (Petran *et al.* 1985*a, b, c*). The apertures are holes or slits near the edge of an opaque, spinning disc, but other methods of scanning aperture arrays are possible.

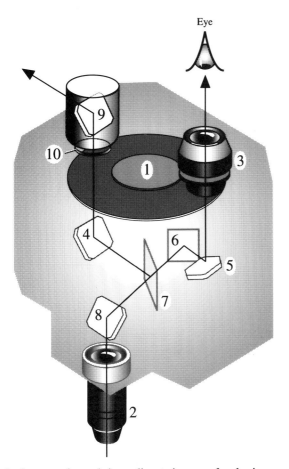

Fig. 2. Layout of a real time, direct view, confocal microscope (a TSM, manufactured in the Czech Republic). Light from a conventional source such as a mercury arc lamp or a tungsten filament is reflected to pass a field lens placed close to a 1% transmissive aperture disc (10 cm diameter), with tens of thousands of 30 μm diameter holes. Light passing the disc is reflected from a beam splitter and is then reflected downwards to enter the 160 mm tubelength RMS objective. Light reflected from, or fluorescent light emanating from, the specimen passes back through the same lens, is reflected by the same final mirror, passes the beam splitter and suffers two more reflections before reaching the observation side of the disc. The last optical component is a Ramsden type eyepiece used to observe the image in the scanning disc. (1) The rotating aperture or Nipkow disc (2) the objective lens (3) a Ramsden type eye-piece focussed on the disc on the image forming side (4, 5, 6, 8 and 9) front surface mirrors (7) an extremely thin beam splitting mirror (10) a field lens.

In the one disc, two sides configuration, pairs of holes on opposite sides and at identical radial distances produce single scanning lines. In early versions of the Plzen TSMs and in the Noran TSM, 1% of the aperture field was open: the 99% solid parts block off the illuminating light. In the Tandem Scanning Corp. TSM, designed to be used only in conjunction with a low light level video

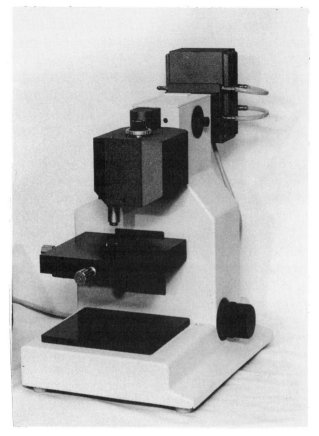

Fig. 3. The confocal 2002 TSM manufactured by JZD Komorno, Czech Republic.

Fig. 4. The layout of holes in a 10 μm copper foil disc, as used in a 1984 TSM manufactured at the Charles University in Pilsen.

camera, the disc is fabricated from chrome on glass, using 20 μm holes and a 0.33% transmission pattern.

Using only one side of a rotating aperture disc for both illumination and observation – the auto-collimation arrangement (1sTSM) – has the advantage that the system requires no alignment. Also the disc may be translated horizontally whilst running, so that several different bands with different aperture or slit sizes and packing densities may be used, or the disc may be removed altogether as in the Technical Instruments model. Similarly, the Newport Instruments design has four bands of apertures in the disc, 1% and 4% holes and 10% and 20% spiral slits: this system uses an additional relay stage employing an extra low power objective (Lichtman & Sunderland, 1989*a*, *b*). With all 1sTSM designs, there is the potential problem that the greater part of the illuminating light will be reflected back from the disc into the viewing channel. This reflected light can be suppressed in various ways, including (a) the use of crossed polars and a quarter wave-plate above or below the objective lens; (b) tilting the disc; and (c) placing a central stop to intercept the reflected rays (see also the method used by Frosch & Korth, 1975). None of these methods may be sufficient when looking at specimens such as living biological tissues, which have an inherently very low level of reflection. Very reflective specimens do not present problems and a 1sTSM design is used exclusively in a silicon wafer evaluation system for completely automated semiconductor production lines (Prometrix Corp., Santa Clara CA-95054-3077, USA).

Since the TSMs give direct view images, they can also be used whilst simultaneously observing the specimen by conventional light microscopy. For example, the specimen is placed on an inverted optical microscope and viewed in transmitted light using the TSM to illuminate the inverted microscope. Alternatively, the translucent specimen can be placed on a conventional microscope illuminator base and viewed via the TSM head using conventional (non-confocal) transmitted brightfield or darkfield illumination.

Single beam, slow scan, digital imaging laser CSLMs

Stationary beam, on-axis scanning

Several different methods of scanning the beam have been adopted in the confocal, unitary beam scanning microscopes. Almost all current models depend on laser light. Minsky's original microscope used a conventional light source, in which the optical beam was stationary and the specimen was scanned past it by vibration and screw driven translation mechanisms. The CRT image was viewed or recorded by photographic means. The BioRad SOM-100 model (1984; successor to the unsuccessful Oxsom) also used specimen scanning (see, for example, Wilson & Sheppard 1984). The precision engineering necessary for high resolution mechanical sample scanning was pioneered by the

Amsterdam group (Van der Voort *et al.*, 1985). These instruments obviously had to use digital data recording of *xyz* datasets.

If the specimen is scanned past a stationary optical beam, the frame speed is limited by the rate at which the specimen can be moved, which depends on its mass. Living biological specimens do not remain stable when scanning at speed. Nevertheless, the unitary beam, specimen scanning approach has the advantage of being 'on-axis' and avoiding all off-axis optical deformations. Specimen scanning is therefore most useful for reconstructing large specimen areas, in the case of stable samples (for example, samples embedded in a solid transparent resin) when acquisition time is unimportant.

Mirror beam scanning

Other methods of scanning had to be adopted to overcome problems with massive, wet or flexible specimens, as well as to increase the frame speed to make it possible to examine moving specimens. Present commercial designs with scan speeds in the range 0.25 to 4 frames per second use galvanometer mirrors for scanning both the line and frame axes. The possible advantages of using the higher scanning speed of the polygonal mirror have been outweighed by other engineering problems and these devices have been abandoned in recent production models. Scanning mirrors can be assembled inside the microscope, or packaged separately from an existing conventional microscope. Such 'black box' external scanning systems usually utilize the conjugate scanning plane located above the eyepiece at the so-called eyepoint. The appeal of such systems is that the normal operational modes of the conventional microscope can be used to locate an interesting field of view in a specimen, before switching to confocal reflection or fluorescence mode. A disadvantage may be that the specimen may have to be configured to fit a normal, conventional microscope.

Video rate, video output, laser scanning instruments

More recent, commercial, laser illuminated CSLM designs have successfully overcome the frame speed limitations of mirror scanning, yet use laser light. These instruments fall into two categories, according to whether the image is initially produced by video techniques (VRCSLMs) or whether, as in the TSMs, a real time, direct view, real colour image is available. In the TSMs the real image is converted to a video signal on being relayed via a video camera (e.g. Meridian's InSight, or BioRad's DVC-250 shown in Fig. 5). All are effectively slit scanning in the fluorescence mode.

The scan speed may be increased by using AOD on the line axis to achieve full video rate, fully confocal operation in reflection, the return beam being descanned via the AOD: this is used in Noran's Odyssey system. However, the fluorescent radiation cannot be descanned by the same device because the

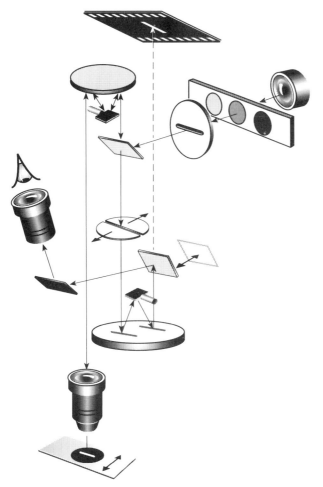

Fig. 5. Layout of components in the BioRad Viewscan DVC-250, direct view, real time, laser confocal fluorescence microscope. Diagram courtesy of BioRad, Hemel Hempstead, Herts, HB2 7TD.

refractive index changes with wavelength. Thus the fluorescence is directed, via a beam splitter, to a slit aperture. In the fluorescence mode, Type I scanning (point illumination, broad detector: Wilson & Sheppard, 1984) occurs in the line direction and Type II scanning (point illumination, point detection, a synonym for confocal: Wilson & Sheppard, 1984) in the frame direction only. The output is either a standard video signal which can be recorded with standard video devices, or the scan pattern can be controlled to give extremely high frame-rate reduced area scans or linear scans for observation of rapid events.

In the Lasertec 1LM series CSLMs, the beam is broadened by a cylindrical lens and AOD is used for the frame scan, reflected light being returned to a linear array of detectors. This very compact He−Ne laser based system is therefore slit or line confocal, and works only in reflection. Although designed for work with reflective materials and especially in the field of surface relief measurement, it has potential applications for work with live cells in the interference reflection mode.

Real time, direct view, laser illuminated CSLMs

In prototype designs published by Brakenhoff & Visscher (1990; 1992) direct laser illumination with a pinhole aperture was scanned, either in both x and y directions by a two-axis scan mirror for fully confocal mode, or, with a slit illuminator; the line confocal mode could be obtained by scanning on one axis only. In both cases, a single mirror was used, the reverse side of the double-sided mirror being used in descanning (as in the Weber patent of 1970) with the output light directed to a linear detector array. In the Meridian InSight system, the laser light is fed via a fibre optic bundle, spread to a line by a cylindrical lens and scanned in the frame axis only: the fluorescent light passes via a slit detector. The BioRad Viewscan DVC-250 is similar except that separate mirrors are used for scanning and descanning (Fig. 5). Because of safety problems with lasers, neither system is yet available for use in other than the fluorescence mode. Both produce real time, direct view, colour images in slit confocal mode.

The images obtained with these new real time, direct view, laser scanning microscopes differ from those of the disc scanning TSMs with conventional light sources mainly in lacking the possibility of using the reflection mode (because of laser safety regulations) and thus retaining a fraction of the reflected light image at wavelengths outside the range of wanted fluorescence in a direct, combined image. They also lack the range of input and output wavelengths available with conventional sources. However, the laser source may be much more intense. As with TSMs, either still photography or TV cameras may be used.

Biomedical applications of CSLM

Confocal scanning eliminates the fog that occurs in conventional light microscopy due to the halo of reflected, scattered or fluorescent light that results from elements in the sample above and below the plane of focus. Confocal mode gives an image of a thin focal plane which changes as the focus is changed. The effect is dramatic and is shown by all confocal microscopes. Its value to the user depends upon the given field of investigation. The improvement over conventional light microscopy in imaging thin sections or thin whole cell preparations may not be too important. The improvement for the examination of the surface layers of bulk samples is nothing short of revolutionary, because both single optical sections and series of sections can be obtained in perfect register. Even if images cannot be obtained through a great depth, it is a great advantage that a thin section does not have to be produced for excellent optical microscopy. A major disadvantage of conventional fluorescence micro-scopy is that detail is obscured by the halo of fluorescent light coming from features above and below the desired plane of focus. It is not possible to find the plane of focus simply from the intensity of the signal in the conventional fluorescence case. A dramatic improvement is secured by eliminating this out-of-focus information in the confocal mode.

Now several years into the era of commercially available and successful CSLMs, it is not surprising that the literature is too large to review in detail. Biological applications have used mostly the fluorescence mode, but of fixed and stabilized specimens, whilst inanimate science has used mostly reflection CSLM. The excellent possibilities for high temporal resolution, vital micro-scopy of living systems have, as yet, been hardly exploited, even though TSM was invented to look inside live tissue.

Real time vital microscopy in reflection or fluorescence

From the outset, the very purpose of high speed CSLMs was regarded as the avoidance or minimization of specimen preparation procedures in biomedical light microscopy. However, access has to be obtained to the layer of interest. Skin and other tissue layers have to be reflected, since only thin intervening layers can be tolerated. In live small animal preparations, where real time or video rate scanning is required, heart muscle cells can be seen through the epicardium. In appropriate species, glomeruli can be seen through the kidney capsule and TSMs have been used to study blood flow through kidney glomeruli (Andrews *et al.*, 1991; New *et al.*, 1991). With the correct objective lens, it is possible to see through the stratum corneum down to the basal, germinative layer in thin human skin. In intact eyes, one can image down to the corneal endothelium and the lens fibres: the Tandem Scanning Corp. TSM has been cleared by the United States Food and Drug Administration for use in clinical ophthalmology. TSMs have been used in humans to study tear film thickness, and all corneal layers down to the corneal endothelium (Lemp, Dilly & Boyde, 1985; Petran *et al.*, 1985c; Petran *et al.*, 1986; Dilly, 1988; Jester, Cavanagh & Lemp, 1988; Xiao, Kino & Masters, 1990). In isolated retinae, one can focus through all the layers (Petran & Sallam-Sattar, 1974; Sallam-Sattar & Petran, 1974). The limits are imposed largely by the transparency of the specimen and only sometimes by the free working distance of the objective.

Thus high speed, confocal imaging makes it possible to study accessible, intact living tissue. In other studies, implantable windows have been allowed to heal in bone, and special objective lenses have been developed to fit the window frame to permit the study of live bone *in vivo*. Outside the living body, the high speed confocal mode has proved to be very useful in the study of rapidly moving living cells. Other applications have included studying the demolition of dental tissues with high speed cutting instruments (Watson, 1990).

The technology is now available to make digital recordings at full TV frame rates, and both confocal reflection and fluorescence images are now good enough to record. Continuous recording requires only a standard video recorder. Movement during the single standard interlaced frame period can be analysed by de-interlacing (Fig. 6). Longer term motion can be analysed by replaying the video tape. This represents the birth of another era in light microscopy where the advantages in spatial resolution of confocal operation are enhanced by the more recently demonstrated improvement in temporal resolution.

Reflection CSLM of live tissues

In specimen preparation for live animal work, the animal is dissected to near the tissue layer to be studied, the tissues are bathed in the appropriate saline or culture medium, and the samples are examined under the microscope using the proper water immersion objective. To make it easy to observe parts of large specimens, some early TSM models were constructed so that the microscope

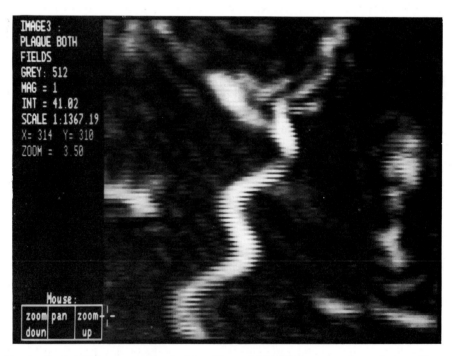

Fig. 6. Single TV frame acquired with a Noran TN-8502 image analyzer from a Noran VRCSLM, showing live, motile bacterial organisms from dental plaque. The centre of the field of view – here zoomed × 3.5 – shows a single spirochaete which has moved during the frame. The extent of the horizontal movement in the 1/50th second between the first field and the second field (half interlace patterns) can be seen as the sawtooth profile of the organism.

head could be moved down to the specimen, rather than a small specimen being moved up under the microscope.

The direct view confocal image of unstained biological objects is superficially similar to phase contrast and interference contrast images, but the contrast stems from refractive index differences at boundaries between constituents and not from the product of these differences and the optical path length, as in phase and interference modes. Some features that are usually easily visible in conventional, fixed, sectioned and stained histological preparations have low contrast in reflection CSLM, but can generally be seen without staining or other preparative treatment. Fixation usually results in a dramatic loss of contrast in reflection confocal microscopy.

Reflection interference contrast for cells on flat substrates

CSLMs give excellent contrast for the interface zone of cells attached to flat substrates such as glass and plastic (Figs. 7 and 8: see Boyde, 1989; Paddock, 1989; Boyde & Jones, 1992a). The contrasts are interpreted as being due to interference in thin layers; either the thin gap between the cell and the substrate, or thin cytoplasm (lamelloplasm). The very low light levels needed for image recording in a TSM plus low light level CCD combination makes this especially suited to the dynamic observation of cell movement phenomena (Boyde & Jones, 1992a). VRCSLMs are also useful for recording very rapid cell organelle movement. Observations of living cells under near optimum culture conditions, with the high spatial and temporal resolution given by a VRCSLM, can give new information about the dynamics of intracellular movements as well as information about rapid changes in transitory structures at the cell periphery, a region where phase contrast images are especially unsatisfactory.

In the author's laboratory, cell cultures maintained at 37 °C have been filmed using a TSM and a low light level camera. Sixteen-bit greylevel images were acquired in 0.1 s and transferred at a resolution of 256×256 pixels to an image analysing computer. Since a TSM is conventional when illuminated non-confocally with another source, the TSM reflection image could be seen combined with the usual phase contrast image of living cells. The Noran TSM, with its piezo-electric focussing control, enables rapid shifts of focus to be made with an accuracy of 0.02 μm. Thus sequences of confocal interference reflection mode images focussed near the plane of contact of cells with a glass coverslip could be interleaved with phase contrast images optimally focussed at 1.25 μm into the cell. Such images were recorded with extremely low (yellow-red) light levels, illuminating the TSM with a 12 V tungsten lamp run at 5 V.

Image recording is simpler, however, with a video rate laser-based system, since the CSLM can then be used as a superior video camera, feeding the signal directly to a standard video recorder. At least in the reflection-scattering mode, VRCSLMs offer an important advantage in temporal resolution compared with

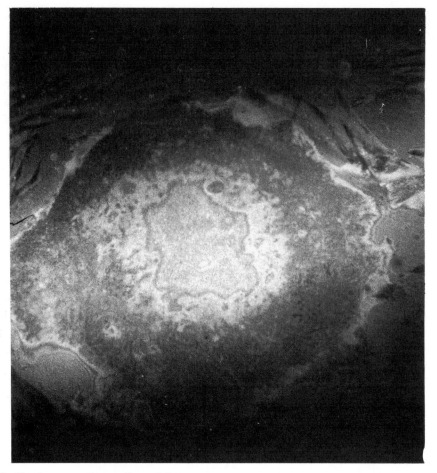

Fig. 7. Tandem scanning, reflected light micrograph of live chick osteoclast on glass. Contrast is principally due to reflection, or frustrated reflection and interference effects at the cell–glass interface. The coverslip is tilted, producing the bright strip at the centre of the field of view. Noran TSM. Nikon × 100/1.4 oil objective. The field height is 100 μm.

even a standard video camera-based light microscope system operating at the same frame rate. The signal deriving from any one pixel location in a video camera is integrated over the entire frame-capture period whilst the corresponding pixel is not being read out. Although it may be limited by 'shuttering', the time resolution for all pixels is usually the standard frame period, 1/25 s. However, in the VRCSLM case, information is read out only while the laser beam is at the corresponding point in the specimen. This means that the time resolution is, for example, 512^2 times faster than standard video in the line direction, and 25 times faster in the frame direction; in a non-interlaced scan it would be 50 times faster in the frame direction. The advantage in temporal resolution combined with the remarkable improvement in spatial resolution

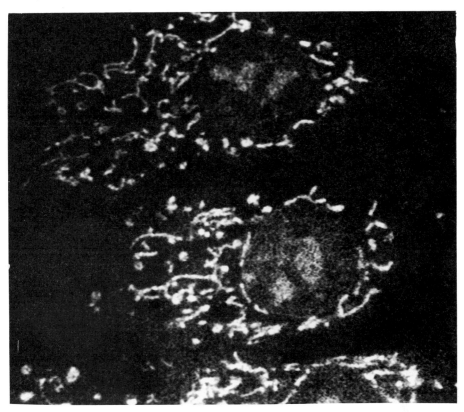

Fig. 8. Confocal fluorescence image of rat intestinal epithelial cells cultured on a coverslip, stained with DASPMI, a mitochondrial marker. Noran VRCSLM. Single frame recorded using a Fenestra image capture system. 488 nm excitation, >515 nm output. Lomo × 70/1.23 water immersion objective. The field height is 83 μm.

enables the detection of rapid movement within cells at 0.2 μm resolution, motion that would normally spoil the spatial resolution.

Conventional slow scan CSLMs for live cell work

Some slow scan CSLMs have problems in reflection mode, though most can also be used to produce excellent, noise free, reflection and interference reflection images of live cells (or, if on a flat substrate, fixed cells; e.g. Fig. 9(a)), either in tissue explants or as grown upon flat glass or plastic substrates. The reflection image may be spoilt by reflections from components elsewhere in the optical train. This problem can be overcome by the use of a quarter wavelength plate, as close to the specimen in the optical train as possible (Francon, 1961). Good reflection images can be obtained in a one-second capture period. If the sample is moving, however, adjacent pixels in the frame direction may be displaced by motion occurring between frames.

In the fluorescence mode, all slow scan CSLMs work well, but the main

168   *A. Boyde*

(*a*)

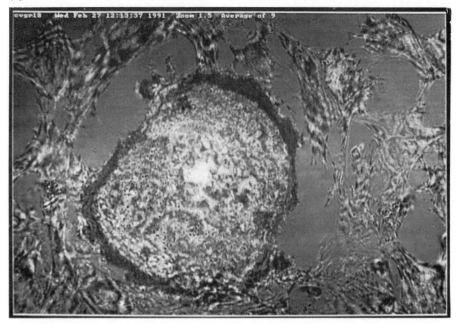

(*b*)

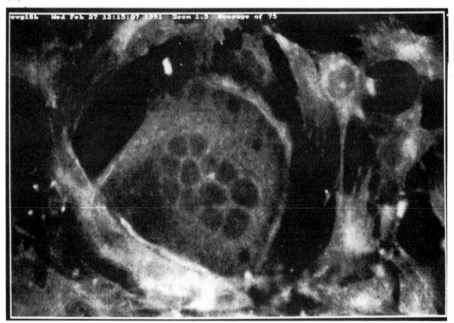

Fig. 9. (*a*) Reflection and (*b*) fluorescence (FITC anti-vinculin staining) confocal images recorded with a BioRad MRC500 Lasersharp CSLM. The specimen is bone derived cells on a glass coverslip, showing an osteoclast at the centre. Oil immersion objective (× 60/1.4), zoom factor × 1.5. Field dimensions are 117 μm by 77 μm.

problem is usually the degradation of the fluorophore due to the intense radiation. The compromise is between reducing this intensity and increasing the need for frame averaging. If the fluorophore does not decay too badly, excellent hard copy static images of fixed tissues and cells can be obtained, obviously far better than single TV rate frames. However, if the sample is alive, the loss in resolution due to sample movement during frame averaging is unacceptable.

Vital fluorescent dyes for high frame rate CSLMs

Now that real time fluorescence CSLMs are available commercially, there is likely to be an even greater interest in the use of the vital dyes developed for other applications, including fluorescence activated cell sorting. (A useful information resource in this field is the Molecular Probes catalogue.) Some examples of well-established dyes tested in real time, fluorescence CSLM include acridine orange, alizarin, calcein, chromomycin, DAPI, Hoechst-Dye No. 33258 (bisbenzimid), rhodamine 123, lucifer yellow, and tetracyclines (Fig. 10).

Particularly recommended dyes for VRCSLM include:

1 DASPMI for mitochondria and nucleoli.
2 Ethidium for DNA (nuclei, nucleoli).
3 Nile red for lipid droplets and as a 'stains-all' (Figs. 11–15). Neutral-red-staining organelles which appear red by transmitted light are black in confocal fluorescence, lipid drops are bright, but the dye stains all at a sufficient intensity and low cost.
4 Evans blue for cell surface.
5 Lissamine rhodamine for mitochondria.
6 Rhodamine B as a stains-all.
7 Fluorescein dextran for extracellular space, cells negative. Fluorescein stains mitochondria, but bleaches very rapidly so that the cells appear in negative contrast. Bodipy, a membrane probe, stains all, but fades like fluorescein; nevertheless, like nile red, it is very good for free-floating motile microorganisms and rapidly motile mammalian cells permitting them to be imaged in confocal fluorescence.

Ion concentration sensitive dyes

Attempts to measure, from images, the concentrations of intracellular ions such as calcium, pH and magnesium are currently a major field of endeavour. The usual ratiometric methods (dual wavelength excitation or fluorescence) are supposedly correct for the greater mass of cell found at its centre. However, there are problems, not the least of which is the lack of axial discrimination in conventional light microscopes. The assumption is usually made that the dye

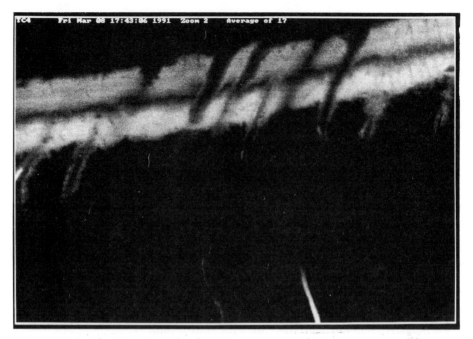

Fig. 10. BioRad MRC500 Lasersharp, confocal fluorescence image of a longitudinally sectioned human permanent molar tooth showing two fluorescent bands due to therapeutic administration of a tetracycline antibiotic. The bulk specimen was cut, ground flat on wet emery paper, washed, covered with glycerin and a coverslip and examined using a × 60/1.4 oil immersion objective, zoom factor × 2. Note the deposition of tetracycline label in peritubular dentine extending deeper into the dentine (towards the lower part of the micrograph) indicating the extent of the delay in mineralization of the peritubular phase. Field dimensions are 87 μm by 57 μm.

(for example, fura-2 for calcium) is uniformly distributed throughout the cytosol, and that cytosolic fluorescence ratios are being recorded. Partition of such dyes into an organelle-dependent distribution can be seen with good conventional optics in many cells, and confocal fluorescence imaging demonstrates an unexpectedly high rate of organellar partition. Confocal fluorescence is, however, also able to demonstrate an apparently uniform cytosol distribution, with the exclusion from organelles such as mitochondria and nucleus, when this occurs. For both reasons, one would conclude that confocal mode would be a good thing. However, the signal level will be reduced in confocal mode, and it is already low in most such applications, so that the favourable choice of excitation wavelengths offered by conventional arc lamp sources (which can be used with a TSM) will be offset by this factor. When one considers the problem of longitudinal chromatic aberration (Fig. 16, and see later for remarks about objective lenses), it is not surprising that the ratio results obtained with conventional light microscopes for thin lamellar regions of well spread cells are dubious: they will be even more so in strictly confocal work.

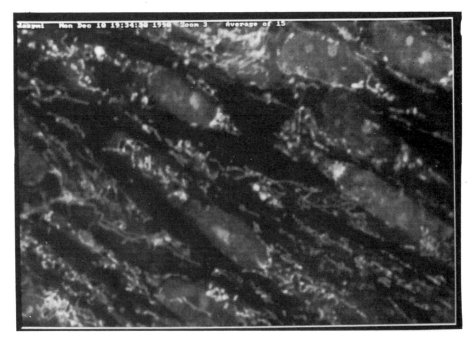

Fig. 11. Live osteoblasts on an opaque ceramic implant material stained with DASPMI to reveal the distribution of mitochondria. The orange fluorescence of DASPMI was excited with the 488 nm laser in a Biorad MRC500 Lasersharp confocal microscope. Nikon × 40/0.55 water immersion objective, zoom factor × 3. The field width is 87 μm.

For several reasons, it is more attractive to employ single wavelength methods with a laser CSLM, and preferably to use a dye, such as fluo-3 for calcium, which is efficiently excited by the most efficiently generated line in the most commonly employed laser, the 488 nm line of the argon ion laser (Hernández-Cruz, Sala & Adams, 1990; Niggli & Lederer, 1990; Williams, 1990), although ultraviolet light from the 325 nm line of a He–Cd laser and dual output wavelengths have been employed with indo-1 (Kuba, Hua & Nohmi, 1991). Because calcium fluxes are so fast and the output data so noisy, this has proved to be a proving ground for '*xt*' scanning, in which the specimen is scanned repeatedly along a single line, the data being formatted as single lines in an *xy* image. For example, 512 repeats of a single line scan (or 512 repeats of averages of several scans along the same line) are seen in one 512 × 512 image. Changes in gradient along the line under investigation are easily appreciated, particularly in pseudocolour or *y*-modulation displays.

Prepared, fixed specimens for CSLM

Fluorescence imaging: real time and slow scan CSLMs

The slow scan CSLMs are now so common that it is important to remember that fluorescence imaging is not only possible in the real time, white light,

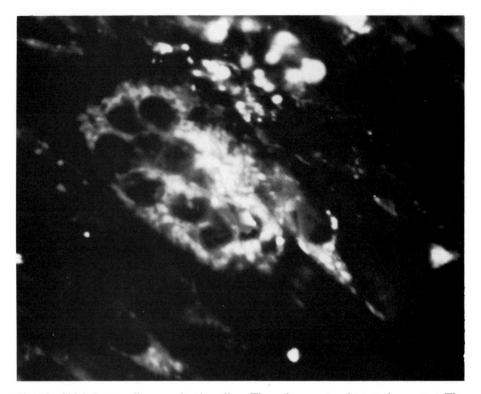

Fig. 12. Chick bone cells on a dentine slice. There is an osteoclast at the centre. The preparation was stained with BODIPY for a few minutes after staining with DASPMI. Noran VRCSLM. Photographed from a TV monitor (live, one second). Lomo ×70/1.23 water immersion objective with 130 μm coverslip. The field height is 83 μm.

direct view instruments, but was demonstrated (in 1984) before any significant work had appeared from the laser CSLMs. Much work has been done, and more could be done, using the direct view and direct photography, real colour fluorescence mode in TSMs (Watson, 1989). For those samples that show insufficient fluorescence intensity to be viewed with the unaided eye or recorded with normal photographic emulsions, a suitably sensitive TV camera is employed. The combination of a TSM with a cooled CCD or silicon intensified target (SIT) camera, or an image intensifier and TV camera, may result in less damage to the sample than the use of a laser CSLM, and one may be able to observe low level fluorescence for much longer periods with this combination. An advantage of the white-light-illuminated TSMs in fluorescence is that any fluorophore excited in the spectral range from the ultraviolet through to the near infra-red range can be chosen, again assuming that the image is detected via a suitably sensitive TV camera and discriminating filters.

A specific area of application of the direct view CSLMs (TSMs) in fluorescence has been in the study of dental restorations and dental and skeletal implant research. Fluorescent markers have been used to study the distribution of bonding agents between composite restorations and tooth tissues. Labelling

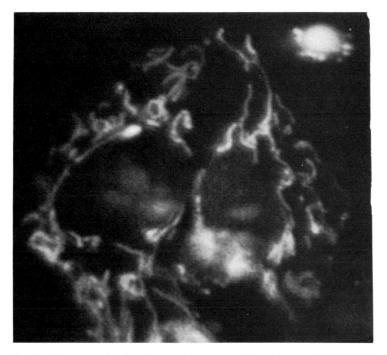

Fig. 13. Chick bone derived cells on a glass coverslip stained with DASPMI to demonstrate mitochondrial distribution. Photographed live (one second) from the display monitor of a Noran VRCSLM. Lomo × 40/0.75 water immersion objective, no coverslip, zoom factor × 2. The field height is 72 μm.

of chemically and light-activated dentine adhesives with fluorescent compounds has been used to improve the visualization of the 3-D dispersal of components at the tooth-restoration interface. The possible artificial disruption from sectioning a tooth after filling can be avoided by placing a restoration after sectioning and using a TSM to examine structure deep to the section surface in both reflection and fluorescence modes, maintaining a normal hydrated environment.

As noted above, the bulk of recently published work using confocal microscopy in biology and medicine has been performed with slow scan laser microscopes, which have an advantage in applications using only fluorescence imaging of stable, prepared biological samples. The high intensity of illumination available from the laser gives a correspondingly higher intensity of fluorescent light. Furthermore, since the returning signal is handled point by point, even very low levels of fluorescence can be successfully imaged using a sensitive photomultiplier.

Fluorescent stains

To date, most biomedical CSLM has used fixed tissue or fixed cells. The most commonly used mode is fluorescence (Fig. 9(*b*)), and the most commonly

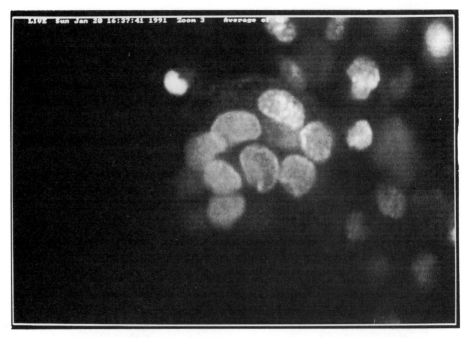

Fig. 14. Human odontoclast on a freshly exfoliated deciduous molar tooth stained with ethidium bromide, showing several of its nuclei at a focus level 20 μm into the cell. Nikon × 40/0.55 water immersion objective, zoom factor × 3. The field height is 57 μm.

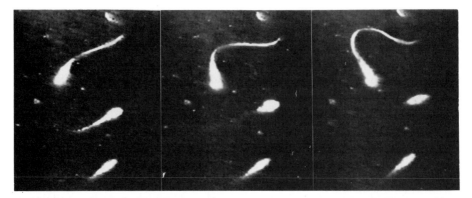

Fig. 15. Live sperm in seminal fluid stained with nile red. Three successive interlaced TV frames were recorded by photographing still frames from a video tape. Noran VRCSLM, combined reflection and fluorescence image (> 515 nm), dominated by the fluorescence signal excited by the 488 nm line of the argon ion laser. Oil immersion objective (× 60/1.4).

employed stains are the fluorescein or rhodamine derivatives, and/or dyes with similar excitation and emission frequencies. The most common applications are in immunofluorescence. Common problems are fluorescence bleaching, the low intensity of the fluorescence – which makes laser CSLM attractive – and

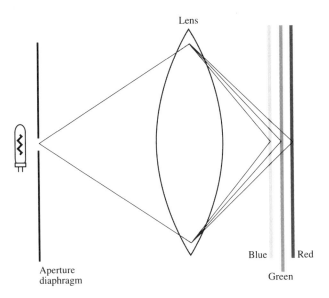

Fig. 16. Chromatic aberration used for colour coding for depth in a white-light-illuminated confocal microscope such as a TSM. The spectral colours passing an illuminating aperture in the intermediate image plane of the objective lens are focussed at different distances in front of the objective lens because of the longitudinal chromatic aberration of that lens. Returning light through the pinhole is maximum in blue, green and red for reflectors lying at the distances indicated by the blue, green and red planes (for the appropriately designed objective).

the need to visualize two or more epitopes simultaneously, an area where considerable improvement in instrumental performance is indicated. Unfortunately, no fluorescence is excited at a unique wavelength. Given the differences in power available at the frequencies of the commonly used lasers, more effort should be devoted to separating the simultaneous output frequencies with a single wavelength of excitation than attempting to excite fluorophores separately with different frequencies.

The most commonly used input wavelength is the 488 nm line of the argon ion laser. This is extremely efficient at exciting dyes such as fluorescein, but fluorescein is relatively unstable and photobleaches or degrades. Longer wavelength lines (e.g. 514 and 529 nm) have much lower intensities, but excite rhodamine-like dyes more efficiently, and such dyes are usually more stable.

Autofluorescence and negative fluorescence

As regards fluorescence imaging for morphology, rather than cytochemistry, the possibilities are excellent in CSLM. First, all tissues fixed in formaldehyde and glutaraldehyde acquire aldehyde-induced autofluorescence, that of glutaraldehyde being more intense. Although glutaraldehyde-induced fluorescence is unstable under 488 nm excitation, it is strong enough and persists for long enough to allow tissue sections to be studied without further staining. It follows that these fixatives need to be avoided where specific fluorescent staining is required.

Many mounting media are autofluorescent (e.g. old-fashioned canada balsam) and can be used as a negative stain in semi-porous solid samples. Here again – as with staining extracellular space with a fluorescent dye when working with live cells and tissues – confocal fluorescent mode has an advantage over conventional fluorescence: it can be used to find the exact plane of focus in a featureless film of fluorescent medium (Kimura & Munakata, 1990).

Amongst non-fluorescent mounting media, polymethylmethacrylate (PMMA) is particularly recommended. It is used in embedding bone blocks, but commonly thought to be unsuitable for use with other tissues because it is hard to cut with a microtome. It also has the disadvantage that it is not suitable for use with immunofluorescent stains, where glycol methacrylate may be preferred. For optical sectioning microscopy, however, it excels. Expensive and unreliable microtomy can be replaced with grinding on fine, wet abrasive papers. The refractive index of PMMA is high and a close match for glycerin, which does not affect the PMMA and can be removed by washing with water. Residual surface roughness effects, which may cause a breakthrough of unwanted reflection detail in fluorescence images very close to the block surface, can be removed by applying a coverslip with glycerin, permitting the use of both dry and oil objectives.

A few years ago, it was still being argued whether there would be any point in building a confocal microscope which worked at a speed significantly greater than one frame per second, because there would never be enough fluorescence signal to be able to image any faster. Today, it can be seen that this is not true, even with vital dyes. There are many stable and intensely fluorescent dyes that permit video rate confocal scanning and can be used with fixed and prepared tissue. All material stained with haematoxylin and eosin using classical histology and histopathology methods can be employed. Eosin is strongly fluorescent and the haematoxylin is a local absorber reducing the fluorescence intensity. The most stable fluorescent dye is brilliant sulphaflavine (Fig. 17). This cheap substance stains all proteins and can even be imaged using cathodoluminescence in a scanning electron microscope.

Fluorophores last longer if the dwell time per pixel is reduced, which is an advantage for rapid scanning microscopes. Some conventional slow scan CSLMs actually dwell longer at each pixel during a single, slower scan in order to achieve better signal averaging. In this case the radiation damage may be high, even though blurring due to the frame averaging of long term movement may be lower.

Reflective stains

Much more could be done with reflective, rather than fluorescent 'stains' – particularly if some of the commercial laser CSLMs were substantially improved in this mode. Many stains are reflective and are valuable for work with

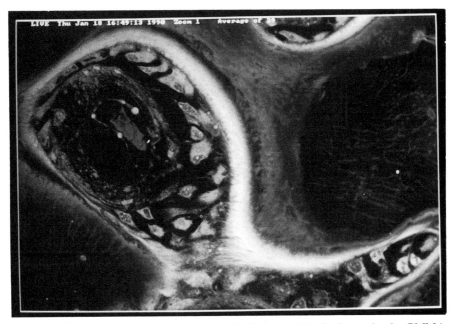

Fig. 17. Confocal fluorescence image of brilliant sulphaflavine-stained, PMMA-embedded rabbit proximal tibia, showing the bone close to a titanium implant (not visible). The yellow-green fluorescence was excited with the 488 nm laser of a BioRad MRC500 Lasersharp confocal microscope. Oil immersion objective ($\times$ 60/1.4). Field dimensions are 175 μm by 115 μm.

all types of CSLM. Obviously, the reactions that deposit metallic silver or gold or insoluble metal salts in, or on, the tissue have the most dramatic effect. Examples of such reactions include the Golgi-type impregnations used by neurocytologists and the immunogold and silver-enhanced immunogold reactions developed in the first instance for electron microscopic immunocyto-chemistry (Figs. 18–21). In fact, the colloidal gold particles are so small that the process should be described as light scattering. However, many commonly used organic dyes are reflective and considerable advances in this area of CSLM application can be expected. For example, toluidine blue increases the reflectivity of fixed cells (Figs. 22 and 23) and of any surfaces to which proteins have attached, as, for example, during cell culture procedures (the reflective colours in a white light CSLM are also outstandingly beautiful). Of particular importance is the diaminobenzidine (DAB) end product (brown in normal transmitted light microscopy) of many immunocytochemical staining reactions, since this is notably reflective.

Reflective coatings

Reflection contrast will be highest in the case of a dry sample viewed in air. Immersion media and objective lenses are used to reduce the relative significance of this surface reflection. However, immersion lenses may also be used in imaging rough surfaces of bone, tooth and implant or prosthesis

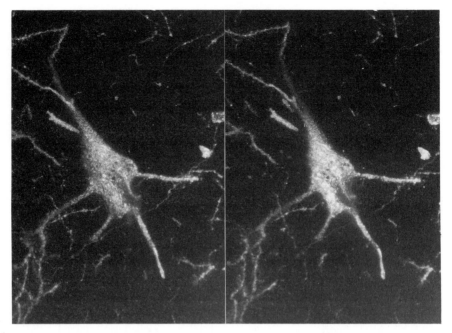

Fig. 18. Cerebral cortex from a 26-day-old cat, from a Golgi preparation made by Santiago Ramon y Cajal, borrowed from the Cajal Museum, Madrid. The images are a stereopair, with a simulated tilt angle difference of 12°, depth range 17 μm. Nikon ×60/1.4 oil immersion objective. Tungsten lamp. Noran TSM with 1990 disc. The field width is 120 μm.

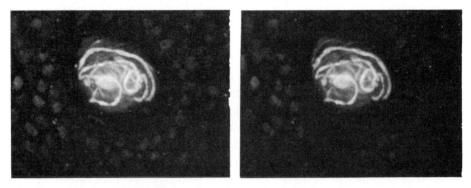

Fig. 19. Reflection TSM images of a silver-stained Meissner's corpuscle in human fingertip skin (section by Prof Novotny). The image was captured using a cooled CCD camera (Wright Instruments Ltd) at a resolution of 512 × 385 pixels and then transferred to a Noran 8502 image analysing computer. These extended focus or range images were recorded during one second for each frame by through-focussing along mutually inclined axes. Photographed from the display monitor.

samples in order to record detail from steeper topographic slopes than can be captured with a dry lens. The reduction in the surface reflection may then be a problem, particularly if there is a good index match between the immersion fluid and the substrate. The reflection image may then be enhanced by

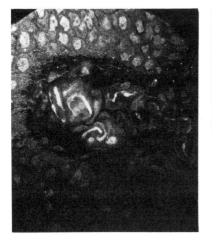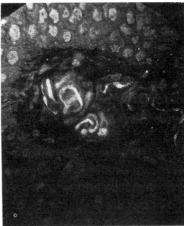

Fig. 20. TSM reflected light stereopair of a silver-stained Meissner's corpuscle in human fingertip skin, directly recorded on black and white photographic film. The original image was highly coloured, the reflection from the surrounding epithelial cells being dominated by the green region of the mercury arc spectrum, whilst the reflections from the coiled nerve ending in the Meissner's corpuscle were yellow. Depth range 8 μm. The simulated tilt angle difference is 7.125°. Oil immersion objective ($\times$100/1.4). The field height is 91 μm.

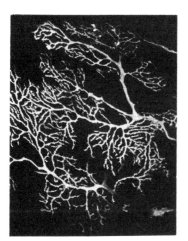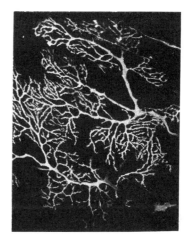

Fig. 21. Purkinje cells in mouse cerebellum stained by the Golgi-Cox procedure. Noran TSM, reflected light. Stereopair, simulated tilt angle difference 10°, depth range 11 μm in 50 μm thick section. Nikon $\times$ 60/1.4 oil immersion objective. The field height is 166 μm.

employing a metallic coating such as is used on scanning electron microscopy (SEM) samples. The information content may be improved by evaporating metals with contrasting colours to code for slopes facing in different directions; for example, the silver colour of aluminium, the green of gold and the red of copper.

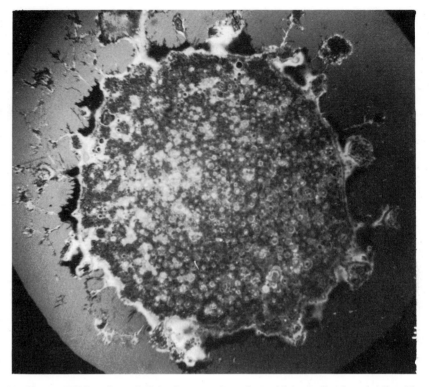

Fig. 22. Noran TSM reflected light image of a glutaraldehyde-fixed, toluidine-blue-stained osteoclast on a glass coverslip. Nikon × 100/1.4 oil immersion objective. The field height is 98 μm.

How low can we go?

Resolution in conventional and confocal light microscopy

Considering first the case of conventional light microscopy, Abbe's formula for the lateral resolution, d, of a light microscope states that:

$$d = 1.22\lambda/(N_c + N_o)$$

where λ is the wavelength of light, N_c is the numerical aperture of the condenser and N_o is the numerical aperture of the objective.

For a reflecting microscope illuminated through the objective via a beam splitter, $N_c = N_o$. As an example, the NA of the best, short working distance dry objectives is 0.95. Therefore, at $\lambda = 0.5$ μm, $d = \pm 0.32$ μm.

For depth resolution, h, Francon (1961) gives:

$$h = \frac{\lambda}{8n \sin^2 (\alpha/2)}$$

where n is the refractive index of the immersion medium and α is the angle of

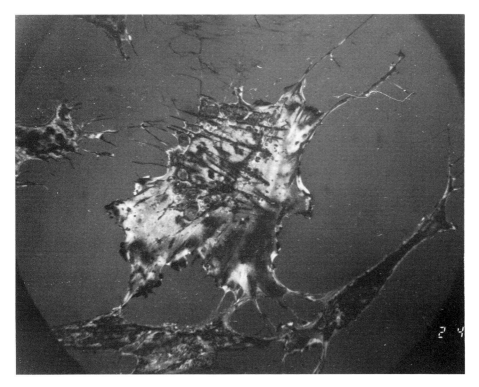

Fig. 23. TSM image of chick bone derived cells on glass, glutaraldehyde-fixed, and stained with toluidine blue. The live reflection image in the TSM of such preparations is brilliantly and strongly coloured. Nikon × 100/1.4 oil objective. The field height is 98 μm.

the half cone of light that enters the objective (NA = $n \sin \alpha$). For a 0.45 NA objective with $\lambda = 0.5$ μm, $n = 1$, $\alpha = 13.4°$ giving $h = \pm 1.168$ μm. For NA = 0.95, with $\lambda = 0.5$ μm, $h = \pm 0.182$ μm.

For confocal microscopy, both the lateral and the depth resolution are improved by a factor of 1.4 (Brakenhoff *et al.*, 1985). For an objective of 0.95 NA therefore, d will reduce to ± 0.23 μm and h to ± 0.13 μm. More important, however, is that the integrated intensity or power falls dramatically in out-of-focus confocal images. Sheppard & Wilson (1978) showed that integrated intensity falls by 2% for a defocus of 0.097 λ for NA = 1, i.e. a measurable change would be found for a change in focus of 0.048 μm for $\lambda = 0.5$ μm. Hamilton & Wilson (1982*b*) made a practical demonstration of a vertical resolution of better than 0.1 μm with an objective of NA 0.5 and $\lambda = 0.633$ μm. With a method that involves the sensitive measurement of the intensity, reproducibility will be 0.05 μm using white light and a 0.95 NA objective. In such a procedure, large numbers of measurements (the number of pixels multiplied by the number of focal planes) are taken and errors even out around the mean value: the observer cannot introduce bias.

Magnification calibration

The magnification of any CSLM must be rigorously checked against a standard. A silicon standard with a repeating grid pattern of 10, 100, and 1000 μm squares, as in a chequer board sold for SEM calibration, can be recommended for this purpose. It will clearly demonstrate non-uniform pixel dimensions in *xy* as well as scan distortions. The CSLM user should have a reference calibration image at hand before considering the worth of any calculations of the size of features, but should also remember that, in measuring widths or areas (or in calculating volumes), the uncertainty due to the finite resolution, irrespective of magnification, is complicated by problems due to finite pixel dimensions in image digitizing systems.

At the highest magnifications, it is useful to have a test object with periodicities at the limit of resolution. Test diatoms are particularly good reflectors, and can be purchased mounted under standard thickness coverslips for use with the usual objective lenses available in biological laboratories (Fig. 24).

Signal strength, absorption, scattering and depth

Nearly all practical CSLMs work in a reflection or epi-illumination configuration. Light paths are twice the depth of penetration into the sample, one of the reasons that the range of depths over which useful images can be obtained is

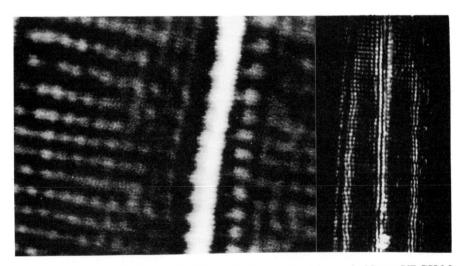

Fig. 24. Diatom, *Amphipleura pellucida*, reflection confocal image in Noran VRCSLM. Photograph of a single frame from a video recording. Oil immersion objective (× 60/1.4), zoom factor × 23. The horizontal line structure has a periodicity of 0.25 μm and the side-to-side dot pattern has a periodicity of 0.2 μm (Inset zoom factor × 2). This standard resolution test is very convenient for checking the width of the field of view in a CSLM at high magnification and is available from Northern Biological Supplies, Ipswich, UK.

rather limited in most preparations. Another is that most real specimens are optically inhomogeneous: the refractive index differences between components give rise to the reflection and scattering necessary to make images in this mode. In most animal tissues, this limits the depth for high resolution work to less than 50 μm, often less. This may sometimes be more in special cases like the eye.

Refractive differences are not usually eliminated in the preparation of specimens for confocal fluorescence work and also spoil the imaging possibilities. Greater efforts could be made by users to 'clear' their specimens, i.e. to replace water with media having high refractive indices matching those of the dry cell solids, glass, and mounting and immersion media for which the objective lenses are designed to function. This brings the additional benefit that the shift in focus level read from the mechanical stage of the microscope will correspond with real axial distance in the specimen.

In fluorescence CSLM, signal strength varies with depth into the sample due to absorption and scattering of the incoming radiation by layers above the current focal plane in the sample, and these need to be modelled in any attempt at a quantitative study of fluorescence (Visser & Brakenhoff, 1990). Light loss with depth is also prominent in reflection imaging in translucent samples, but the only quantitation likely here is that based on the determination of the height at which the maximum signal strength is returned from the reflective or scattering element.

About objective lenses

In practice, one finds that most biological CSLM installations are equipped only with dry objectives corrected for 170 μm coverslips, and oil immersion objectives for which the refractive index of the immersion oil should match that of the glass coverslip. The thickness of the coverslip is then unimportant optically with oil immersion lenses, though it may be a nuisance physically in preventing close range working with certain macroscopically rougher specimens. It is, however, possible simply to omit the coverslip, or to use a very thin one or a thin sheet of plastic film as appropriate to avoid collisions.

The common dry objectives in medical and biological laboratories are not corrected for the examination of dry specimens in which surface topography is to be examined. Special no-coverslip dry objectives need to be acquired, but good, high numerical aperture lenses are hard to find for the standard 160 mm tubelength light microscopes. When dry objectives are used with translucent samples to image internal reflective or fluorescent features, the focus increment is read incorrectly (usually by a factor close to 1.5 for mounted samples), yet one rarely finds that this factor has been taken into account in publications which show CSLM section series or 3-D reconstructions.

Oil immersion objectives are used for all high resolution microscopy in medicine and biology, yet only the oil and the glass are designed for the job.

Unless the sample is mounted in a medium of the same refractive index, resolution in depth will be spoilt by spherical aberration, the relative depth increment will again be read incorrectly and the depth range over which useful results can be obtained will suffer badly (Visser, Oud & Brakenhoff, 1992). In most cases, the specimen will be mounted in water or glycerin or a glycerin-based medium (e.g. Citifluor). Special glycerin immersion objectives are available and would be correct for most fluorescence work in practice, but they require special care in maintenance.

Water immersion objectives should be considered as indispensable in the biological CSLM laboratory for all work with living cells and tissue, or fixed tissue mounted in water. These lenses should be available both for use with no coverslip, and with a coverslip thickness correction collar. Special objectives need to be developed for many areas of application of confocal microscopy. In clinical ophthalmology, $\times$ 30/0.38 (BioOptics, Japan) applanating (tissue contact) objectives are in everyday use.

Differences in the performance of copies of the same objective from the same manufacturer occur in practice. It is strongly recommended that the lens on the confocal microscope be tested before purchase.

Axial chromatic aberration

Using a white light CSLM, such as a TSM, to look at a reflecting surface reveals the existence of chromatic aberration of the objective lens. Even the best lenses have some axial (longitudinal) chromatic dispersion, so that the microscope will not be focussed at the same axial distance for all wavelengths simultaneously (Fig. 16). A single image of a non-flat surface recorded in colour at one focus level in a TSM gives rise to a coloured map of the specimen surface, features in the same colour being at the same distance from the objective. This information can be used for rapid surface mapping (Browne, Akinyemi & Boyde, 1992). (This should not be confused with the pseudocolour coded topographic maps which can be computed from the reflection signal obtained when *xyz* scanning is performed with any kind of CSLM).

With a laser CSLM, longitudinal chromatic focussing problems may be assessed by finding the height difference at focus for the laser wavelengths provided. It may be possible to tune a slow scan CSLM to be confocal at the same plane at the excitation and several emission wavelengths for a given part of the field of a given objective lens used under ideal circumstances, i.e. when working with a fluorescent specimen of uniform refractive index. The practical problems will be most important where morphological identification of cell types and tissue layers in a semi-bulk sample is required: then the reflection image must derive from exactly the same plane as the fluorescence image.

In dual labelling fluorescence work, it is again important to be sure that both signals are maximized at the same focal level. A workmanlike solution would be for the manufacturers of objective lenses to offer specific designs for single and dual wavelength applications. Thus lenses with the same focal length at the most commonly used 488 nm line of the argon ion laser and the emission maxima of fluorescein and rhodamine (or texas red) would have widespread application in modern cell biology.

Extended focus or range images

The shallow depth of field of all the CSLMs may sometimes be a disadvantage and one may want to combine the improvement in lateral resolution with a controlled increase in the depth of field. Using the fact that the signal level is very low for out-of-focus planes, a set of images representing different focal planes in the specimen is acquired and they are summed to make an in-focus image for all the levels scanned. Extended focus or range images can be acquired by averaging the frames whilst changing the focus, or by through-focussing when photo-recording a single frame in the real time, direct view instruments (Figs. 18–21). If separate digital images of the stack are recorded, the maximum intensity at each pixel can be displayed, which usually gives a visual improvement over the image of the simple sum. In processing fluorescence image series, Van der Voort and colleagues (1985) have shown that more complex image processing routines may translate the image information into a more easily understood form, for example, by showing the object with a computed shadow, using an assumed direction of illumination. Two or more sets of discrete information, such as reflective features or fluorescence from one or more fluorophores, for example, can be combined in one 3-D image using pseudocolours.

Stereo imaging

A stereoscopic view of a slice can be produced by reconstructing two mutually inclined, extended focus views through the same through focus stack. Multiple views can be reconstructed to generate rotating or oscillating displays, but they are of little use without video or cine display. They are also computationally expensive.

For the simple case of stereo images and the direct view (real image) CSLMs, it is only necessary to scan through focus while recording two separate photographs, the z axes being inclined at a suitable angle (Figs. 18, 20, 21). This results in beautiful, real colour stereos that exploit the resolution and the enormous data storage capacity of the photographic emulsion (Boyde, 1985a).

Any type of CSLM image can be processed in a frame store. One stereo view can be reconstructed by simply summing the individual focal plane images, and the other by shifting each component image sideways to simulate an oblique view through that volume. Shifting each component of the summed image laterally in opposite senses gives symmetrical oblique viewing. In this way 3-D images can be generated after a single through-focus pass, the stereoscopic view being available soon after the focussing has been completed.

Stereo images are acquired more rapidly by frame averaging fast scan images. With disc scanning TSMs, the images are conveniently summed in a slow readout, cooled CCD camera (Fig. 19). With VRCSLMs, the images are summed in the computer frame store. In either case, excellent 3-D images are acquired in periods of the order of one second per view for 10 to 40 μm layers.

A real time, direct view stereo imaging system was described by Baer in a confocal slit microscope (Baer, 1970; Courtney-Pratt, 1986). We have recently constructed a similar system for real time CSLM (Maly & Boyde, 1994). New objective lenses have been computed with a deliberately large, but linear longitudinal chromatic dispersion. The TSM is illuminated with a flat spectrum (xenon arc) lamp. Reflective specimens appear coloured according to their distance along the optical axis within the range of focal distances covered by the colours of the visible spectrum. This coloured image is viewed by a special binocular viewing head with complex prismatic elements that disperse the spectral colours in opposite senses for each of the two eyes. Thus the colour information is converted to stereo parallax and seen as the corresponding height.

When 3-D images are reconstructed by summing individual focal planes from any CSLM, they have parallel projection geometry, as distinct from the perspective or central projection geometry of conventional light optics. A possible method for 3-D reconstruction from recorded stereo pairs would be via x, y and delta-x (parallax) coordinate measurements as in scanning electron microscopy photogrammetry, for which special measuring and analytical equipment is available. Such an approach would, however, be cumbersome in comparison with the direct analysis of surface morphology available by rapid through-focus mapping.

Confocal surface mapping

Mapping surfaces by determining reflection maxima in xz (profile) or xyz (map) digital datasets was pioneered by Cox, Hamilton, Sheppard & Wilson in Oxford. In our laboratories, a Noran TSM interfaced via a Cohu 4710 CCD TV camera (Cohu Inc, San Diego, CA, USA) to a TN8502 image analysing computer has been used extensively for such studies (Fig. 25). The objective lens of the TSM could be focussed by piezo-electric devices controlled by the computer to a positional accuracy of 0.0125 μm (Boyde et al., 1990).

The Lasertec 1LM11 VRCSLM has a control system designed for the rapid acquisition of extended focus maximum intensity and map images. Each focus plane is imaged once at full video rate, so that a 256 greylevel (256 contour level) map is available for analysis. The simplest analysis involves the use of cursor lines to define xz profiles from which the vertical range and width of

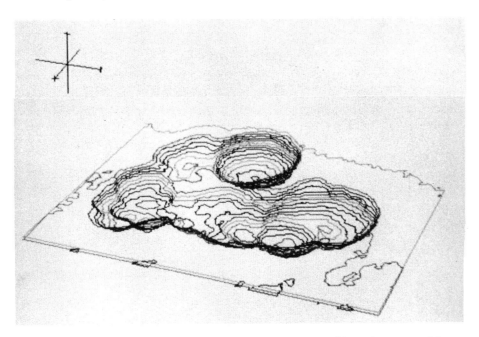

Fig. 25. Reconstruction of the surface of a slice of dentine with a pit excavated by an osteoclast which differentiated from the long bone marrow of a pre-hatch chick (preparation by Prof. S. J. Jones). The data were acquired by through-focussing, determining the focus value at which the greatest signal intensity was returned, using a Noran TSM interfaced to a Noran 8502 image analysing computer. The resultant z-map was contoured at 1 μm intervals and is displayed from an oblique viewpoint.

features are recovered (Fig. 26). More advanced software allows the interactive or semi-automatic definition of areas from which volumes of outlined features are recovered: the volume is the integral of all the pixel values (depths or heights) corrected by subtracting the mean pixel value in the surrounding flat surface. This system has been used to measure the 3-D resorptive capacity of osteoclasts as the volume of the pits that they excavate when seeded on flat slices of compact bone and dentine (Boyde & Jones, 1992*a*, *b*). Here, speed and efficiency depend on the means adopted to process the information from the surrounding unaltered surface, which may be both rough and tilted. CSLM mapping can also be used to measure the heights and volumes of cells on flat substrates prepared as SEM specimens by freeze drying or critical point drying and the application of a metallic, reflective coating.

Stereology and other uses of image processing

Stereology

Stereology is concerned with recovering 1-, 2- or 3-D information from 2-D sections. Most is based upon the study of single flat cuts through bulk samples.

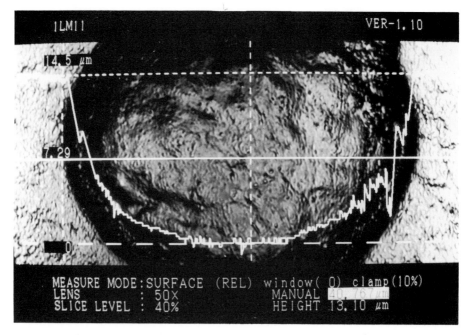

ILMI1   VER-1.10

14.5 μm

7.29

0

MEASURE MODE:SURFACE (REL) window(0) clamp(10%)
LENS   : 50X   MANUAL 40.76μm
SLICE LEVEL : 40%   HEIGHT 13.10 μm

Fig. 26. Surface profiling with the Lasertec Corporation 1LM11 VRCSLM with He-Ne laser, a line confocal system optimized for the measurement of feature width and depth. In the background, the confocal range image of a pit made in sperm whale dentine by a chick osteoclast can be seen. Superimposed on this is the trace of a profile through the surface taken along the central white line. Two horizontal cursor lines indicate the level of the original top and bottom surface of the pit, giving the depth, in this case 13.1 μm. Vertical cursors crossing each edge of the feature give the width as 40.76 μm. Photographed from a curved TV monitor display.

Confocal scanning optical microscopy has the advantages that a translucent object can be sampled in depth and sections obtained in exact register.

Precise estimates of number density can be obtained from single pairs of sections (e.g. Howard *et al.*, 1985). Features are counted if they are present in one section plane, but not the next. With digital images, one needs only to subtract one from the next, a procedure that automatically provides a shading correction for all local but repeatable scan anomalies. All regions that are the same in two successive image planes will appear grey. Those occurring in one plane but not the next are white, and those in the second plane but not the first are black. Either the black or the white features are counted.

Much useful work can be done by thresholding individual image planes to produce series of binary images that hold only the positions of the contours of phases or regions within the microscopic object. These binary images have the advantage over those derived from serial physical sections that they are in perfect register. They can be used with many of the commercial software packages sold for 3-D reconstruction, most of which are actually concerned mainly with improving 3-D visualization. The 3-D surface map image is a special case of the 3-D dataset where only one piece of information is retained at each xy address, namely the z coordinate at which the brightest return signal was obtained. Sequential binarisation of map images results in sequential contours, and it is often helpful to view these from an oblique projection (Fig. 25). Subtracting a smoothed map image from the original gives a version that demonstrates local relief (Boyde & Fortelius, 1991).

Other uses of image processing

Any kind of image processing or analysis which is possible with other images can be applied to CSLM images. Measurements of area and intercept, methods of edge enhancement, shade correction and spatial filtering (for further noise reduction) are all applicable.

Processing to accentuate highlights can be very important in combining reflection and fluorescence images. The immunofluorescence image of a probe for a particular protein can be processed to enhance and to retain only local and significant maxima, and this image can be added to a version of the reflected light image (or a background, non-specific fluorescence image) with a reduced image histogram to provide a morphological image with the super-imposed, specific immunochemical information.

Fast Fourier transform (FFT) routines can be applied to determine periodici-ties in single image planes. By applying a mask to the FFT in the reverse FFT process, certain spatial frequencies can be enhanced or removed. This pro-cedure may be valuable not only in analysing the structure of the object plane, but also in reducing periodic lines due to imperfections in the scanning process in the CSLM image, for example, TV or disc scanning artefacts.

All slow scan CSLMs use frame averaging to reduce noise. Users of these systems will wish to store multiple digital images on a temporary basis, for later image enhancement, 3-D analysis and reconstruction and single image analysis. Much of the data analysis work of the system is best done off-line in order to permit the digital data collection system to be used as such. Spare PCs with good image processing and analysis capabilities are therefore essential. These could be based on an extra frame store card in the host PC and software from any number of suppliers (e.g. PC_IMAGE from Foster-Findlay Associates and Fenestra from Kinetic Imaging Ltd, Liverpool). The cheapest to date uses the hard disk of the PC for image storage and processing (Cyclops from Kinetic Imaging Ltd, Liverpool).

Choosing the type of CSLM

The choice of CSLM will be based upon the conflicting requirements of the need to scan large fields and the means to record images. Scanning over a lot of material to find a field of interest or to obtain a general overview dictates that scanning should be as rapid as possible. It may be very difficult to gain a good impression of a range of appearances in a sample if one has to wait several seconds per frame per focus level. High temporal resolution is, therefore, desired for this reason alone, but compulsory for all but slowly moving live samples.

Although the TSMs and the line laser CSLMs which work without image reconstruction on a display monitor are presently the best in temporal resolution, slow scan CSLMs have their own advantages. The disc scanning TSMs currently have much higher frame speeds than even the relatively fast VRCSLMs or the line confocal, laser scanning systems. They are so fast that image formation for direct visual inspection is, for all practical purposes, the same as a conventional microscope.

The on-axis, laser based instruments in which the specimen is scanned mechanically past a fixed beam are the slowest but the most confocal, and show the highest resolution in x, y and z planes with the least image degradation. A mechanically scanned sample, laser based instrument would be chosen if ultimate resolution in either reflection or fluorescence was the sole requirement, although they are difficult to obtain commercially. Such instruments would be inappropriate for bulk samples, living samples, or samples which change with time.

The mirror scanning, off-axis laser instruments, as already noted, have higher frame speeds than the on-axis microscopes, but there is still a delay while a frame builds up on a conventional TV display. The fastest scanning rates for full resolution are about one frame per second, but at reduced pixel resolution it is possible to increase this frame speed to, say, four frames per second for rapid scanning to locate a plane of interest. In most cases, however, sequential frame averaging is employed to reduce noise in image recording, especially in the fluorescence mode. A scanned beam type of microscope, preferably the kind in which the beam is injected into an existing microscope from a 'black box', would be satisfactory if the standard transmission and reflection methods of optical microscopy are to be combined with the advantages of confocal imaging. This kind of microscope can also be used for slowly moving, live biological objects. The high intensity of illumination for a sensitive biological sample may be a problem with any of the laser based instruments.

The fastest frame rates in TSMs, VRCSLMs or direct view laser CSLMs are best for observing large samples, for working with live samples, for studying fast interactions, or for searching large areas and at a lot of depths. The TSMs always have an advantage in reflection work or if real colour (in natural reflection or fluorescence) is a requirement. Some TSMs have been configured to look at even very large samples: all form an image in real colour as well as in real time.

Type I and Type II scanning

New users of commercial CSLMs are often unaware that the system may not be confocal unless they make it so. The degree to which the signal is discriminated from layers outside the ideal focus plane clearly depends both on the NA of the objective lens and on the size of the confocal detection pinhole. The novice working in the fluorescence mode, however, is impressed by the fact that the rate of decay of the fluorescent radical dictates the need for some compromise: by increasing the area of the confocal detection aperture, a much less noisy image is acquired in a much shorter time and the specimen is saved. Increasing the aperture to the limit, however, turns the system into a Type I scanning microscope as defined by Wilson & Sheppard (1984), i.e. one in which either a broad source of illumination or a broad detector is used. That this is so frequently done – and done in ignorance of the fact that the system is no longer confocal or Type II (as defined by Wilson & Sheppard, 1984) – depends upon the fact that the sample is itself very thin and that the out-of-focus fluorescence halo is sufficiently reduced by this circumstance alone. Given that the ultimate aim of most biological fluorescence confocal microscopy is to produce a 3-D reconstruction of a thin subsample, direct recording of stereo fluorescence images by conventional means would be faster, easier, and produce much less noisy data (Osborn *et al.*, 1978).

Much work currently performed on so called CSLMs is not done in the confocal mode and really only exploits the advantages of the intensity of the laser, the ability to control the power input to the sample field and the limitation of the sample field in the *xy* plane. If radiation damage depends only on the total dose delivered, then it is easy to see that, because all focal planes above and below the ideal plane covered by the field of view receive the same radiation dose, fluorescence fading will occur at the same rate in all the z planes contained within the scanned field (a disappointment and a great disadvantage). However, there is no illumination outside the field and those areas will be saved, which represents a substantial advantage. A further advantage of the CSLM is that image recording is rapid and reliable and that only the images needed to illustrate a report need be converted from digital data.

Confocal microscopes may not be required for work with thin samples. If further improvement is needed, deconvolution procedures such as those pioneered by Agard and colleagues (Chen, *et al.*, 1990; Carrington *et al.*, 1990) and Fay *et al.* (1989) and available as commercial software from Microtome may provide the solution. The equipment required then only amounts to a personal computer, frame store card, and a good CCD camera.

Acknowledgements

The TSM1 project was supported by the MRC, TSM3 by SERC and the Noran Odyssey by The Wellcome Trust. Recent work with confocal microscopy has also been supported by Research Into Ageing and the Horserace Betting Levy Board. None of this work would have been possible without the help and collaboration of Prof Sheila J Jones. The author is grateful to Roy Radcliffe and Maureen Arora for technical assistance.

References

Andrews, P. M., Petroll, W. M., Cavanagh, H. D. & Jester, J. V. (1991). Tandem scanning confocal microscopy (TSCM) of normal and ischemic living kidneys. *American Journal of Anatomy*, **191**, 95–102.

Åslund, N., Carlsson, K., Liljeborg, A. & Majlöf, L. (1983). PHOIBOS, a microscope scanner designed for microfluorimetric applications, using laser induced fluorescence. *Proceedings of the Third Scandinavian Conference on Image Analysis*, pp. 338. Lund: Studentliteratur.

Baer, S. C. (1970). Optical apparatus providing focal-plane specific information. US patent 3,547,512; priority 16.04.68, patented 15.12.70.

Bille, J. (1986). Gerät zur Wafer-Inspektion. EP 168 643; priority 14.06.84 DE, published 22.01.86.

Boyde, A. (1985a). Stereoscopic images in confocal (tandem scanning) microscopy. *Science*, **230**, 1270–2.

Boyde, A. (1985b). Tandem scanning reflected light microscopy (TSRLM) Part 2 – Pre-MICRO 84 applications at UCL. *Proceedings of the Royal Microscopical Society*, **20**, 131–9.

Boyde, A. (1989). Combining confocal and conventional modes in tandem scanning reflected light microscopy. *Scanning*, **11**, 147–52.

Boyde, A., Dillon, C. E. & Jones, S. J. (1990). Measurement of osteoclastic resorption pits with a tandem scanning microscope. *Journal of Microscopy*, **158**, 261–5.

Boyde, A. & Fortelius, M. (1991). New confocal LM method for studying local relative microrelief, with special reference to wear studies. *Scanning*, **13**, 429–30.

Boyde, A. & Jones, S. J. (1992a). Real time confocal microscopy. *Binary Computing in Microbiology*, **4**, 119–23.

Boyde, A. & Jones, S. J. (1992b). Surveying surfaces at sub-micrometre resolution: the measurement of osteoclastic resorption lacunae. *Photogrammetric Record*, **14**, 59–84.

Boyde, A. & Petran, M. (1990). Light budgets, light and heavy losses: one or two sided tandem scanning (real-time direct view confocal) microscopy. *Journal of Microscopy*, **160**, 335–42.

Boyde, A., Petran, M. & Hadravsky, M. (1983). Tandem scanning reflected light microscopy of internal features in whole bone and tooth samples. *Journal of Microscopy*, **132**, 1–7.

Brakenhoff, G. J. (1979). Imaging modes in confocal scanning light microscopy (CSLM). *Journal of Microscopy*, **117**, 233–42.

Brakenhoff, G. J., Barends, P. & Binnerts, J. S. (1981). High-resolution confocal scanning light-microscopy (CSLM) as applied to living biological specimens. *Scanning Electron Microscopy*, 1981/2, 131–8.

Brakenhoff, G. J., Blom, P. & Barends, P. (1979). Confocal scanning light microscopy with high aperture immersion lenses. *Journal of Microscopy*, **117**, 219–32.

Brakenhoff, G. J., van der Voort, H. T., van Spronsen, E. A., Linnemans, W. A. & Nanninga, N. (1985). Three-dimensional chromatin distribution in neuroblastoma nuclei shown by confocal scanning laser microscopy. *Nature*, **317**, 748–9.

Brakenhoff, G. J. & Visscher, K. (1990). Novel confocal imaging and visualization techniques. *Transactions of the Royal Microscopical Society New Series*, **1**, 247–54.

Brakenhoff, G. J. & Visscher, K. (1992). Confocal imaging with bilateral scanning and array detectors. *Journal of Microscopy*, **165**, 139–46.

Browne, M. A., Akinyemi, O. & Boyde, A. (1992). Confocal surface profiling utilizing chromatic aberration. *Scanning*, **14**, 145–53.

Carlsson, K. S. (1986). Method and apparatus for microphotometering microscope specimens. US patent 4,631,581; priority 15.03.84 SE, granted 23.12.1986 US, EP 155 247, published 18.09.85 EP.

Carlsson, K., Danielsson, P. E., Lenz, R., Liljeborg, A., Majlof, L. & Åslund, N. (1985). Three-dimensional microscopy using a confocal laser scanning microscope. *Optics Letters*, **10**, 53–5.

Carrington, W. A., Fogarty, K. E., Lifschitz, L. & Fay, F. S. (1990). Three-dimensional imaging on confocal and wide-field microscopes. In *Handbook of Biological Confocal Microscopy*, ed. J. B. Pawley, pp. 151–61. New York: Plenum.

Chen, H., Sedat, J. W. & Agard, D. A. (1990). Manipulation, display, and analysis of three-dimensional biological images. In *Handbook of Biological Confocal Microscopy*, ed. J. B. Pawley, pp. 141–50. New York: Plenum.

Courtney-Pratt, J. S. (1986). Avoiding unwanted scattered light in microscopy. *Scanning*, **8**, 251–2.

Cox, I. J. & Sheppard, C. J. R. (1983). Digital image processing of confocal images. *Image and Vision Computing*, **1**, 52–6.

Cox, I. J., Sheppard, C. J. R. & Wilson, T. (1982a). Improvement in resolution by nearly confocal microscopy. *Applied Optics*, **21**, 778–81.

Cox, I. J., Sheppard, C. J. R. & Wilson, T. (1982b). Super-resolution by confocal fluorescent microscopy. *Optik*, **60**, 391–6.

Davidovits, P. & Egger, M. D. (1972). Scanning optical microscope. US patent 3 643 015; priority 19.06.70 US, published 15.02.72.

Dilly, P. N. (1988). Tandem scanning reflected light microscopy of the cornea. *Scanning*, **10**, 153–6.

Egger, M. D., Gezari, W., Davidovits, P., Hadravsky, M. & Petran, M. (1969). Observation of nerve fibers in incident light. *Experentia (Basel)*, **25**, 1225–6.

Egger, M. & Petran, M. (1967). New reflected-light microscope for viewing unstained brain and ganglion cells. *Science*, **157**, 305–7.

Fay, F. S., Carrington, W. & Fogarty, K. E. (1989). Three-dimensional molecular distribution in single cells analysed using the digital imaging microscope. *Journal of Microscopy*, **153**, 133–49.

Francon, M. (1961). *Progress in Microscopy*, Row Peterson, Evanston, IL.

Frosch, A. & Korth, H. E. (1975). Method of increasing the depth of focus and or resolution of light microscopes by illuminating and imaging through a diaphragm with pinhole apertures. US patent 3,926,500; priority 02.12.74 US, patented 16.12.75 US.

Goldstein, S. R. (1988). Confocal scanning laser microscope having no moving parts. WO 88/08550; priority 29.04.87 US, published 03.11.88 WO.

Goldstein, S. R., Hubin, T., Rosenthal, S. & Washburn, C. (1990). A confocal video-rate laserbeam scanning reflected-light microscope with no moving parts. *Journal of Microscopy*, **157**, 29–38.

Hamilton, D. K. & Sheppard, C. J. R. (1982). A confocal interference microscope. *Optica Acta*, **29**, 1573–7.

Hamilton, D. K. & Wilson, T. (1982a). Surface profile measurement using the confocal microscope. *Journal of Applied Physics*, **53**, 5320–2.

Hamilton, D. K. & Wilson, T. (1982b). 3-Dimensional surface measurement using the confocal scanning microscope. *Applied Physics B Photophysics and Laser Chemistry*, **27**, 211–13.

Hernández-Cruz, A., Sala, F. & Adams, P. R. (1990). Subcellular calcium transients visualized by confocal microscopy in a voltage-clamped vertebrate neuron. *Science*, **247**, 858–62.

Horikawa, Y. (1988). Two dimensional scanning photo-electric microscope. US patent 4 734 578; priority 27.03.85 JP, patented 29.03.88 US.

Horikawa, Y. (1990). Scanning optical microscope. US patent 4 893 008; priority 09.06.87 JP, patented 09.01.90 US.

Houpt, P. M. & Draaijer, A. (1988). (Nederlandse Organisatie vor Toegepast Natuurwetenschappelijk) Confocal laser scanning microscope. EP 0284,136; priority 13.03.1987 NL, published 28.09.88 EP.

Howard, C. V., Reid, S. A., Baddeley, A. & Boyde, A. (1985). Unbiased estimation of particle density in the tandem scanning reflected light microscope. *Journal of Microscopy*, **138**, 203–12.

Jester, J. V., Cavanagh, H. D. & Lemp, M. R. (1988). In vivo confocal imaging of the eye using tandem scanning confocal microscopy (TSCM). *Proceedings of the Electron Microscopy Society of America*, **46**, 56–7.

Kelderman, H. F., Fein, M. E., Loh, A. E., Adams, A. & Neukermans, A. P. (1989). Confocal measuring microscope with automatic focusing. US patent 4,884,617; priority 20.01.88 US, patented 04.07 89 US.

Kimura, S. & Munakata, C. (1990). Depth resolution of the fluorescent confocal scanning optical microscope. *Applied Optics*, **29**, 489–94.

Koester, C. J. (1979). Scanning microscope apparatus with three synchronously rotating surfaces. US patent 4,170,398; priority 03.05.78 US, patented 09.10.79.US.

Koester, C. J. (1980*a*). Scanning optical system for incrementally generating a composite image of a strip-scanned object. US patent 4,241,257; priority 24.05.79 US, patented 23.12.80 US.

Koester, C. J. (1980*b*). Scanning mirror microscope with optical sectioning characteristics: applications in ophthalmology. *Applied Optics*, **19**, 1749–57.

Kuba, K., Hua, S. Y. & Nohmi, M. (1991). Spatial and dynamic changes in intracellular Ca^{2+} measured by confocal laser-scanning microscopy in bullfrog sympathetic-ganglion cells. *Neuroscience Research*, **10**, 245–59.

Lemp, M. A., Dilly, P. N. & Boyde, A. (1985). Tandem-scanning (confocal) microscopy of the full-thickness cornea. *Cornea*, **4**, 205–9.

Lichtman, J. W. & Sunderland, W. J. (1989*a*). Kit for converting a standard microscope into a single aperture confocal scanning epi-illumination microscope. US patent 4,884,880; priority 14.09.88 US, patented 05.12.89.

Lichtman, J. W. & Sunderland, W. J. (1989*b*). Single aperture confocal scanning epi-illumination microscope. US patent 4,884,881; priority 14.09.88 US, patented 05.12.89.

Lukosz, W. (1966). Optical systems with resolving powers exceeding the classical limit. I. *Journal of the Optical Society of America*, **56**, 1463–72.

Lukosz, W. (1967). Optical systems with resolving powers exceeding the classical limit. II. *Journal of the Optical Society of America*, **57**, 932–41.

Maly, M. & Boyde, A. (1994). Real time stereoscopic confocal reflection microscopy using objective lenses with linear longitudinal chromatic dispersion. *Scanning*, **16**, 187–192.

McLachlan, D. (1968). Microscope optical system to increase depth of observation. US patent 3,398,634; priority 27.08.64 US, patented 27.08.68 US.

Mellors, R. C. & Silver, R. (1951). A microfluorometric scanner for the differential detection of cells: application to exfoliative cytology. *Science*, **114**, 356–60.

Mendez, E. R. (1982). Speckle in confocal scanning-transmission optical microscopes. *Optics Communication*, **43**, 318–22.

Mendez, E. R. (1985). Speckle statistics and depth discrimination in the confocal scanning optical microscope. *Optica Acta*, **32**, 209–21.

Minsky, M. (1961). Microscopy apparatus. US patent 3,013,467; priority 07.11.57 US, granted 19.12.61 US.

New, K. C., Petroll, W. M., Boyde, A., Martin, L. B., Corcuff, B., Leveque, J. L., Lemp, M. A., Cavanagh, M. D. & Jester, J. V. (1991). In vivo imaging of human teeth and skin using real-time confocal microscopy. *Scanning*, **13**, 369–72.

Niggli, E. & Lederer, W. J. (1990). Real-time confocal microscopy and calcium measurements in heart muscle cells: towards the development of a fluorescence microscope with high temporal and spatial resolution. *Cell Calcium*, **11**, 121–30.

Nipkow, P. (1884). Elektrisches Teleskop. Patentschrift 30105 (Kaiserliches Patentamt, Berlin), patented 06.01.1884.

Osborn, M., Born, T., Koitsch, H.-J. & Weber, K. (1978). Stereo immunofluorescence microscopy. I. Three dimensional arrangement of microfilaments, microtubules and tonofilaments. *Cell*, **14**, 447–88.

Paddock, S. W. (1989). Tandem scanning reflected light microscopy of cell-substratum adhesions and stress fibres in Swiss 3T3 cells. *Journal of Cell Science*, **93**, 143–6.

Petran, M., Benes, J., Boyde, A. & Hadravsky, M. (1986). In vivo microscopy using the tandem scanning microscope. *Annals of the New York Academy of Sciences*, **483**, 440–8.

Petran, M. & Hadravsky, M. (1968*a*). Zpusob a zarizeni pro zlepseni rozlisovaci schopnosti a kontrastu optickeho mikroskopu. (Methods and arrangement for improving the resolving power and contrast of an optical microscope.) CES 128937; priority 05.12.1966 CES; see also US 3,517,980; patented 30.06.1970 US.

Petran, M. & Hadravsky, M. (1968*b*). Zpusob a zarizeni pro omezeni rozptylu svetla v mikrokroskopu pro osvetleni shora. (Method and installation to restrict scatter of light in a microscope with illumination from above.) CES 128936; priority 05.12.1966 CES.

Petran, M. & Hadravsky, M. (1970). Method and arrangement for improving the resolving power and contrast. US patent 3,517,980; priority 05.12.1966; patented 30.06.1970.

Petran, M. & Hadravsky, M. (1974). Employment of tandem scanning microscope in morphological research of living sensory systems. *Activitas Nervosa Superior (Praha)*, **16**, 289.

Petran, M., Hadravsky, M., Benes, J., Kucera, R. & Boyde, A. (1985*a*). The tandem scanning reflected light microscope. Part 1 – The principle, and its design. *Proceedings of the Royal Microscopical Society*, **20**, 125–9.

Petran, M., Hadravsky, M. & Boyde, A. (1985*b*). The tandem scanning reflected light-microscope. *Scanning*, **7**, 97–108.

Petran, M., Hadravsky, M., Boyde, A. & Muller, M. (1985*c*). Tandem scanning reflected light microscopy. In *Science of Biological Specimen Preparation*, ed. M. Muller, R. P. Becker, A. Boyde & J. Wolosewick, pp. 85–94. SEM Inc, AMF O'Hare, Chicago IL.

Petran, M., Hadravsky, M., Egger, M. D. & Galambos, R. (1968). Tandem scanning reflected light microscope. *Journal of the Optical Society of America*, **58**, 661–4.

Petran, M. & Sallam-Sattar, M. (1974). Microscopical observations of the living (unprepared and unstained) retina. *Physiologia Bohemoslovenica*, **23**, 369.

Reed, S. F. (1962). Automatic camera. US patent 3,052,168168; priority 17.01.58 US, granted 04.09.62 US.

Roberts, C. W. (1982). Wide field specular scanning device. US patent 4,323,299; priority 03.08.80 US, patented 06.04.82 US.

Sallam-Sattar, M. & Petran, M. (1974). Dynamic alterations accompanying spreading depression in chick retina. *Physiologia Bohemoslovenica*, **23**, 373.

Schmidt, W., Müller, G., Weber, K. & Wilke, V. (1983). Method and apparatus for light-induced scanning-microscope display of specimen parameters and of their distribution. US patent 4 407 008; priority 08 10 80 DE, patented 27.09.83 US.

Sheppard, C. J. R. & Wilson, T. (1978). Depth of field in the scanning microscope. *Optics Letters*, **5**, 115–17.

Sheppard, C. J. R. & Wilson, T. (1979). Imaging properties of annular lenses. *Applied Optics*, **18**, 3764–9.

Sheppard, C. J. R. & Wilson, T. (1981). The theory of the direct-view confocal microscope. *Journal of Microscopy*, **124**, 107–17.

Slomba, A. F., Wasserman, D. E., Kaufman, G. I. & Nester, J. F. (1972). A laser flying spot scanner for use in automated fluorescence antibody instrumentation. *Journal of the Association for Advanced Medical Instrumentation*, **6**, 230–4.

Van der Voort, H. T. M., Valkenburg, J. A. C., Brakenhoff, G. J. & Nanninga, N. (1985). Design and use of a computer-controlled confocal microscope for biological applications. *Scanning*, **7**, 66–78.

Visser, T. D. & Brakenhoff, G. J. (1990). Absorption and scattering correction in confocal microscopy. *Transactions of the Royal Microscopical Society*, **1**, 223–6.

Visser, T. D., Oud, J. L. & Brakenhoff, G. J. (1992). Refractive index and axial distance measurements in 3-D microscopy. *Optik*, **90**, 17–19.

Watson, T. F. (1989). A confocal optical microscope study of the morphology of the tooth/restoration interface using Scotchbond-2 dentin adhesive. *Journal of Dental Research*, **68**, 1124–31.

Watson, T. F. (1990). The application of real-time confocal microscopy to the study of high-speed dental-bur tooth-cutting interactions. *Journal of Microscopy*, **157**, 51–60.

Webb, R. H. (1988). Double scanning optical apparatus and method. US patent 4,765,730; priority 17.09.85 US, patented 23.08.88.

Webb, R. H. & Wornson, D. P. (1989). Scanning optical apparatus and method. EP 307,185; priority 10.09.1987 US, published 15.03.1989 EP.

Weber, K. (1970). Device for optically scanning the object in a microscope. US patent 3,518,014; priority 10.08.66 DE, patented US 30.06.70.

White, J. G. (1987). Confocal scanning microscope. GB patent 2,184,321; priority 17.12.85 GB, published 17.6.87.

Wijnaendts van Resandt, R. W., Marsman, H. J. B., Kaplan, R., Davoust, J., Stelzer, E. H. K. & Stricker, R. (1985). Optical fluorescence microscopy in three dimensions: microtomoscopy. *Journal of Microscopy*, **138**, 29–34.

Williams, D. A. (1990). Quantitative intracellular calcium imaging with laser-scanning confocal microscopy. *Cell Calcium*, **11**, 589–97.

Wilson, T. & Sheppard, C. J. R. (1984). *Theory and Practice of Scannning Optical Microscopy*. London: Academic Press.

Xiao, G. Q. & Kino, G. S. (1987). A real-time confocal scanning optical microscope. *Proceedings of the Society of Photo-Optic Instrumentation Engineers*, **809**, 107–13.

Xiao, G. Q., Kino, G. S. & Masters, B. R. (1990). Observation of the rabbit cornea and lens with a new real-time confocal scanning optical microscope. *Scanning*, **12**, 161–66.

Young, J. Z. & Roberts, F. (1951) A flying-spot microscope. *Nature*, **167**, 231.

11

Transmission electron microscopy

F. GRACIA-NAVARRO, A. RUIZ-NAVARRO,
S. GARCÍA-NAVARRO and J. CASTAÑO

Introduction

Classical electron microscopic studies in histology provide qualitative descriptions of structural and ultrastructural features of cells and organelles. More recently, number, size, shape and position measurements, amongst others, have become essential in order to avoid subjective errors. Moreover quantitative approaches are necessary to assess changes in the ultrastructural features of cells under physiological and experimental conditions. Earlier quantitative studies involved the use of manual methods for determining morphological parameters (e.g. diameter, size) of such organelles as mitochondria, secretory granules, lysosomes, etc., methods which were time consuming and scarcely accurate or repeatable. Counting and measuring the size, shape and other similar properties of given objects in an image are all quite affordable by microcomputers, which can perform these tasks quite rapidly and reproducibly. However, computers cannot replace humans in recognizing objects, since this frequently involves examination of incomplete or unusual images, and is difficult to accomplish through computer software. On the other hand, computers are highly useful tools for measuring objects which have been previously identified by human operators, as is the case with electron microscopic image analysis, where the best results are achieved through an interactive process between the computer and operator. With manual methods, reproducibility tests on the same images typically reveal large variations between the results obtained by different observers or those measured by a single observer at different times. This is not the case with computer based measurements, which are subject only to statistical fluctuation patterns, so errors are predictable and, in many instances, controllable.

Image analysis has scarcely been used in electron microscopic studies. Below we describe a general procedure of varied uses in quantitative electron microscopy that is commonly employed at our laboratory to study cell organelles in various types of biological samples under physiological and experimental conditions.

Processing of electron microscopic images

Image analysis and measurement involve a number of steps in a sequence including image production, image acquisition, greyscale image processing, discrimination, image editing and measurement. While not all situations involve every one of these steps, each may be used to solve special problems.

Image production and acquisition

In most systems, image analysis is based on a discrimination process using greylevels. Because of the nature of electron microscopy, only monochrome images can be obtained in which different intensities are essentially the result of the contrast process, so high contrast images are required for ready recognition of cell organelles and image processing. Therefore, with few exceptions, osmium post-fixed material embedded in a hydrophobic resin such as araldite or Epon is to be preferred. The use of hydrophilic resins such as Lowycril or non-osmicated material should be limited to specific studies where preservation of antigenicity or of temperature-sensitive compounds is more important than image quality.

Once the material has been prepared for obtaining high quality images, an appropriate sampling procedure must be designed in order to obtain a representative number of images for measurement. A detailed description of different methods used for this purpose is given in Chapter 8.

The images observed under the electron microscope must be transferred to a computer for processing and quantification. This can be done by using photographic prints, negative films or by electronic means. Photographic prints are expensive and time consuming to use, but allow the quality of low grade images to be improved by darkroom processing. Negative films are cheaper to use than photographic prints but allow for no image improvement by themselves. Computer storage media (magnetic diskettes, portable hard disks, CD-ROMs, etc) are the least expensive alternative as they are re-usable; however, they require substantial investments in hardware, because the electron microscope must be fitted with a special video camera and monitor, both of which are usually expensive, and the computer must be interfaced to a system for storing the images. In any case, the storage methods should be selected according to specific needs and resources.

Stored images must be acquired by the computer in order to start the image analysis procedure proper. This can be done by using a video camera or by retrieving the required data from a storage medium, depending on the system used.

Greyscale image processing

Most currently available image analysis software converts the original greyscale image into an electronic image composed of a matrix of 512 × 512 pixels each of 256 greylevels. The brightness of each individual picture point can be changed depending on its original value and/or the values of neighbouring points or other points in the same or a different image. By using different electronic filters and convolutions, described in other chapters of this book, one can enhance the original image. The following process is recommended for electron microscopic images:

1 Shading correction. Electron microscopic images may pose two problems arising from illumination and the sample thickness and density. In many cases, the illumination provided is not uniform or strikes the object at an angle; also, the video camera or alternative device used to record the image may not provide a uniform response. In other cases, the problem arises from the sample itself: many specimens are not uniform in density or thickness as viewed under the electron microscope. The net result in both cases is a non-uniform recorded image that precludes direct determination of features from absolute brightness values. This problem can be addressed in a number of ways, of which the most expedient and straightforward is described: a control or background image is measured by acquiring an image from a reference greycard or the light source itself; subsequently, the sample image is corrected by subtracting the background image pixel by pixel or using the ratio between the two. A number of software packages include code for some type of shadow correction.

2 Inversion. Negative images should be turned into positive images for easier visual identification of cellular structures. This can be performed by virtually all software packages.

3 Contrast enhancement. One of the most interesting features of image analysis as applied to electron microscopy is the ability to enhance the contrast and brightness of the original images. The most common way of boosting image contrast involves thresholding of the greylevel histogram. This image operation, known as histogram stretching (Russ, 1990), samples the image in order to determine its lowest and highest greylevels, and then loads the lookup table of the image processor to convert each incoming greyvalue to a new value. This operation ensures maximum image contrast and hence the highest possible intensity resolution.

4 Image sharpening. Sharpening filters are used to accentuate high-frequency signals in the images such as those of colloidal gold particles in immunocytochemistry or membrane profiles in classical transmission electron microscopy. The overall appearance of an image after sharpening is very similar to that of the original, but small details stand out better, so that closed structures can be readily distinguished.

5 Image discrimination. A binary image is different from a greyscale image because each point in the former is either white or black. Greyscale images are usually converted to binary format by interactively selecting a range of greyvalues that correspond to the structures of interest which are then made white, whereas the remainder are turned into black. This

process can be performed automatically by selecting the maximum and minimum greylevels of a reference image.

6 Binary image processing. Binary images themselves may require further processing before they can be measured. There is a broad range of filters and convolution procedures available for smoothing outlines, isolating overlapping regions, etc. One of the chief aims here is to eliminate automatically the objects that are not to be measured, which can be done by implementing an erode-dilate procedure to remove small particles or the background. Even after automatic processing, the image may still included unwanted objects that must be removed interactively by the operator.

7 Measurement. At the final stage, measurements of either of two types of parameters (that is, object parameters such as areas, perimeters, diameters, etc., and field parameters such as numbers of objects, total area fraction in the image, etc) are made.

Fig. 1 illustrates the different steps of the general procedure: Fig. 1(a) shows the original image and Fig. 1(b) the result after shading correction, contrast enhancement and sharpening. Fig. 1(c) shows the binary image obtained on discrimination of the image in Fig. 1(b). Finally, Fig. 1(d) was obtained from Fig. 1(c) after an erode-dilate process.

Quantification of cell organelles

This section deals with the use of image analysis at the electron microscopic level for studying cell organelles under physiological and experimental conditions as a useful tool for solving biological problems related to histology.

Image analysis of chromatin patches in interphasic nuclei

Chromatin in mammalian cells reportedly undergoes condensation–decondensation cycles beyond mitosis (Mazia, 1963). Plant cells with high levels of DNA permanently display a nuclear phenotype characterized by large patches of dense chromatin that contain heterochromatin and variable amounts of temporally inactive chromatin. Transcriptional activity during the cell cycle can also be explained by the condensation–decondensation cycle of distinct chromosomal regions (de la Torre *et al.*, 1975; de la Torre & Navarrete, 1974). Because of those considerations, *Allium cepa* L. meristematic cells are specially suitable for studying changes in the condensation pattern of chromatin in relation to both the quiescence to proliferation shift and to interphase progression. Image analysis of electron microscopic photographs of cell nuclei has allowed examination of the condensation cycle of dense chromatin at the interphase of onion meristematic cells as well as the response to inhibition of protein synthesis (Guerrero *et al.*, 1992). For this purpose, meristems with

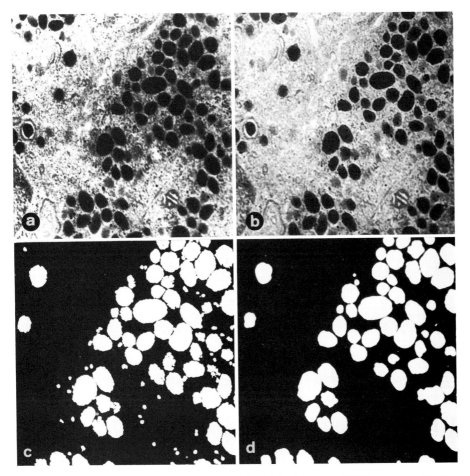

Fig. 1. Processing of a pituitary cell image. (*a*) Original image. (*b*) The same cell after shading correction, sharpening and contrast enhacement. (*c*) Discrimination of secretory granules. (*d*) Elimination of small objects by an erode-dilate process.

binucleate cells synchronized by the caffeine method (Gimenez-Martín *et al.*, 1965) were fixed with glutaraldehyde and post-fixed in osmium tetroxide at different times of the cell cycle. Also, root cultures in cycloheximide were fixed in order to study the effect of protein inhibition on the chromatin cycle. After dehydration, the roots were embedded in Epon. Finally, sections were stained with uranyl acetate and lead citrate according to the method of Reynolds (1962).

Electron microscopic photographs of binucleate cells were taken and subsequently analysed using an IBAS system (Kontron, Germany) to determine two stereological parameters for chromatin patches: volume and surface densities. Magnification of photographs was selected in order to include the complete nuclear profile in the photographic area. Nuclear chromatin was quantified by automatic image analysis of electron microscopic photographs or negatives. Image processing involved the following steps: shading correction, contrast enhancement, sharpening, interactive selection of nuclear area to be measured as reference area (Fig. 2(*a*)), discrimination – which had to be interactively selected by the operator owing to variations in image contrast (Fig. 2(*b*)) – and measurement of the following parameters: object area and perimeter, and reference area.

The results obtained showed the early G1 phase to be characterized by a transient period of rapid condensation of chromatin followed by a decondensation step that peaked at the G1 to S transition. The first half of the S period was characterized by further condensation of chromatin, dense chromatin being 1.7 times more abundant at mid-S phase than at the replication onset. The amount of dense chromatin increased sharply again in G2. Finally, condensation of chromatin appeared to be dependent on labile proteins since cycloheximide reversed it, whatever the cell position at the interphase (Guerrero *et al.*, 1992).

This type of study can be conducted not only to investigate the chromatin condensing cycle, but also to evaluate the effect of different natural, experimental or pathological situations on the chromatin phenotype of a given cell type. Thus, Komitowski & Zinser (1985) and Komitowski *et al.* (1986) used image analysis of chromatin to study the effect of toxic substances and the neoplastic process. Also, Komitowski *et al.* (1988) examined the effect of chronic low stress on the structure of chromatin in pituitary cells. Other parameters, such as the number and position of chromatin patches, could also be determined.

In the examples above, image analysis has proved clearly superior to manual methods, which do not allow the observation of small changes in chromatin structure (Panno & Nair, 1986).

Evaluation of nucleolar components

Nucleoli are major nuclear structures that reflect the activity and/or differentiation of each cell (Hernandez-Verdun, 1986). Conventional transmission electron microscopic techniques allow various nucleolar components, including fibrillar centres, the dense fibrillar component, the granular component, the nucleolar vacuoles or interstices and the nucleolar associated chromatin, to be observed in most cells (Goessens, 1984; Jordan, 1984; Risueño & Medina, 1986). These components can be used as morphological measures of nucleolar activity. Nucleolar organization in a specific cell type is given by the distribution, shape and size of the different nucleolar components: such organization is dynamic and varies with the physiological or experimental conditions. In 1989, Moreno *et al.* studied changes in nucleolar components under physiological conditions of proliferation and quiescence. For this purpose, they combined the use of a cytochemical technique to show the positions of the nucleolar organizer region, where ribosomal genes were located, with a morphological

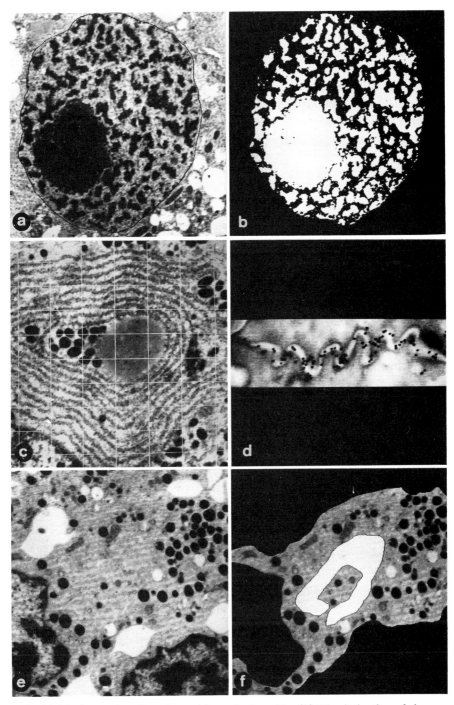

Fig. 2. (*a*) Meristematic cell nucleus with marked profile. (*b*) Discrimination of chromatin patches shown in (*a*). (*c*) Improved electronic image of endoplasmic reticulum with a grid superimposed. (*d*) Constant area frame selected to evaluate labeling density of membrane glycoproteins marked with colloidal gold conjugated lectin. (*e*) Improved electronic image of a pituitary cell. (*f*) Selection of cytoplasmic profile and Golgi-complex area to evaluate volume density of Golgi-complex.

quantitative study using electron microscopic image analysis. Nucleolar components were quantified stereologically on photographic plates of nucleoli that were randomly chosen from ultrathin silver-stained sections. Photographic magnification was selected to include the complete section area of the nucleolus covering most of the plate. The image processing procedure used was similar to that described for chromatin patches, with the sole exception that the nucleolar area was used as reference. The results showed that quiescent cells have a diminished nucleolar size compared to proliferating cells. However, the ratio of the silver-stained area to the nucleolar area (fibrillar component) remains constant under both physiological conditions (Moreno *et al.*, 1989).

Similar methods were used by Mirre & Knibiehler (1984), who investigated the potential relationship between the number and volume of fibrillar centres and the nucleolar organizer activity, as well as by Bessone & Seite (1985) who studied daily changes in nucleoli of supraoptic neurons. As with chromatin, the use of image analysis to quantify nucleolar components allows small changes that go undetected for classical techniques to be rapidly and effectively revealed.

Ultrastructural changes in the synthetic machinery

Endoplasmic reticulum and Golgi complex are cellular organelles involved in the biosynthetic process of the cell. In secretory cells, this biosynthetic machinery is well developed so quantitative study of these organelles is very important to understand changes or modifications in cell function (Alberts *et al.*, 1983).

The use of image analysis for quantifying the endoplasmic reticulum and Golgi complex is somewhat limited. While image processing can be used to enhance image quality, quantification of morphological and stereological parameters of organelles calls for manual methods. We have used this approach extensively to evaluate ultrastructural changes in amphibian pituitary cells under physiological and experimental conditions (Gracia-Navarro *et al.*, 1984, 1986, 1990, 1991; Malagón *et al.*, 1991*a*, *b*; Castaño *et al.*, 1992). Thus we obtained electron microscopic negatives of different pituitary cell types identified by colloidal gold immunocytochemistry. Photographs were taken at the lowest magnification that guarantees a high representative sample of the cytoplasm with enough resolution to identify cellular structures. Images were acquired by the computer by using a video camera and later processed by using the following procedures: image inversion, contrast enhancement and sharpening. We thereby obtained substantially improved images in terms of brightness and sharpness. At this point, for quantification of the rough endoplasmic reticulum, the computer superimposed a grid (Fig. 2(*c*)) designed to estimate volume and surface densities by using point counting methods (Weibel, 1979). Finally, the operator marked the points hitting the cisternae of the endoplasmic reticulum and the computer automatically calculated the stereological parameters.

For the Golgi complex, we used the same image processing procedure but the operator used a pointing device to bound both the cytoplasmic reference area and the Golgi complex area (Fig. 2(*e*) and (*f*)) that included dictiosomal cisternae and vesicles. Finally, the computer calculated the stereological parameters by using the area analysis method (Weibel, 1979).

We have used this methodology to assess changes in the biosynthetic machinery of pituitary gonadotrope and corticotrope cells subjected to environmental stressing conditions for different lengths of time (Gracia-Navarro *et al.*, 1984, 1986). The results obtained showed changes in the environmental conditions to cause hypertrophy of the biosynthetic machinery in both types of cells. In another set of experiments we used these techniques to evaluate the time course of changes in thyrotrope, prolactin, growth hormone, corticotrope and gonadotrope pituitary cells after stimulation with hypothalamic factors, both *in vivo* and *in vitro* (Gracia-Navarro *et al.*, 1990, 1991; Malagón *et al.*, 1991*a*, 1991*b*; Castaño *et al.*, 1992). The results revealed that stimulation with the hypothalamic factors occasionally induced hypertrophy of both the rough endoplasmic reticulum and the Golgi complex, even though the time course and intensity of the response depended on the secretagogue used and the cell type concerned. All the above studies have shown image analysis to be extremely useful for assessing development of biosynthetic machinery as an estimate for cell activity. Thus, even though methods for quantification of the endoplasmic reticulum and Golgi complex cannot be automated in full, image analysis provides more reproducible results which can be obtained more rapidly and economically. This type of study could equally be aimed at solving other histological problems related to biosynthetic cell activity or dynamic relations between organelles of the endomembrane system (Hidalgo *et al.*, 1992).

Image analysis of secretory granules and lysosomes

Secretory granules and lysosomes are cytoplasmic, vacuolated structures that contain secretory products and hydrolytic enzymes, respectively, so quantification of these organelles may provide interesting information on the secretory or lytic activity of cells (Alberts *et al.*, 1983).

These organelles appear as highly electron-dense bodies when stained using a classical technique, thus permitting virtually automatic processing of their images by greylevel discrimination. Secretory granules and lysosomes can be quantified on electron microscopic photographs or negatives. Magnification was selected to obtain a picture of a large part of the cytoplasmic area. For this purpose, the electronic image is subjected to the following steps: image inversion (when negative plates are used), shading correction (a critical step in as much as it facilitates automatic discrimination of these organelles), contrast enhancement and image sharpening, automatic discrimination, erode-dilate convolution, image editing to delete and/or select objects to be measured, and measurement of the object area and diameter and of two stereological parameters (volume and numerical densities). In estimating numerical density it is of the utmost importance to edit the image, in order to separate objects that appear fused after discrimination, by cutting along the overlapping profiles. One further problem may arise if the cell contains both secretory granules and lysosomes. In such a case, it is difficult to distinguish between the two types of organelle on the basis of greylevels alone, so measurements must be performed in a selecting mode where the operator marks the profiles corresponding to lysosomes or secretory granules with the aid of a pointing device. The computer is used to calculate the corresponding parameters for each type of object separately.

This method has been used to evaluate development of secretory granules in pituitary endocrine cells by calculating their volume and numerical densities as an indirect measure of secretory activity, as well as the amount of hormone remaining within the cells. This strategy has been employed to study the effect of hypothalamic factors on pituitary cell types (Gracia-Navarro *et al.*, 1984, 1986, 1990, 1991; Malagón *et al.*, 1991*a*, *b*; Castaño *et al.*, 1992). The results showed that different hypothalamic factors induce a diminution in secretory granule number of corresponding cells; the time course and intensity of response depend on the cell type and the secretagogue tested. At the time these experiments were carried out, radioimmunoassays for homologous amphibian hormones had not been developed, so quantitative histology was the only way of determining the direct effect of hypothalamic factors on amphibian pituitary cells. This method provides additional valuable information on ultrastructural changes in endocrine cells that is unaffordable by classical physiological methods.

Image analysis of colloidal gold probes

The use of gold probes in cytochemistry allows quantification of staining intensities, at the electron microscope level, as relative concentration measures of a given substance. When cytochemistry is used to localize small amounts of substances, measurement of staining intensities in different cellular compartments is necessary to distinguish specific labelling from the background. Size of the gold particles may interfere with specific and background staining in quantifying gold probes; however, this is outside the scope of this book and the reader is referred to a paper by Gu & D'Andrea (1989) for further information. On the other hand, labelling efficiency is dependent on 3-D particle distribution (Posthuma *et al.*, 1987); in fact, differential penetration of gold probes into non-embedded sections results in differences in labelling efficiency between various cell structures, and labelling densities can be used to evaluate changes only within a given organelle (Slot *et al.*, 1989). On the other hand, gold particles do not penetrate the whole tissue thickness in embedded sections

(Bendayan & Zollinger, 1983), so this method prevents the variable dependent on 3-D particle distribution.

Image analysis is very useful for quantifying labelling intensity in the electron microscope when colloidal gold probes are used. Image processing in this case involves the following steps: image acquisition, inversion (if necessary), sharpening, interactive drawing of labelled organelles (Plate 4(a)) discrimination of colloidal gold particles and estimation of gold particle density per organelle section area. This requires using low contrast images, which do not interfere with the black colour of the gold particles, since very bright images usually hinder measurement of gold particles. A representative sample of organelles at high magnification must be obtained to facilitate the analysis of colloidal gold particles. As for secretory granules and lysosomes, fused gold particles must be separated interactively by the operator. This can be facilitated by having the computer assign an arbitrary colour to each isolated object (Plate 4(b)), after which the fused particles can be readily identified because they are all of the same colour. This methodology has been used to quantify pancreatic enzymes localized by immunocytochemistry (Posthuma *et al.*, 1986); GnRH-binding sites detected by avidin–gold in rat pituitary cells (Childs *et al.*, 1989), and to study relative gonadotrope hormone storage in secretory granules of amphibian pituitary that were doubly immunostained for both gonadotropins (Gracia–Navarro & Licht, 1987).

One possible application of this methodology is in measuring the amount of a specific protein in the plasma membrane: the protein is marked immunocytochemically or by lectin cytochemistry with colloidal gold. For this purpose, after the image has been processed, the operator places a rectangular frame of constant area with the longer side parallel to the plasma membrane profile (Fig. 2(*d*)) and then the computer calculates the gold density in relation to this area as an estimate for the labelling density (Navas *et al.*, 1987; Villalba & Navas, 1989).

Hardware and software

A host of software packages for general image analysis is currently available. All of them can be used to assess electron microscopic images. Examples of such packages include: Fenestra, from Kinetic Imaging Ltd. (UK); Aequitas, from Dynamic Data Links (UK); JAVA, from Jandel Scientific (Germany); PC—Image, from Foster Findlay Associates Limited (UK); Visilog 4, from Noesis SA (France); and MCDI M1 and M2, from Imaging Research Inc. (Canada). Although this commercially available software is usually very powerful and includes real-colour image analysis, monochrome versions (if available) are more than adequate for the purpose; also, a fairly small number of functions is enough for electron microscopic image analysis. The minimum hardware requirements for performing image analysis are a personal computer equipped with a 286, 386 or 486 microprocessor, 2 MBytes or more of RAM memory and a VGA colour display. The computer must have enough space and electric power to support a video digitizing board connected to the video source (usually a camera). A standard video monitor in addition to the computer monitor is also necessary for displaying the video image. Finally, a pointing device (a mouse or a digitizing tablet) is required to control cursor movement. The particular system requirements (amount of expanded memory, type of graphic adapter and video digitizing board, etc.) depend on the software to be run. One other possibility is to develop one's own software to solve specific problems (Nysen *et al.*, 1982; Peachey, 1982; Silage & Gil, 1984; Russ & Russ, 1984). SIVA, the computer research group of the University of Cordoba, have developed the program IMAGO for general image analysis which meets most of the requirements for analysing electron microscopic images. Most of the work reported in the present review has been carried out using this program.

Acknowledgements

We wish to acknowledge Dr J. M. Villalba for the lectin membrane marked Figure. Financial supported from the Spanish Junta de Andalucia (Group 3087) and Dirección General de Investigación Científica y Técnica (Project no PB91-0844) is gratefully acknowledged by the authors.

References

Alberts, B., Bray, D., Lewis, J., Raff, M., Roberts, K. & Watson, J. D. (1983). *Molecular Biology of the Cell*. New York: Garland Publishing Inc.

Bendayan, M. & Zollinger, M. (1983). Ultrastructural localization of antigenic sites on osmium-fixed tissue applying the protein A-gold technique. *Journal of Histochemistry and Cytochemistry*, **31**, 101–9.

Bessone, R. & Seite, R. (1985). Daily fluctuations of nucleoli in neurosecretory cells of the rat supraoptic nucleus. An ultrastructural and stereological study. *Cell and Tissue Research*, **240**, 393–6.

Castaño, J.-P., Ramirez, J.-L., Malagón, M. M. & Gracia-Navarro, F. (1992). Differential response of amphibian PRL and TSH pituitary cells to *in vitro* TRH treatment. *General and Comparative Endocrinology*, **88**, 178–87.

Childs, G. V., Yamauchi, K. & Unabia, G. (1989). Localization and quantification of hormones, ligands, and mRNA with affinity-gold probes. *American Journal of Anatatomy*, **185**, 223–35.

De La Torre, C., Sacristán-Gárate, A. & Navarrete, M. H. (1975). Structural changes in chromatin during interphase. *Chromosoma*, **51**, 183–98.

De La Torre, C. & Navarrete, M. H. (1974). Estimation of chromatin patterns at G1, S and G2 of the cell cycle. *Experimental Cell Research*, **88**, 171–4.

Gimenez-Martín, G., González-Fernández, A. & López-Sáez, J. F. (1965). A new method of labelling cells. *Journal of Cell Biology*, **26**, 305–9.

Goessens, G. (1984). Nucleolar structure. *International Reviews of Cytology*, **87**, 107–58.

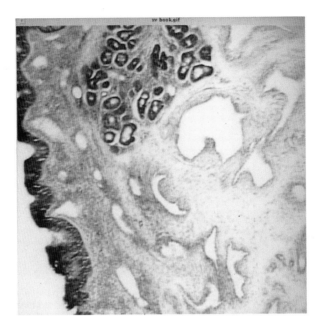

Plate 1. A 512 × 512 pixel,16-bit colour image of a (10μm) section of nasal mucosa. The tissue was stained with haematoxylin and eosin.

(a)

(b)

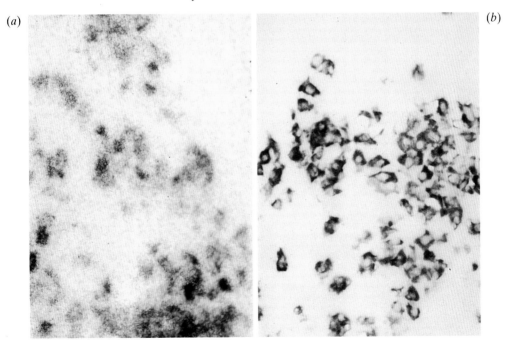

Plate 2. *In situ* hybridization to detect mRNA for thyroid-stimulating hormone in rat pituitary using radioactive and non-radioactive probes. A strong signal is seen in thyrotrophs with both labels: (a) ^{32}P detected by autoradiography, (b) digoxigenin detected by alkaline phosphatase conjugated antibody. The staining with the enzyme label is clearer and less diffuse than the autoradiograph, but the technique is less sensitive.

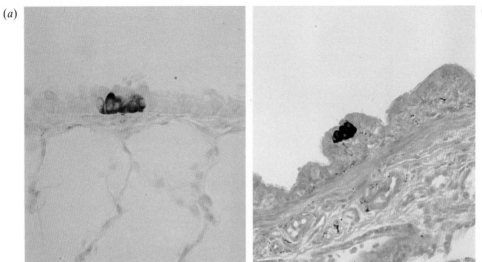

(a)

(b)

Plate 3. Immunostaining of the vasodilator peptide calcitonin gene-related peptide in bronchiolar epithelial endocrine cells of rat lung. Sections stained by (a) the avidin-biotin complex method with peroxidase label and (b) the indirect immunogold method with silver enhancement.

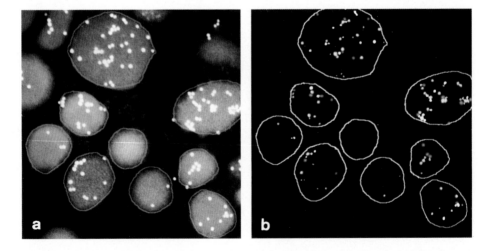

Plate 4. Electronic images of colloidal gold immunostained secretory granules. (a) Negative image of secretory granules, the profiles of which are marked in green. (b) After discrimination of colloidal gold particles, and arbitrary colour is assigned by the computer to each discrete particle.

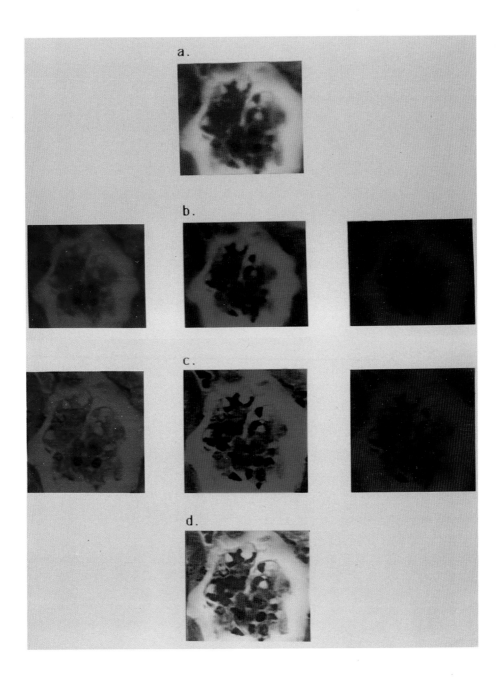

Plate 5. True colour deconvolution: low power transmitted light images of a kidney glomerulus stained with Masson stain. Oil objective (x40, NA 1.0), image width 85 μm, z-slice interval 0.5μm. Three original 24-bit RGB images were taken and resolved into three triplets of red, green and blue images. These were used with the NNA to produce three focussed red, green, and blue images which were then recombined to make the final composite focussed image (*d*). (*a*) The original RGB image of the central slice.

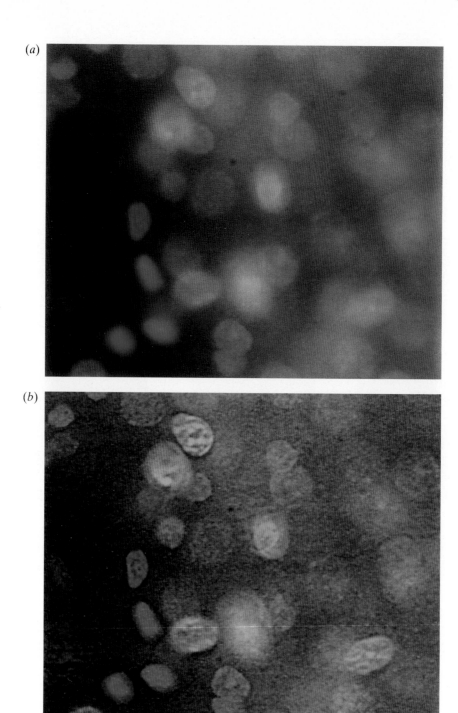

(a)

(b)

Plate 6. Mouse hippocampus stained with Hoescht and ethidium bromide.
Epifluorescence data obtained with a monochrome camera and interference filters for the
emission frequencies of the two dyes. Oil objective (x40, NA 1.0), z-interval 0.5μm.
(*a*) Before and (*b*) after deconvolution with 90% haze removal.

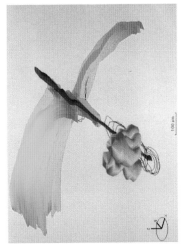

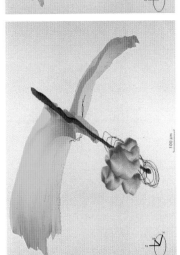

Plate 7. Stereo pair showing surface rendering of the spread of orf virus down a hair follicle on ovine skin. The orf virus (orange) is shown partially cut away to reveal the hair shaft (purple) in the hair follicle (blue outline only) and the lobes of the sebaceous glands (green). Image created with MacStereology software.

(a)

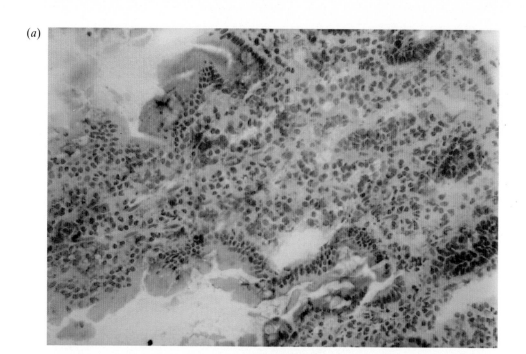

(b)

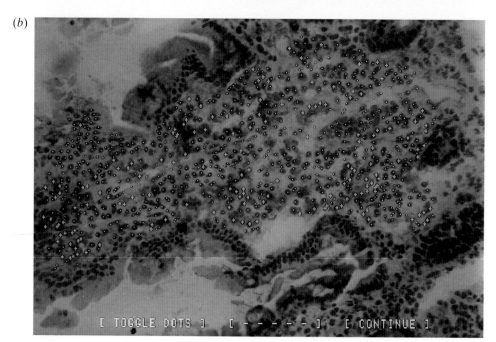

[TOGGLE DOTS]   [- - - - -]   [CONTINUE]

Plate 8. (*a*) Intestinal lymph tissue stained for CD3 lymphocytes. (*b*) A frame was drawn free hand around a region of the image. Within this area, cells have been counted positive (crosses superimposed) or negative (dots superimposed) on the basis of the intensity of local cytoplasmic labelling. Cells are located using pattern recognition techniques.

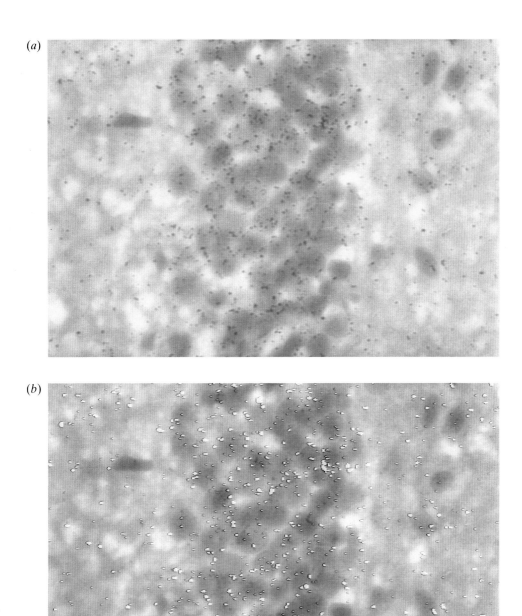

Plate 9. (*a*) Rat dentate gyrus labelled autoradigraphically using a cRNA antisense probe complementary to rat GR. (*b*) Yellow marks show detection of silver halide grains.

Gracia-Navarro, F. & Licht, P. (1987). Subcellular localization of gonadotrophic hormones LH and FSH in frog adenohypophysis using double-staining immunocytochemistry. *Journal of Histochemistry and Cytochemistry*, **35**, 763–69.

Gracia-Navarro, F., Castaño, J.-P., Malagón, M. M. & Torronteras, R. (1991). Subcellular responsiveness of amphibian growth hormone cells after TSH-releasing hormone stimulation. *General and Comparative Endocrinology*, **84**, 94–103.

Gracia-Navarro, F., García-Navarro, S. & García-Herdugo, G. (1986). A morphometric study of subcellular responses in frog pituitary corticotropic cells to constant environmental conditions. *Biology of the Cell*, **57**, 153–60.

Gracia-Navarro, F., Porter, D., Malagón, M. M. & Licht, P. (1990). Stereological study of gonadotropes in the frog, *Rana pipiens*, after GnRH stimulation in vitro. *Cell and Tissue Research*, **262**, 171–6.

Gracia-Navarro, F., González-Reyes, J. A., García-Navarro, S. & García-Herdugo, G. (1984). Subcellular responses in frog pituitary gonadotrophic cells to constant environmental conditions: a morphometric study. *Biology of the Cell*, **51**, 87–96.

Gu, J. & D'Andrea, M. (1989). Comparison of detecting sensitivities of different sizes of gold particles with electron-microscopic immunogold staining using atrial natriuretic peptide in rat atria as a model. *American Journal of Anatatomy*, **185**, 264–70.

Guerrero, F., De La Torre, C., Gracia, F. & García-Herdugo, G. (1992). Condensation of chromatin in the interphase of meristem cells depends on labile proteins. *Cytobios*, **71**, 141–9.

Hernandez-Verdun, D. (1986). Structural organization of the nucleolus in mammalian cells. *Methods and Achievements in Experimental Pathology*, **12**, 26–62.

Hidalgo, J., Garcia-Navarro, R., Gracia-Navarro, F., Perez-Vilar, J. & Velasco, A. (1992). Presence of Golgi remmant in the cytoplasm of Brefeldin A-treated cells. *European Journal of Cell Biology*, **58**, 214–27.

Jordan, E. G. (1984). Nucleolar nomenclature. *Journal of Cell Science*, **67**, 217–20.

Komitowski, D. & Zinser, G. (1985). Quantitative description of chromatin structure during neoplasia by the method of image processing. *Analytical and Quantitative Cytology and Histology*, **7**, 178–82.

Komitowski, D., Muto, S., Weiss, J., Schmitt, B. & Taylor, G. T. (1988). Structural changes in nuclear chromatin in rat pituitary after chronic stress of low intensity. *Anatomical Record*, **220**, 125–31.

Komitowski, D., Schmezer, P., Schmitt, B. & Muto, S. (1986). Image analysis of hepatocyte nuclei in assessing Di(2-ethylhexyl)phthalate effects eluding detection by conventional microscopy. *Toxicology*, **41**, 11–19.

Malagón, M. M., Castaño, J. P., Dobado-Berrios, P. M., García-Navarro, S. & Gracia-Navarro, F. (1991*a*). Human pancreatic growth hormone-releasing factor (1–44) stimulates GH cells in an anuran amphibian (Rana perezi). *General and Comparative Endocrinology*, **84**, 461–9.

Malagón, M. M., Ruiz-Navarro, A., Torronteras, R. & Gracia-Navarro, F. (1991*b*). Effects of ovine CRF on amphibian pituitary ACTH and TSH cells *in vivo*: a quantitative ultrastructural study. *General and Comparative Endocrinology*, **83**, 487–97.

Mazia, D. (1963). Synthetic activities leading to mitosis. *Journal of Cell Comparative Physiology*, **62**, 123–40.

Mirre, C. & Knibiehler, B. (1984). Quantitative ultrastructural analysis of fibrillar centers in the mouse: correlation of their number and volume with nucleolar organizers-activity. *Protoplasma*, **121**, 120–8.

Moreno, F. J., Rodrigo, R. M., Gracia-Navarro, F. & García-Herdugo, G. (1989). Nucleolar component behaviour in plant cells under different physiological conditions. A morphological, cytochemical and quantitative study. *Biology of the Cell*, **65**, 67–74.

Navas, P., Villalba, J. M., Buron, M. I. & García-Herdugo, G. (1987). Lectins as markers for plasma membrane differentiation of amphibian keratinocytes. *Biology of the Cell*, **60**, 225–34.

Nysen, M., Cornelis, A., Maes, L. & De Zanger, R. (1982). A system to acquire and process scanning transmission electron microscopic images. *Ultramicroscopy*, **8**, 429–36.

Panno, J. P. & Nair, K. K. (1986). Effects of increased lifespan on chromatin condensation in the adult male housefly. *Mechanisms of Ageing and Development*, **35**, 31–8.

Peachey, L. D. (1982). A simple digital morphometry system for electron microscopy. *Ultramicroscopy*, **8**, 253–62.

Posthuma, G., Slot, J. W. & Geuze, H. J. (1986). A quantitative immunoelectron microscopic study of amylase and chymotrypsin in peri- and tele-insular cells of the rat exocrine pancreas. *Journal of Histochemistry and Cytochemistry*, **34**, 203–7.

Posthuma, G., Slot, J. W. & Geuze, H. J. (1987). Usefulness of the immunogold technique in quantitation of a soluble protein in ultra-thin sections. *Journal of Histochemistry and Cytochemistry*, **35**, 405–10.

Reynolds, E. S. (1962). The use of lead citrate at high pH as an electron opaque stain in electron microscopy. *Journal of Cell Biology*, **17**, 208.

Risueño, M. C. & Medina, F. J. (1986). The nucleolar structure in plant cells. *Cell Biology Reviews*, **7**, 1–140.

Russ, J. C. (1990). *Computer-Assisted Microscopy. The Measurement and Analysis of Images*. New York: Plenum Press.

Russ, J. C. & Russ, J. C. (1984). Image processing in a general purpose microcomputer. *Journal of Microscopy*, **135**, 89–102.

Silage, D. A. & Gil, J. (1984). Methods in laboratory investigation. Digital reversal and enhancement of negatives in video-based interactive morphometry. *Laboratory Investigation*, **51**, 112–6.

Slot, J. W., Posthuma, G., Ghang, L. Y., Crapo, J. D. & Geuze, H.J. (1989). Quantitative aspects of immunogold labeling in embedded and in nonembedded sections. *American Journal of Anatomy*, **185**, 271–81.

Villalba, J. M. & Navas, P. (1989). Polarization of plasma membrane glycocojugates in amphibian epidermis during metamorphosis. *Histochemistry*, **90**, 453–8.

Weibel, E. R. (1979). *Stereological Methods*, Vol. 1 *Practical Methods for Biological Morphometry*. London: Academic Press.

12

Television cameras and scanners

P. M. GAFFNEY

Introduction

Television cameras and scanners have been used to advantage both qualitatively and quantitatively in conjunction with optical microscopy. They have proved invaluable as teaching aids and video enhanced microscopy has found widespread acceptance. Most modern cameras will perform adequately for qualitative applications and they are straightforward to use. However, despite substantial improvements in technology in recent years, many television (TV) cameras are unsuitable for quantitative image analysis. The high standards of performance required across a broad range of characteristics are not necessary for most commercial uses to which cameras are put, so that great care must be exercised in making a selection for a particular experiment. Published specifications often fall short of providing adequate information from which to make judgement and often empirical measurement of performance against standards is necessary. In this Chapter, I will introduce the available camera and scanner technologies and will focus on the practical application of these tools to biological image analysis. Particular consideration will be given to errors introduced into measurement as a consequence of technological limitations.

Brief history

The advent of the vidicon camera in 1950 paved the way for the introduction of closed circuit TV into education, medicine and industrial inspection (Zworykin *et al.*, 1958). Video microscopy permitted observation over an extended spectral range, from infra-red, through visible wavelengths, to ultraviolet. A limited amount of contrast enhancement was possible, and the early cameras found widespread acceptance in teaching. In parallel with the utilization of tube camera technology, flying spot scanners were introduced to microscopy. The flying spot scanner was developed principally for the conversion of cine film to video. In 1951 Young & Roberts demonstrated that a sensitivity improvement of two orders of magnitude relative to the photographic film of the day was possible. Image intensifiers were developed and applied to low light microscopy in the early 1960s (Reynolds, 1964; Eckert & Reynolds, 1967; Reynolds, 1972). Improvements in sensitivity to light, achieved through continuous development of the image intensifier for military use as an aid to night vision, made fluorescent microscopy possible. The use of solid state photosensors began in the 1960s and the demonstration of the first charge coupled device (CCD) cameras in 1969 were major milestones. Both the resolution and signal-to-noise performance were steadily improved thereafter. In addition, specialist cameras, such as the cooled and integrating types, have extended observation to extremely low light levels. Stability has improved to the point at which optical densitometry can be performed by cameras to the same standard as flatbed scanning microdensitometers. In the 1980s CCD camera development followed two main paths: medium resolution (less than 1500×1500 pixels) monochrome and panchromatic 2-D arrays were developed for use in conventional TV cameras. In addition, high resolution (more than 5000 pixels) linear arrays were developed for use in scanners, e.g. facsimile machines and document scanners.

Video generation and errors

A vacuum tube video camera generates a voltage signal by sweeping an electron beam across a photoconductive or photoresistive surface onto which is focussed an optical image. A solid state camera generates the signal by reading out the charge stored at fixed locations on a semiconductor array onto which an image is focussed. At each point in the scan, the voltage produced is proportional to the intensity of illumination falling onto that point. The camera scans the top line of the image sequentially across the screen and then moves down to the next line. This is repeated until the bottom line of the image is scanned, whereupon the whole process restarts. Timing information defining the position within the scan is added to the analogue voltage produced by the sensor to form a composite video signal which is suitable for display on a monitor or as an input for an image analysis system. However, no TV camera is capable of converting the optical image into an exact electrical analogue. The reason for diversity in cameras and scanning devices is that no single technology so far developed has proved capable of performing well in all applications. It remains necessary to match the characteristics of the camera to the conditions under which it is to be used.

The electronic representation of an image

A more detailed understanding of the process of converting an optical image into an electrical signal will aid appraisal of the practical limitations which directly impinge on measurement accuracy and experimental design. Errors in conversion occur both in the reproduction of illumination levels and in the spatial accuracy within the array. Consider first the problems related to reproducing electronically a light intensity at a remote observation point. Only three components are required, a photoelectric sensor, an amplifier and a display device capable of turning an electrical input signal into a proportional light output. Even in a system as simple as this the accuracy with which the output light intensity matches the input intensity is determined by several factors.

An ideal light sensor, when completely covered, should always output the same noise-free voltage. This voltage should increase in a linear fashion with increasing illumination. In practice, all light sensors deviate from this ideal. Their output will be influenced by temperature, noise, past exposure to light and ageing effects. The linearity may deviate from the ideal, most noticeably at low and high levels of illumination. At some maximum illumination, the sensor will enter saturation, where a further increase in illumination will not generate a further increase in voltage. The rate of change of output voltage with respect to the rate of change of light intensity will also be constrained by a maximum value, above which linear proportionality will fail.

The output of an ideal amplifier would be related to the input by a fixed and determined gain. In practice, the gain varies with the rate of change and amplitude of the input signal and with temperature. As with the sensor, a saturation level will be reached above which further increase in input voltage will not cause a proportional change in output. A variable offset voltage dependent on temperature will be added to the output signal. The amplifier will add certain noise to the signal, further degrading the output.

The display device can also suffer from most of these defects, although because its output is viewed by imperfect human eyes, its performance is much less critical. In quantitative studies, it would be replaced by the analogue-to-digital converter in the imaging system and would be separately characterized. By using an array of sensors each capable of reproducing the intensity of a point source it is possible to build up an image of a 2-D scene. If a lens (microscope) is used to focus an optical image onto an array of 10 × 10 sensors such that each conveys only the light intensity falling on it to the corresponding display device, a low resolution picture depicting the scene would be produced. Each sensor in the array will be subject to the limitations described already. In addition, no matter how good the production techniques, it will not be possible to make each sensor exactly the same. This spread in characteristics will produce a shading in the image causing the greylevel to be measured differently according to where in the picture the intensity is measured.

To be useful many more sensors are required to produce a picture which will do justice to the image formed by a modern microscope. A 35 mm slide has the equivalent resolution of an array of 4000 × 3000 picture elements (pixels). Only very high quality scanners and cameras are capable of this resolution, it being more usual to work at an array size of less than 1000 × 1000. It is clearly

impractical to expand this simple TV model by increasing the number of
sensors and amplifiers. Microscopes usually produce a small projected image,
typically under 18 mm across. The sensors must therefore be very small,
making the task of individually connecting them to amplifiers and display
devices impractical. (This has been done in the past with special purpose
sensors for very high speed imaging but is not of general applicability.) An
alternative approach is therefore required to the parallel array. Almost all
modern TV systems sample each sensor sequentially. This works because the
human eye exhibits a phenomenon known as persistence of vision, namely, that
the brain perceives light for a short period after a visual stimulus has ceased. A
human observer is not able to detect light modulation at a frequency in excess
of 50 Hz. If the entire image is scanned in less than 1/50th of a second the
image will appear to be displayed continuously as though it were from a
parallel system. Although there are now no technical difficulties associated
with operating at speeds well in excess of those at which flicker would be
noticeable, almost all TV cameras and broadcast systems operate at speeds
where some flicker is present.

Scanning and synchronisation

Sequential scanning of the photosensitive surface introduces yet further sources
of variability and inaccuracy into video derived measurements. In order to
produce an image on the remote display array, it is essential that there is a
means of ensuring that the intensity being sampled by a sensor in the array is
being displayed by the corresponding display element. By convention, the
array is scanned from the top left to the bottom right, the complete scan being
called a raster. To maintain synchronization between the scanning of the
sensors and the display, synchronizing or sync pulses are added to the signal
representing change in intensity. Two pulses are generally used, one to signify
the start of a horizontal scan, and one to signal the start of a vertical scan. They
are respectively termed line sync and field sync. Timing information between
horizontal sync pulses is not usually transmitted, reliance being made on linear
interpolation between the pulses. The stability of timing in the camera and the
accuracy of synchronization are therefore critical, since any drift or non-
linearity will cause errors in both linear measurement and intensity measurement. Good design will minimize these errors, but it will not usually be
possible to determine this from manufacturers' data sheets. If high accuracy is
required, it is essential that the camera be calibrated against traceable
standards with calibrated test equipment. In all cameras accuracy of synchronization timing will, to some extent, be temperature dependent and care should
be taken to ensure that as far as possible the camera is always allowed to reach
normal operating temperature before being used for measurement. This can
often take 30 minutes after switching it on.

Performance of video cameras

Resolution

Spatial resolution is a measure of the ability of a camera to resolve fine detail. It is determined by the properties of the photosensor, for example the number of pixels, the processing electronics and the connections to the imaging system. The overall performance will only be as good as the weakest element. In order to have a means of comparing cameras that have different-sized sensors, spatial resolution is normally expressed as the total number of black and white lines that can be resolved over a distance equal to the height of the active picture area. By imaging a series of successively finer lines, a point will be reached where the individual black and white lines become indistinguishable. Many cameras do not have identical spatial resolution in vertical and horizontal directions. Consequently, it is usual to define horizontal and vertical resolution separately. By convention, the horizontal resolution is measured in a central zone of the picture over a width equivalent to the height of the active picture area. The vertical resolution is measured through the centre of the picture for the active height of the picture. In tube cameras, resolution decreases towards the edges and corners of the picture. Spatial resolution is highly subjective and unless the conditions of measurement are precisely defined will be of limited value in comparing cameras. A more useful indication is given when spatial resolution is referenced to the generation of an image with adequate reproduction of contrast. As finer black and white lines are imaged, the electrical signal they produce will decrease from 100% modulation. A camera which shows discernible lines at 600 per screen height (from the data sheet) is likely only to be able to resolve 250 black and white lines for accurate intensity measurement. The same camera would have useful resolution at up to 350 lines when used for morphometry. Dependent on the noise levels and sensor design, point counting could be performed almost to the stated resolution of the camera.

One of the major advantages of camera technology compared to scanners is that it is possible to change the actual sample space that is scanned by each TV line by altering the optical magnification. Therefore, with a usable resolution of 350 black and white lines for morphometry the sample resolution will be 286 μm for an image 100 mm across or 2.86 μm for an image 1 mm across. The corresponding limiting resolutions for optical density measurement would be 400 μm and 4 μm. These resolutions should be achievable with a good quality camera.

Contrast

The ability of a camera to distinguish contrast is also dependent on the size of the object. Sensitivity is high for objects that cover a large part of the sensor, but decreases as objects cover smaller areas. If nine squares of a black and white chequer board were to be projected onto the entire area of the sensor and the resulting video signal assigned a value of 100% modulation, it would be found that if the magnification were to be reduced such that more squares were visible, the greylevel difference value would decrease. The white squares would appear darker and the black squares lighter. Consequently, the accuracy of densitometric measurements would decrease as objects become smaller relative to the scanned area. An optical magnification should be selected to ensure that any image features to be measured cover at least four pixels on a good quality camera. The modulation transfer function (MTF) of a camera relates the modulation of the output signal to the incoming signal at various frequencies. For example, if a sinusoidal signal with an amplitude modulation of 60% is input to a piece of video equipment and is output with an amplitude modulation of 20%, the modulation transfer ratio is $20/60 = 33\%$. The transfer ratio varies as a function of frequency. When two or more pieces of video equipment are cascaded the overall modulation transfer ratio is the product of the individual MTFs.

Linearity and dynamic range

In the simple model presented for reproducing a given illumination level through the use of a sensor, an amplifier and a display device, it was stated that an ideal sensor would give a linear increase in output for a corresponding increase in illumination. Below the dark threshold of the sensor, low levels of light will not produce measurable output. Above saturation level of the sensor, a further increase in illumination will not give rise to an increase in signal level. The difference in response between the dark threshold and the saturation threshold represents the dynamic range of the sensor.

Optical density (O) is defined as:

$$O = -\log_{10}(L_\mathrm{t}/L_\mathrm{i}),$$

where L_t is the transmitted light and
L_i is the incident light (Fig. 1).

High quality video cameras may be used to measure optical densities within the range 0 to 2.1, typically. Linescan cameras, cooled solid state cameras, and slow rate scanners can yield up to two orders of magnitude greater dynamic range.

The relationship between incident illumination and signal output is:

$$I = K L^\gamma,$$

where I is the signal current,
K is a constant,
L is the level of illumination and
γ is a constant, known as the gamma ratio.

For a linear transfer characteristic, the constant (gamma) will be 1. Many

(a)

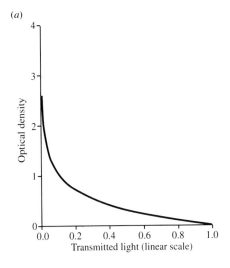

(a)

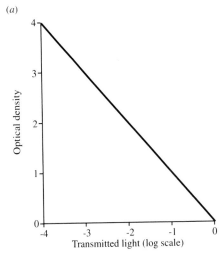

Fig. 1. Optical density and its relation to transmitted light on (*a*) linear and (*b*) logarithmic scales.

cameras will be supplied with gamma set to 0.65 or an arbitrary value. The phosphors available for use in early monitors did not have a linear output characteristic. The camera gamma was selected so that the overall gamma of the system appeared to be unity. For optical density studies, it is essential that the camera be correctly set for unity gamma. Newvicon tubes, Chalnicon tubes and solid state sensors all have an intrinsic gamma of 1. However, the cameras into which they are fitted may modify the apparent gamma through the use of non-linear amplifiers. If the pedigree of a camera is not known absolutely it should not be used for optical density work unless facilities exist for full characterization against known optical standards.

Signal-to-noise ratio

A camera viewing a uniformly illuminated scene will not output a single video level, but will produce a series of values distributed about a mean. The scatter about the mean is determined both by the type of sensor and by the conditions of operation. The level of noise will determine the accuracy to which objects of interest may be separated from their background using greylevel thresholding techniques. The sensor-related noise will be considered when each type of camera is treated in turn. Generally, good quality cameras will offer a signal-to-noise ratio (SNR) of 45–60 dB for an individual pixel. The SNR has improved substantially with each new model of camera released to the market. This improvement, together with improvements in linearity and dynamic range warrant consideration of upgrading all cameras more than two years old in any but the least demanding applications. The overall measurement accuracy of an imaging system is determined by the weakest component. There is no point in investing in a high performance imaging system if the camera produces images of poor contrast and high noise.

Using video cameras in biological experiments

So far, the limitations inherent in all types of image sensor have been described. In addition, there are further error mechanisms specific to particular types of sensor. As most available cameras have some advantages, it is necessary to put the errors into perspective.

There is no single camera technology which is better in all applications. It is not possible to predict all possible uses to which a camera may be put. In the following examples, many types of imaging problem have been classified generically and appropriate camera technologies suggested. There will be occasions when these general rules do not apply. In these cases it is likely that extensive qualification will need to be performed.

Coupling the camera to the microscope

Although many investigations will be performed using a macro viewer, the majority of images will be collected through a microscope. Regardless of the camera technology adopted, it will be necessary to interface the camera to the microscope. As this problem is common to most applications, the problems involved will be considered before specific examples.

The microscope image can be projected by the ocular lenses directly onto the photosensitive surface of the camera. An alternative is to use a special camera lens focussed to infinity to produce a focussed image on the camera target. It is generally preferable to minimize the amount of glass in the optical path and the first method will usually give better results.

Most monochrome cameras and single CCD colour cameras have a standard 'C' mount. This is a female, one-inch fine thread that will mate with a range of microscope adaptors for all common microscopes. Specialist companies will produce custom adaptors for older or less common microscopes. Depending on the microscope, the adaptor will either be a simple connecting tube or will contain one or more lenses. Particularly for fluorescence work, where the available light is restricted, better results will be obtained with straight-through adaptors. Some three chip colour cameras require the use of proprietary bayonet adaptors which will often require the use of additional lenses. These adaptors are almost always specific to a particular model of microscope and camera and will frequently be available from the camera manufacturer. The trend is towards standardization on the 'C' mount, and it is likely that the expensive variants will become less common. Adaptors are available for most camera formats.

The diagonal dimension of the solid state array used in modern cameras is likely to be $\frac{2}{3}''$, $\frac{1}{2}''$ or $\frac{1}{3}''$. The $\frac{2}{3}''$ sensor has been the most common device offering good resolution. With improving technology, the $\frac{1}{2}''$ and $\frac{1}{3}''$ sensors are gaining popularity. A different adaptor is required for each format to ensure that the size of the focussed image matches the scanned area of the sensor. It is usually the case that the image displayed from a TV system will cover a smaller field of view than that observed in the microscope eyepieces. If this is likely to be a nuisance, care should be exercised in selecting the appropriate adaptor.

It is essential that there be good electrical continuity between the 'C' mount thread of the camera and the body of the microscope. A problem occurs where poor connection results from oxide build up on some 'C' mount adaptors or from a film of oil. The typical symptom will be random interference on the televised picture, often observed as sloping bright lines drifting through the picture. In extreme cases if this cannot be cured by cleaning, a separate earth wire should be run from the camera to the microscope body.

It is essential when using CCD cameras with microscopes to ensure that illumination at unwanted wavelengths is prevented from reaching the sensor. In particular, most cameras will respond to infra-red illumination unless they contain internal filters. Because the tungsten light source used in most microscopes emits significant energy in the infra-red spectrum, a strong image will be produced by the camera in addition to that produced by visible wavelengths. This will lead to serious degradation of the image. The centre of the screen will appear brighter than the edges as a result of the different focus of the condenser for infra-red illumination. The image will have less contrast, because differently stained tissues will often have similar transmissivity to infra-red and lastly, a sharp focus will be impossible to obtain as a result of mixing of images of substantially different wavelengths. An infra-red cutoff filter should be placed in the optical path as close to the camera faceplate as is practical. In many microscopes it will be possible to fit a suitable filter above the 'C' mount adaptor. The penalty for using a strong infra-red cutoff filter is reduced sensitivity to the wanted wavelengths. However, the improvement in image quality is usually spectacular if adequate light is available.

Matching the camera to the experiment

Point counting

When attempting to count point objects such as silver grains or colonies on agar, success will be determined mainly by the sophistication of the image analysis routines used. However, the camera plays an important role in determining the size of object that will be detectable. The parameters of importance are the modulation transfer ratio, spatial resolution, SNR and the physical characteristics of the sensor. The first three parameters have a direct proportionality to cost. Modern, high quality, solid state cameras are typically substantially better than their older tube counterparts and should be used in most cases. However, for detecting very small objects the vidicon tube camera may well perform better than even the most expensive solid state camera. Vidicon cameras are available with very high resolution. Their resolution is limited only by the size of the scanning electron beam spot and properties of the photosensitive target rather than by discrete isolated pixels as in the case of the solid state camera. If the electron beam spot profile is correctly adjusted such that there are no gaps between scanned lines, the limiting particle detection will usually be determined by the SNR of the video system.

Until recently, simple vidicon cameras have outperformed even the best solid state cameras where repeatability of counting point colonies on agar has been required. If the plate was rotated and recounted, the variance was less than 2% on a plate with 350 colonies. This was not achievable with solid state cameras where the variance was more than 7%. This change in detectability is primarily due to the image of the colonies being small with respect to the size of the pixel sensors. As the plate was rotated the object image covered varying numbers of pixels. Adjacent pixels in the array have often slightly different sensitivities. If it is required to make measurements other than simple counting, a high resolution monochrome solid state camera would be the better choice in almost all circumstances.

Morphological measurements

Most morphological measurements made by an imaging system are made on objects which have been discriminated from their background by greylevel thresholding techniques. It is therefore necessary to choose a camera which will introduce least error when this type of discrimination is used. Shading, rise time (frequency response), greylevel stability and SNR will determine the threshold accuracy. The errors introduced will be minimized if the experiment is arranged so that there is high contrast between the objects of interest and the background. This can be achieved through staining techniques in conjunction with narrow band filters, monochromatic light or simply utilizing the spectral response curve of the camera sensor. The information on spectral response may well not be included with the camera but will be obtainable from the manufacturer. Care should be taken to ensure that auxiliary filters are not fitted in the camera that are not considered in the data sheet. Measurement errors will be small if the number of pixels (or scanned area) is large with respect to the projected object size. This can be ensured by selecting a suitable optical magnification. The best choice of camera for morphological measurements would be a solid state camera with as high a resolution as is affordable. Remember that the MTFs of cascaded video equipment (the imaging system has its own modulation transfer ratio) are multiplicative and generally the larger the number of pixels in the array, the better the transfer ratio. In general monochrome cameras have lower resolution and SNRs than colour cameras and may therefore be used at higher magnifications. Where objects of only one or two distinct colours are of interest, a monochrome CCD camera with narrow band filters or monochromatic illumination would be the best choice.

Optical density measurements

Many investigative techniques are being developed that require optical density to be measured accurately for objects or areas within an image. This is a technically demanding application and, unless all parameters are controlled (this applies as much to the experimental conditions and protocols as to the camera technology), results will be unacceptable. The main application for TV cameras is to allow a human observer to view a scene remotely. The markets that have allowed the rapid development of the technology have been security and observation. The performance required for optical density measurement is not required in these applications. All image analysers performing optical density measurements will allow correction for shading and lighting variation. However, it is not possible to correct fully the gross errors that are developed by tube cameras. By nature, the shading in a tube camera is variable and will change in the course of an experiment. Any stray magnetic fields in the laboratory will further change the shading in an unpredictable fashion. For this application, a tube camera should not be used as it has been completely superseded by the solid state camera. Not all solid state cameras will match the performance of a modern image analyser. The arguments limiting the resolution discussed earlier should be considered. The principal error which will cause poor repeatability is drift in the black level within the camera. When the camera is covered and no light falls on the sensor, the output should be zero. Most cameras will output video with an imprecisely defined and unstable black level. To cure this problem it is necessary to define a reference level which the sensor generates when it is known to be covered. This may be done either with an external metal mask or preferably by scanning a row of dummy sensors which are covered within the solid state device. The video signal generated while the sensor is covered will track changes in performance with temperature and long term drift.

Fluorescence microscopy

Low light level imaging will generally require the use of specialized cameras. Significant differences will be found in the image brightness from the same samples in different microscopes. Four experimental constraints will affect the choice of camera: the colour of the emitted light, whether counting or intensity measurement is required, the speed with which the measurements need to be made and, lastly, the available budget. Most camera technologies have poor sensitivity to short wavelength (blue) illumination and have a peak response at longer wavelengths in the visible to infra-red regions. It will often be necessary to normalize spectral response curves before direct comparisons of absolute sensitivity can be made at the wavelengths of interest. Fluorescence microscopy will almost certainly require the use of integrating (asynchronous) solid state cameras or image intensifier technology. Both means of working at low light levels have advantages and disadvantages.

An integrating camera, typically under the control of the imaging system, will collect light for a longer period than the normal 1/50th or 1/60th second used in video cameras. The limit to the integration period and therefore the maximum achievable sensitivity is determined by fixed pattern and dark current noise generated by the CCD array. This noise is temperature related and substantial improvements can be made by cooling the sensor. This is done in peltier cooled cameras with a solid state cooler and in cryogenic cameras with liquid nitrogen. The peltier cooled cameras have applications in general microscopy. However, the liquid nitrogen cooled cameras are too inconvenient for any but the most demanding of applications. Cooled cameras are available in both video rate and slow rate versions. An advantage of slow rate cameras is that very high quality images of large dynamic range may be obtained, albeit taking several seconds to acquire. Normally, the eight-bit resolution of conventional cameras and analysers is more than adequate in the context of the biological accuracy obtainable.

When high sensitivity together with fast response time is required a different type of technology must be used. Microchannel plate photomultipliers allow real time operation at very low levels of illumination. These devices couple the advantages of the gain of a photomultiplier with the ease of use of a normal camera, although they can be easily damaged by exposure to bright light. Their principal disadvantages lie in the typically high noise content of the output signal which makes object discrimination more difficult and the instability of gain and shading. In addition, the image is frequently marred by a fixed pattern noise phenomenon often described as a 'chicken wire' effect across the entire image. Some later variants of this technology whilst not being universally improved have eliminated this effect. Care should be taken to select an intensifier with the right gain for the application or one whose gain is adjustable, as the noise increases with gain. The variability of gain and shading makes quantification with the intensifier extremely difficult and investigations should be confined to relative measurements made within a short time interval. Intensifier gain changes significantly with age and the instrument should therefore be calibrated against standards within each experiment.

Colour imaging

Colour image processing is a powerful tool when used with good quality colour cameras. There are numerous types of colour cameras available. Vacuum tube cameras are not suitable for quantitative image analysis. Of the solid state technologies available, the best results (at a cost) are obtainable from 'three chip' cameras in which a separate sensor is used for the red, green and blue information. The optical image is split into the three primary colours by prisms and focussed on the three sensors. The extra glass in the optical path together with the colour filters reduces the amount of light reaching the sensors, decreasing the sensitivity when compared to monochrome cameras. The three, separate, colour video signals may be used individually with a monochrome imaging system, or more usefully with a full colour image analyser. The resolution and noise performance of the three colour channels will not be identical and this must be borne in mind if the results of image segmentation are not to be biased. This will become more of a problem as the magnification is reduced resulting in smaller detected areas of colour. The cameras allow the ratio of the outputs of the three channels to be modified to correct for illumination colour temperature. Ideally these controls should not be accessible and should certainly not be altered for quantitative work. Similarly other external controls, for example, peaking, aperture correction and shutter speed, should be set to fixed values. It is rare for these controls, which affect image appearance, to benefit an image analyser's ability to discriminate objects and make measurements. They will however, result in worthless data being obtained if indiscriminately adjusted. The microscope lighting must be stabilized because the manufacturer's lamp supply is usually inadequate. The lamp must always be operated at the same brightness. Changes in the level of received illumination caused by microscope setup, sample thickness, appearance and staining should be compensated by the use of an iris or by use of neutral density filters.

An alternative to the three chip camera is a camera with a single, solid state sensor in which the necessary filtering is integral to the chip. These cameras are capable of acceptable performance and are substantially cheaper than their three chip counterparts. Additionally some may be operated in an integrating mode allowing them to be used for fluorescence applications. Only a small proportion of the available three chip cameras have this facility. The principal disadvantage of the single chip technology is the relatively low resolution which limits the applications to which it can be put. All solid state cameras suffer from beat effects caused by discrete sampling when viewing patterns with repetitive features whose size is similar to that of the pixels. This aliasing appears as a moiré pattern across the image when certain scenes are imaged. It will be more noticeable in images from the single chip colour camera. Applications in which fine colour discrimination is required, or where the objects of interest appear with different hues and intensities, will benefit from the use of colour cameras and full colour image analysis.

Which camera?

Almost every experiment will produce images with subtly different imaging problems. For general use a high resolution, monochrome, solid state camera would be the best choice. If the image analysis system is capable of driving the camera correctly it is possible to obtain one which will produce excellent optical density measurements. This allows non-cooled image integration, thus making fluorescence analysis possible. These features should be available at very little extra cost compared to a standard camera. Cameras are available calibrated against international measurement standards and should be used and kept in calibrated condition. Finally, the camera should be tested with the actual samples to be imaged on the actual microscope in the experimental conditions envisaged for its use. By the use of known calibrated samples (available from the image analysis supplier) total confidence can be obtained in the use of this technology.

References

Eckert, R., & Reynolds, G. T. (1967). The subcellular origin of bioluminescence in Noctiluca miliaris. *Journal of General Physiology*, **50**, 1429–58.

Reynolds, G. T. (1964). Evaluation of an image intensifier system for microscopic observations. *IEEE Transactions on Nuclear Science*, **11**, 147–51.

Reynolds, G. T. (1972). Image intensification applied to biological problems. *Quarterly Reviews of Biophysics*, **5**, 295–347.

Zworykin, V. K., Ramberg, E. A., & Flory, L. E. (1958). *Television in Science and Industry*. New York: Wiley.

PART 3

Image processing

13

Segmentation

A. K. C. WONG

Introduction

Histology involves the study of microscopic structures of animal and plant tissues. These studies relate to several levels of structural organization in multicellular organisms: (1) the cell, (2) the tissue which is an aggregation of cells and their intercellular substances and (3) the organ, a larger structural unit, usually visible to the naked eye. In order to use computer vision to assist in histological studies, the image analysis system must be able to handle different levels of microscopic information in images obtained from optical or electron microscopes.

In image analysis, segmentation means partitioning an image into meaningful regions or marking regions that belong to an object (or the background) in some special way. A region is a group of connected pixels or an area of the image which has common properties. In the early days, the majority of work in segmentation was based on greylevel values (Weszka, 1978). More recently segmentation has involved regions with homogeneous texture (Raafat & Wong, 1988).

At the cellular level, a machine vision system should be able to segment cells, identify the nucleus, and classify intracellular substances, etc. At the histological level, it can help to segment the aggregation of cells and various types of intercellular substances. Finally, at the level of the organ, it should be able to segment and classify regions made up of various parts of the organ. Hence, the segmentation of objects from their background and the segmentation of various regions of homogeneous tissue structures (textures) are equally important.

In general, segmentation techniques can be categorised into two major groups: point dependent techniques and region dependent techniques. Point dependent techniques label pixels according to the greylevel of the individual pixels. To reduce local noise, low pass filtering can be applied to the image before segmentation. Commonly used techniques are histogramming and thresholding. Region dependent techniques involve region segmentation based on the properties of the regions, e.g. Gaussian distribution of the greylevel and/or other context dependent information, such as textures. There are two major approaches for the region dependent methods: boundary establishment based on gradients or other second-order statistics, and point by point (or cell by cell) class labelling based upon region properties or neighbouring characteristics. In this chapter, only a brief description of selective methods will be given to illustrate various problems and approaches. For a more detailed description of these methods and others, refer to Sahoo *et al.*, (1988), Haddon & Boyce (1990), Raafat & Wong (1988), Mao & Jain (1992). Although not all the examples chosen are directly related to histology, they cover a variety of tasks required for various levels of histology applications.

Thresholding methods

A popular approach in image segmentation is thresholding. Its objective is to segment an image into two regions, one of which represents object(s) of interest and the other represents the background. For instance, in a microscopic image, cells could be segmented from their background. In general, a thresholding method is one that determines the threshold value (t^*) for two-level partitioning based on a particular criterion. If t^* is determined solely from the greylevel of each pixel, then the thresholding is point dependent. If it is determined from some local property, for example the greylevel distribution of a group of pixels in the neighbourhood of each pixel, then the threshold method is region dependent.

Point dependent methods

Ostu's method

Ostu's method is a popular thresholding method based on discriminant analysis (Ostu, 1978). It partitions the pixels of an image into two classes at some greylevel t. An optimum threshold t^* is determined by minimizing one of the following objective functions with respect to t:

$$\lambda = \frac{\sigma_B^2}{\sigma_W^2}, \; \eta = \frac{\sigma_B^2}{\sigma_T^2}, \; \kappa = \frac{\sigma_T^2}{\sigma_W^2},$$

where σ_W^2 is the within class variance,
σ_B^2 is the between class variance and
σ_T^2 is the total variance.

Each of these is a function of t. In practice it is simplest to minimise η.

Entropy method

An entropy based method proposed by Kapu, Sahoo & Wong (1985) provides an alternative algorithm for finding t^*. In this method, two probability distributions (e.g. object distribution and background distribution) are derived from the original greylevel distribution of the image as follows:

$$\frac{p_0}{P_t}, \frac{p_1}{P_t}, \ldots, \frac{p_t}{P_t},$$

and

$$\frac{p_{l+1}}{1 - P_t}, \frac{p_{l+2}}{1 - P_t}, \ldots, \frac{p_{l-1}}{1 - P_t},$$

where p_i is the probability of occurrence of grey level i, grey level 0 is the darkest, greylevel $l - 1$ is the lightest, t is the threshold value and

$$P_t = \sum_{i=0}^{t} p_i.$$

Define the entropies as:

$$H_b(t) = -\sum_{i=0}^{t} \frac{p_i}{P_t} \log_e \left(\frac{p_i}{P_t}\right),$$

$$H_\omega(t) = -\sum_{i=t+1}^{l-1} \frac{p_i}{1 - P_t} \log_e \left(\frac{p_i}{1 - P_t}\right).$$

The optimum threshold is the greylevel which maximizes $H_b(t) + H_\omega(t)$.

Examples of point dependent thresholding

Fig. 1 gives the results of thresholding an image of a photograph by the Ostu method and the entropy method. In both cases, the threshold selected is not exactly in the valley region of the greylevel histogram. The thresholding algorithm maps the greylevel image with 256 greylevels into a binary image.

Region dependent methods

Co-occurrence method

The co-occurrence method is based on the concept of a co-occurrence matrix introduced by Haralick *et al.*, 1973. In general, a co-occurrence matrix $M_{(d,\phi)}$ is one whose (i,j) entries are the relative frequency of occurrence of two neighbouring pixels with greylevels i and j, separated by distance d and with orientation ϕ. Ahuja & Rosenfeld (1978) define the greylevel co-occurrence matrix (M) as:

$$M = M_{(1,0)} + M_{(1,\Pi/2)} + M_{(1,\Pi)} + M_{(1,3\Pi/2)}$$

That is, the (i,j) element of M is the frequency that greylevel i occurs as a 4-connected neighbour with greylevel j.

Because of homogeneity, pixels interior to the objects or background should contribute mainly to the near-diagonal entries of M whereas those near an edge should contribute mainly to the off-diagonal entries (close to the corners)

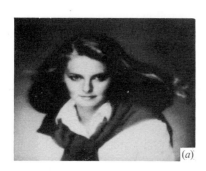
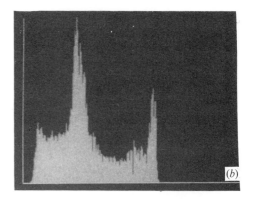

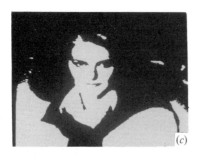
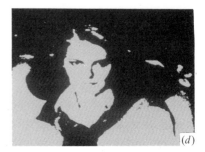

Fig. 1. Thresholding examples: (a) original image with 256 greylevels; (b) histogram of the original image; (c) segmentation results by Ostu's method; (d) segmentation results by the entropy method.

of M because of the greater greylevel change (difference between i and j) near an edge. From M two new histograms can be constructed. One is based on the near-diagonal entries of M. It should have a valley between the object and the background greylevels. Another is based on the off-diagonal entries of M. It should have a sharp peak between the object and the background greylevels. A threshold for the image can then be chosen in the valley of the former and on the peak of the latter.

Fig. 2 shows the segmentation result when the co-occurrence method is applied on a chromosome image and a cloud cover image. In both co-occurrence matrices (Fig. 2(c) and (f)), the bimodal form of the near-diagonal distribution of co-occurrent events is visible (Fig. 2(d) and (e)). Note that, in each case, the threshold position depicted by the peak of the off-diagonal histogram obtained from 1% of all entries in M (Fig. 2(g) and (h)) coincides with the valley region of the near-diagonal histogram.

Relaxation method

The idea of relaxation was first introduced by Southwell (1946) to improve the convergence of a recursive solution for systems of linear equations. In image

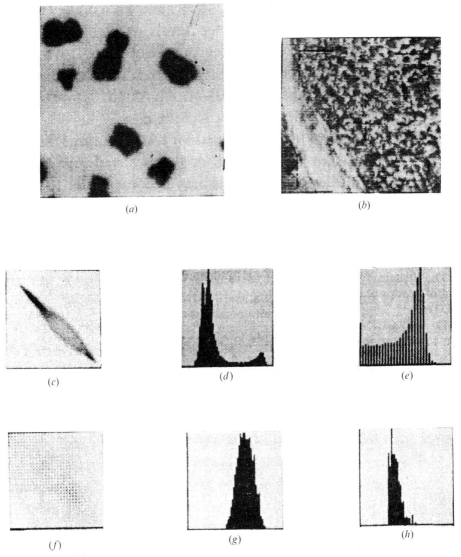

Fig. 2. Segmentation by the co-occurrence method: (*a*) a chromosome image; (*b*) a cloud cover image; (*c*) and (*f*) the co-occurrence matrices of (*a*) and (*b*); (*d*) and (*g*): the near-diagonal and off-diagonal histograms of *M* for (*a*); (*e*) and (*h*) the near-diagonal and off-diagonal histograms of *M* for (*b*). (Adapted from Ahuja & Rosenfeld, 1978).

segmentation, relaxation is applied as follows. The pixels of an image are first classified probabilistically as 'light' or 'dark', (p_{light} or p_{dark}) based on their greylevels. Then the probability of each pixel is adjusted according to the probabilities of the neighbouring pixels.

For the initial classification of the pixels, Rosenfeld & Smith (1981) suggested that if the greylevel of the *i*-th pixel (g_i) was greater than the mean greylevel (μ), the probability of its being classified 'light' was:

$$p_{i,\text{light}} = \frac{1}{2} + \frac{1}{2} \frac{g_i - \mu}{l - \mu},$$

where l is the lightest greylevel.

If the i-th pixel was less than or equal to the mean greylevel, then:

$$p_{i,\text{dark}} = \frac{1}{2} + \frac{1}{2} \frac{\mu - g_i}{\mu - d},$$

where d is the darkest greylevel.

The updating process then adjusts the probability of each pixel based on neighbouring probabilities. An updating formula was proposed by Peleg (1980).

Fig. 3 gives the segmentation results when the relaxation method is applied to the chromosome and the cloud cover images shown in Fig. 2. Note that, in both cases, as iterations progress the peaks heighten whereas the valleys deepen. In the meantime both images are being transformed towards binary images.

Multiple homogeneous region segmentation

The Wang & Haralick method

In a recursive technique proposed by Wang & Haralick (1984), pixels are first classified as edge pixels or non-edge pixels. Each of them is then classified, on the basis of its neighbourhood, as being relatively dark or relatively light. A histogram of the greylevels is then obtained for those pixels that are edge pixels and relatively dark, and another histogram is obtained for those pixels that are edge pixels and relatively light. A threshold is selected based on the greylevel intensity value corresponding to one of the highest peaks from the two histograms. To obtain multiple thresholds, the procedure is applied recursively, first using only those pixels whose intensities are lower than the threshold and then using only those pixels whose intensities are greater than the threshold.

Segmentation using region and boundary information

A two-stage image segmentation method that attempts to unify region and edge segmentation based on greylevel occurrence matrices was introduced by Haddon & Boyce (1990). It applies essentially similar concepts to those proposed in Ahuja & Rosenfeld (1978) and extends them to multiple thresholding.

If an image consists of several regions each of which is characterized by Guassian statistics, the co-occurrent events in the homogeneous regions would be reflected by the near-diagonal peaks in M (Figs. 2 and 4) and the boundary

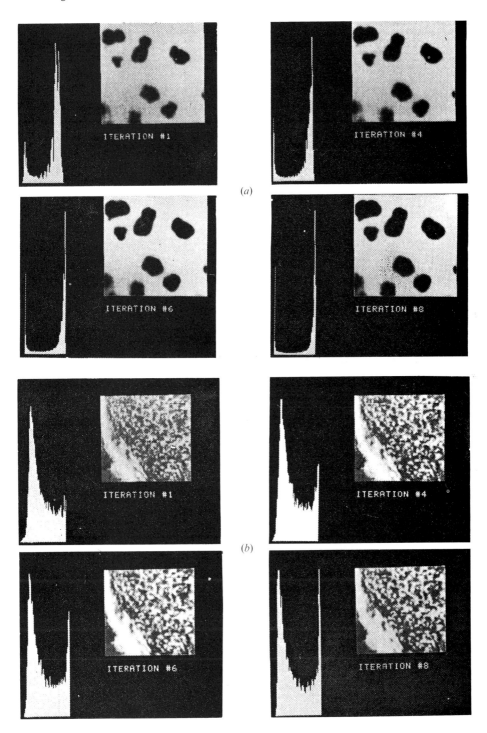

Fig. 3. Segmentation by the relaxation method: (*a*) the relaxation result of the 1, 4, 6 and 8 iterations of the chromosome image given in Fig. 2(*a*) and (*b*) the result of 1, 4, 6 and 8 iterations of the cloud cover image given in Fig. 2(*b*). Adapted from Peleg (1980).

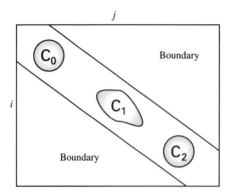

Fig. 4. A diagrammatic illustration of a co-occurrence matrix in a multi-thresholding case.

events by the off-diagonal peaks (see the section on the co-occurrence method above). This structure allows M to serve as a feature space.

The segmentation algorithm consists of two stages: an initial segmentation based on the location of the intensities of each pixel and its neighbours within M followed by a refinement process taking account of the assignment of nearby pixels via relaxation labelling (see the section on the relaxation method above). The compatibility coefficients are derived from M thereby ensuring consistency between the two stages. Similar to the region initiation in Section 4 of the study by Raafat & Wong (1988), the initial segmentation is determined by the global properties of the image. Instead of using a region splitting and growing process based on an information and texture distance measure (Raafat & Wong, 1988), this method uses the relaxation labelling to impose local consistency of pixel labelling during the segmentation by minimizing the entropy of local information, whereas region information is expressed via conditional probabilities that are determined *a priori*. The method roughly segments an image into homogeneous areas and generates an edge map using the Canny edge operator (Canny, 1986).

Fig. 4 illustrates the multi-modal distribution of the near-diagonal entries in the co-occurrence matrix of a multi-thresholding image. From the distribution, homogeneous regions could be initiated.

Segmentation of texture regions

In histology, the microscopic structure (or textures) in image regions may furnish more information than multiple thresholded regions. A method for image segmentation and region classification based on the texture content of different regions in an image has been developed (Raafat & Wong, 1988). It uses an information measure for initiating texturally homogeneous core regions and a texture distance measure to direct the growth of various homogeneous regions. Since the texture information measure reflects both the local and global properties of an image, this segmentation process is highly adaptable to various images.

The algorithm consists of three stages:

1 Initiation of texturally homogeneous regions.
2 Growing of texturally homogeneous regions.
3 Fine tuning of textural region boundary.

In region growing, cores or seeds of regions are initiated first. To describe the local texture content, image blocks (texture elements) are used. A resolution dependent measure (the *I*-measure), derived from the analysis of Wong & Vogel (1977), indicating the typicality of an image block with respect to other blocks in the image is used for region initiation.

First, windows of different resolution sizes are used to extract the primitive features such as average greylevels and gradient vectors within an image neighbourhood of different sizes. Let $w^{(m)}$ be an observation window of resolution level m; $b^m(x, y)$ be the neighbourhood specified by $w^{(m)}$ with the centre positioned at (x,y) and $B^{(m)} = \{b^{(m)}(x,y)\}$ be the set of all possible neighbourhoods observed through w(m) placed on the image. Let $E_t = \{k \mid k = 0, 1, 2, \ldots, K_{t-1}\}$ be the finite set of discretized values where K_t is the number of distinct events for feature t. Then the feature extraction scheme is defined as the mapping of the specified feature content inside the neighbourhood onto the set E_t

$$f_t^{(m)}: b^{(m)}(i,j) \rightarrow E_t.$$

E_t is used to denote feature values in 1- or 2-D space depending on the feature used. It is also possible to extend it to the 3-D case for CT images.

The texture content of a block can be represented by histograms for the feature events defined in E_t. Those corresponding to greylevel are known as scalar histograms and those corresponding to gradient events are known as vector histograms (Fig. 5). The basic concept of *I*-measure is to reflect the local information with respect to the global information of an image. Let $p_{tk}^{(m)}$ be the probability (relative frequency) of the k-th event of type t with resolution m. The total information estimated for an $n \times n$ image block $b_n(x,y)$ is defined as:

$$I_t^{(m)}(x,y) = -\sum_{k=0}^{K'_t} q_{tk}^{(m)}(x,y) \log p_{tk}^{(m)}.$$

The total *m*-resolution *I*-measure at (x,y) is given by:

$$I^{(m)}(x,y) = \frac{I_s^{(m)}(x,y) + \alpha I_v^{(m)}(x,y)}{1 + \alpha},$$

where s and v signify the scalar and the vector features respectively, and α is a factor. It was found that $\alpha = 2$ yields very good results.

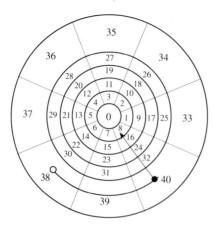

Fig. 5. A 2-D discretized gradient space and distances between gradient events. The distance between events '8' and '38' is 6 (a total of 2 radial and 4 circumferential unit distances).

The total texture information measure $I(x,y)$ at pixel (x,y) is given by:

$$I(x,y) \doteq \frac{1}{R} \sum_{m=1}^{R} I^{(m)}(x,y),$$

where R is the number of resolution levels used. $I(x,y)$ measures the surprise of all the textural events observed in $b_n(x,y)$. For blocks whose texture characteristics are one of the typical types in the image, the $I(x,y)$ value is relatively low due to the high probability value of the texture events observed in the block. Hence, $I(x,y)$ can be used for selecting blocks in homogeneous texture regions during region initiation.

For classifying texture and directing region growing, a texture distance measure between texture blocks is used. Let H_t^a and H_t^b be the histograms of t-feature events for image blocks a and b respectively. Let $c_t(p,q)$ be the distance between event p in H_t^a and q in H_t^b and $K_t' = K_t - 1$. Let $C_t = \{c_t(p,q) | p = 0, 1, 2, \ldots, K_t'\}$ be a set of all possible event distances between events in H_t^a and those in H_t^b. The event distance $c_s(p,q)$ between p and q for the greylevel feature is defined to be $c_s(p,q) = |p - q|$ for all $p,q \in E_s$. For gradient vector histograms, the event distance $c_v(p,q)$ is defined as follows.

Let (r_p,ϕ_p) and (r_q,ϕ_q) be the polar coordinates of the two gradient events p and q, respectively (say events '8' and '38' in Fig. 5). The event distance between them is defined as:

$$c_v(p,q) = \begin{cases} F.r_p & \text{if } p \neq 0 \text{ and } q = 0, \\ F.r_q & \text{if } p = 0 \text{ and } q \neq 0, \\ 0 & \text{if } p = q = 0, \\ F|r_p - r_q| + \min(|\phi_p - \phi_q|, N - |\phi_p - \phi_q|) & \text{otherwise} \end{cases}$$

where F is a normalization factor. The distance between event '8' and '38' is therefore 6 if the unit cost between adjacent cells in the vector histogram is 1.

The total cost obtained from the sum of distances of paired events between the two histograms H_t^a and H_t^b can be expressed as a distance function:

$$d_t^m(a,b) = \sum_{p=0}^{K'_t}\sum_{q=0}^{K'_t} c_t(p,q)x(p,q),$$

where $x(p,q)$ is the number of counts of event p in block a to be paired with event q in block b. Thus the texture event set distance $D_t^m(a,b)$ between H_t^a and H_t^b with respect to resolution level m is defined as the minimum of $d_t^m(a,b)$ with respect to the constraints:

$$\sum_{q=0}^{K'_t}x(p,q) = h_p^a \text{ for } p = 0, 1, \ldots, K'_t$$

$$\sum_{q=0}^{K'_t}x(p,q) = h_q^a \text{ for } q = 0, 1, \ldots, K'_t,$$

and $x(p,q) \geqslant 0$ for all $p,q \in E_t$ and h_p^a and h_t^q are the event frequency of event $p,q \in E_t$ respectively.

$D_t^m(a,b)$, being the minimal cost of matching the events accounted for in the two histograms, is the unique distance between them. It has been proved as a metric (Raafat & Wong, 1988). Any linear programming problem of this form is of the transportation problem type (Hillier & Lieberman, 1990). The total texture event set distance between two image blocks a and b is defined as:

$$D(a,b) = \frac{1}{R}\sum_{m=1}^{R} D^{(m)}(a,b)$$

where R is the number of resolution levels.

Having introduced the I-measures and the texture distances, a texture based segmentation algorithm is as follows:

1 Region initiation. Any two or more 8-connected blocks having low I-measure and small texture distances to each other are selected as the core blocks of a region.

2 Region growing. A block is considered as part of a region if it is 8-connected to any of the blocks of the region and is closer in textural distance to that region than any other region. Region merging is allowed.

3 Region merging. Two regions are merged if they are 8-connected and if their inter-region mean textural distance is within one standard deviation of each of the two intra-region mean textural distances.

4 Region boundary refinement. Boundaries are refined in a similar manner to region growing, but at the sub-block level. Region merging is allowed.

Fig. 6 is an earlier application of segmentation of various regions inside a cell. For region growing and boundary formation, the dotted lines in Figs. 6(*c*) and (*d*) represent the boundary generated by the algorithm based on 9×9 block

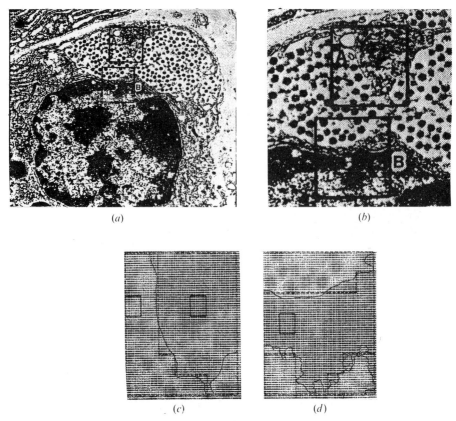

Fig. 6. Region segmentation example from an electron microscope image of a cancerous cell: (*a*) an image of cancerous cell; (*b*) an enlarged portion of the image for segmentation experiments; (*c*) segmentation of area A and (*d*) segmentation of area B.

boundary formation process. In this experiment, no boundary fine tuning is involved.

In another experiment (Fig. 7(*a*)) a photograph of a fish with body texture closely matching that of the surrounding ocean floor was analysed. The segmentation achieved after boundary refinement is shown in Fig. 7(*b*). Note that the segmentation results are good and conform to human expectation. It should also be mentioned that during the region initiation, all the core blocks represent the typical texture characteristics of their corresponding regions.

Conclusion

In this chapter, I have described various image segmentation methods and have illustrated their applications to histology. Most of the methods are based on low level vision where *a priori* knowledge of the image is not required. In practice, these methods can help to identify valuable information for detailed

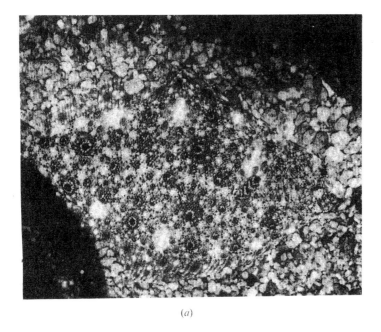

(*a*)

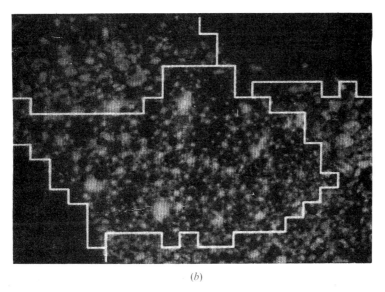

(*b*)

Fig. 7. Region segmentation example: (*a*) the fish (photograph courtesy of B. Saidel and Dr J. Lettvin du Buf) and (*b*) the segmented image.

histological studies. With the advent of computing and system integration, the potential and the capacity of this technology is obvious. To advance this significant and cost effective technology further, more research will have to be pursued.

References

Ahuja, N. & Rosenfeld, A. (1978). A note on the use of second-order gray-level statistics for threshold selection. *IEEE Transactions on Systems, Man and Cybernetics*, **SMC-8**, 895–9.

Canny, J. F. (1986). A computational approach to edge detection. *IEEE Transactions on Pattern Analysis and Machine Intelligence*, **PAMI-8**, 679–98.

Haddon, J. F. & Boyce, J. F. (1990). Image segmentation by unifying region and boundary information. *IEEE Transactions on Pattern Analysis and Machine Intelligence*, **PAMI-12**, 929–48.

Haralick, R. M., Shanmugam, K. & Dinstein, I. (1973). Texture features for image classification. *IEEE Transactions on Systems, Man and Cybernetics*, **SMC-3**, 610–21.

Hillier, F. & Lieberman, G. (1990). *Introduction to Operation Research* (3rd edition). San Francisco: Holden-Day.

Kapu, J. N., Sahoo, P. K. & Wong, A. K. C. (1985). A new method for gray-level picture thresholding using the entropy of the histogram. *Computer Vision, Graphics and Image Processing*, **29**, 273–85.

Mao, J. & Jain, A. K. (1992). Texture classification and segmentation using multiresolution simultaneous autoregressive models. *Pattern Recognition*, **25-2**, 173–88.

Ostu, N. (1978). A threshold selection method from gray-level histogram. *IEEE Transactions on Systems, Man and Cybernetics*, **SMC-8**, 62–6.

Peleg, S. (1980). A new probabilistic relaxation scheme. *IEEE Transactions on Pattern Analysis and Machine Intelligence*, **PAMI-2**, 362–9.

Raafat, H. M. & Wong, A. K. C. (1988). A texture information-directed region growing algorithm for image segmentation and region classification. *Computer Vision, Graphics and Image Processing*, **43**, 1–21.

Rosenfeld, A., & Smith R. C. (1981). Thresholding using relaxation. *IEEE Transactions on Pattern Analysis and Machine Intelligence*, **PAMI-3**, 598–606.

Sahoo, P. K., Soltani, S. & Wong, A. K. C. (1988). A survey of thresholding techniques. *Computer Vision, Graphics and Image Processing*, **41**, 233–60.

Southwell, R. V. (1946). *Relaxation Methods in Theoretical Physics*, London: Oxford University Press.

Wang, S. & Haralick, R. M. (1984). Automatic multithreshold selection. *Computer Vision, Graphics and Image Processing*, **25**, 46–67.

Weszka, J. S. (1978). A survey of threshold selection techniques. *Computer Vision, Graphics and Image Processing*, **7**, 259–65.

Wong, A. K. C. & Vogel, M. A. (1977). Resolution-dependent information measures for image analysis. *IEEE Transactions on Systems, Man and Cybernetics*, SMC-7, **1**, 49–61.

14

Edge detection in microscope images

M. Y. JAISIMHA and R. M. HARALICK

Introduction

One of the central problems in biological and biomedical imaging in general, and in cytological imaging in particular, is the automatic determination of the boundaries of objects of interest. The problem of edge detection in cytological images is further compounded by the wide variety of images that can be obtained. In addition, the greylevel characteristics of the extraneous objects in the images are often very similar to those of the objects of interest. If no prior knowledge is available about the nature of the image, it is then necessary to analyse the greylevel characteristics of the objects of interest, the extraneous objects and the background adjacent to the boundaries of interest. These factors have to be taken into account in order to design a successful image analysis procedure. As we show in this chapter, it is sometimes impossible to perform the desired delineation purely on the basis of domain-independent greylevel spatial information. Some cytological knowledge may have to be incorporated to perform good edge detection.

A large number of image analysis tools are available to the researcher in order to perform an analysis of the greylevel and shape properties of an image. Many of these tools were first developed for machine vision applications and some were developed for cytological image analysis. A judicious combination of some of these procedures can be used for analysing cytological images. Expositions on the vast body of image analysis procedures can be found in Haralick & Shapiro (1991) and in Rosenfeld & Kak (1982). In this chapter, we review briefly the most significant tools used in edge detection in cytological images.

Applying a pure edge detection procedure, such as the facet edge detector (Haralick, 1984) or the Prewitt detector (Prewitt, 1970), to a cytological image directly can have disastrous consequences in terms of the quality of the boundaries detected. A general approach is to apply iterations of conditioning and labelling to the images. Conditioning is based on a model suggesting that the observed image is composed of an informative pattern modified by uninteresting variations that typically add to or multiply the informative pattern.

Conditioning estimates the informative pattern on the basis of the observed image. Thus conditioning suppresses noise, which can be thought of as random unpatterned variations affecting all measurements. Conditioning can also perform background normalization by suppressing uninteresting systematic or patterned variations. Conditioning is typically applied uniformly and is context independent.

Labelling is based on a model that suggests that the informative pattern has structure as a spatial arrangement of events, each spatial event being a set of connected pixels. Labelling determines the kinds of spatial events each pixel participates in. For example, if the interesting spatial events of the informative pattern are events only of high valued and low valued pixels, then the thresholding operation can be considered a labelling operation. Other kinds of labelling operations include edge detection, corner finding, and identification of pixels that participate in various shape primitives. Mathematical morphology is used in both the conditioning and labelling phases of the algorithms.

Thresholding is a process of labelling a greylevel image on the basis of the greylevel value. Thresholding transforms a greylevel image into a binary image. Once an image has been thresholded, the binary image can be analysed to identify the various distinct, yet connected, entities that make it up. The process of identifying connected entities in a binary image is referred to as connected components analysis. The basic theory behind thresholding and connected components analysis is presented in the next section. Before thresholding or other edge detection procedures can be applied to an image, the image has to be conditioned to mitigate the effects of noise or extraneous objects. After thresholding, the shape properties of the objects have to be analysed. The tools of mathematical morphology can be used to perform these tasks and a somewhat qualitative introduction to this subject is given in a section below. A brief introduction to the facet model and edge detection based on this model is also provided.

Some objects of interest in cytological images have a boundary that is composed of components with fairly distinct greylevel characteristics. It is also possible for some edge detection procedures to perform relatively well in detecting certain components of the boundaries without being able to detect all of them. An obvious step is to use the results of each edge detection procedure where it works best. The procedures we describe in this chapter employ this principle. We present procedures that use a combination of thresholding, morphology, facet model-based edge detection and region property analysis for edge detection in four different cytological images.

Thresholding and connected components

Thresholding is the process of labelling the pixels in a greylevel image based on their greylevel values. It has been used extensively as a first step in binary machine vision. Thresholding can be used to distinguish pixels that have a lower greylevel value from those having a higher greylevel value. Pixels having a value higher than the threshold value are associated with one label (say a binary 1) and those lower than the threshold value are associated with another label (typically a binary 0).

Procedures exist for automatically determining the threshold based on the histogram of the pixels in the image (Haralick & Shapiro, 1991). If the objects of interest occupy a significant fraction of the image and have a greylevel value sufficiently different from the background, the greylevel histogram that results is bimodal with a fairly deep valley between the two modes. Automatic thresholding procedures attempt to identify this valley and place the threshold value at this location. Unfortunately, in cytological images the objects of interest quite often satisfy neither of the two assumptions that automatic procedures depend on for their functioning. Threshold selection thus has to be done manually. This is not unduly restrictive in practice since the threshold value depends to a large extent on a knowledge of the nature of the image. A complete system for cell image segmentation would require *a priori* knowledge to determine the threshold value.

Once the image has been thresholded, a connected components operator (Lumia *et al.*, 1983) can be used to group the binary 1 pixels into maximally connected regions which are referred to as connected components. Two pixels are said to be connected if there is a path between them lying entirely on binary 1 pixels and where each pixel on the path is connected to one of its binary 1 neighbours. If the path is restricted to turns in the four cardinal compass directions (north, south, east and west), the pixels are said to be 4-connected. If the intermediate compass directions are allowed, the pixels are called 8-connected. A thresholded image is used as input to the connected components algorithm and the output consists of a symbolic image where the label assigned to each pixel is an integer that uniquely identifies the connected component on which the pixel lies. Once the connected component image has been generated, the region properties can be computed. A full description of these properties is given in Haralick & Shapiro (1991). In this chapter, the following properties are used to distinguish between the various components and perform edge detection:

1 The mean and variance of the greylevel value of the pixels that contribute to a given component.
2 The size of the component.
3 The circularity measure of the component.

Mathematical morphology

Mathematical morphology is a powerful algebraic system of operators which has been extensively used in shape analysis (Haralick & Shapiro, 1991; Giardina & Dougherty, 1988; Haralick *et al.*, 1987). Using the basic morphological operators of dilation, erosion, opening and closing (defined below), shape primitives can be extracted from images and contaminating structures discarded. The contaminating structures could either be random noise or shapes with characteristics that differ from those of the shapes of interest. In a typical morphological image processing algorithm the image is operated on by a relatively small kernel or structuring element which is selected to achieve the intended effect.

Dilation, as the name implies, results in expansion or swelling of the image. In set notation, the dilation of the two sets A and B is denoted by $A \oplus B$ and is defined as:

$$A \oplus B = \{c \in E^N | c = a + b \text{ for some } a \in A \text{ and } b \in B\}$$

The above definition holds for binary (two level) images that might, for example, be obtained from the output of a thresholding operation.

Erosion results in a contraction of the image. In set notation, the erosion of the two sets A and B is denoted by $A \ominus B$ and is defined as:

$$A \ominus B = \{x \in E^N | x + b \in A \text{ for every } b \in B\}$$

The opening of two sets A and B can be defined in terms of the dilation and erosion operators as follows:

$$A \bigcirc B = (A \ominus B) \oplus B$$

The closing of two sets is defined as:

$$A \bullet B = (A \oplus B) \ominus B.$$

Binary openings can be used to eliminate additive noise in the background and closings can be used to eliminate subtractive noise in the foreground of binary images. In the case of greylevel images, the definition of the dilation (erosion) operator is modified in terms of maxima (minima) of sums (differences) of the structuring element and image greylevel values in the domain of the structuring elements. Greylevel closings can be used to fill 'dark pits' and greylevel openings can be used to eliminate 'bright hills' in images. A complete introduction to the theory and applications of mathematical morphology can be found in the studies of Giardina & Dougherty (1988), Haralick & Shapiro (1991), Haralick *et al.* (1987) and Costa (1990).

The facet model

A common strategy for edge detection in the machine vision literature has been to model edges in the images as being derived from a step change (or blurred versions of a step) in the greylevel value. Pixels are then labelled as edge pixels if the change in greylevel value, or the gradient, is high enough. A gradient magnitude edge detector that can be used is the second directional derivative edge detector described by Haralick (1984) and Haralick & Shapiro (1991). The edge detector uses the facet model to estimate the gradient magnitude at each pixel location in the image. The facet model considers a digital image as being derived by sampling a continuous underlying greylevel intensity surface.

Each neighbourhood of this surface can be represented by a low degree polynomial, usually quadratic or cubic. In the cubic case, the polynomial or 'facet' is:

$$f(r,c) =$$
$$k_1 + k_2 r + k_3 c + k_4 r^2 + k_5 rc + k_6 c^2 + k_7 r^3 + k_8 r^2 c + k_9 rc^2 + k_{10} c^3,$$

where k_i are the polynomial coefficients,
    r are the row co-ordinates and
    c are the column coordinates.

The first step in the edge detection sequence is the computation of the polynomial coefficients by performing a local surface fit over a neighbourhood centred around each pixel in the image. The coefficients $\{a_i\}$ are computed by minimising:

$$e^2 = \sum_{r \in R} \sum_{c \in C} [I(r,c) - \sum_{n=0}^{K} a_n P_n(r,c)],$$

where R and C are the set of row and column coordinates respectively that
    belong to the neighbourhood,
    $I(r,c)$ is the pixel intensity at coordinate (r,c) and
    $P_n(r,c)$ is the set of Chebyshev polynomials, used as basis polynomials.

The gradient direction is given in terms of the polynomial coefficients as arctan (k_3/k_2) and the gradient magnitude is given by $(k_2^2 + k_3^2)^{1/2}$. The second directional derivative in the direction of the gradient and the contrast can also be obtained in terms of the facet polynomial coefficients (Haralick, 1984).

The centre pixel of the neighbourhood is labelled as an edge pixel if the second directional derivative in the direction of the gradient has a negatively sloped zero crossing within a threshold radius of the centre of the pixel and if the edge contrast exceeds a threshold value. That is, an edge is detected at (r,c) if:

1   $f'(r,c) \neq 0$
2 $f''(x,y) = 0$ for some (x,y) within a threshold radius of (r,c)
3 $f'''(x,y) < 0$

where f', f'' and f''' denote the first, second and third directional derivatives of the facet polynomial. Increasing the size of the window permits the detection of relatively flat-sloped edges. Increasing the degree of the polynomial approximation to the image neighbourhood improves the ability of the detector to detect relatively sharp edges.

Boundary detection in cell images

Boundary detection and/or segmentation of cell images is usually the first step in an image understanding system where a high level module utilizes the output of a low level boundary extraction and region characterization procedure to perform quantitative and qualitative measurements. Boundaries in cell images are usually of two types:

1 Boundaries of relatively small spatial extent characterized by 'cliffs' between regions of different greylevel intensity, similar to the 'frontier' boundaries described by Garbay (1986).

2 Boundaries of relatively large spatial extent are characterized by a particular greylevel intensity or intensity pattern. That is, there are 'moats' that are characterized by regions of relatively lower greylevel intensity and 'walls' that are characterized by relatively higher greylevel intensities.

Gradient based edge detectors and region growing operators can be used to identify cliff boundaries. Moat and wall boundaries can be identified either by thresholding or gradient based edge operators. In most cases, the boundaries in real cell images are not perfect cliffs, moats or walls. In addition to noise in the images, there are also extraneous objects whose boundary characteristics are indistinguishable from the objects of interest (whose boundaries are to be identified). In addition, there may be objects that touch and hence have to be grouped together in the boundary delineation step.

In order to contend with the problems of real cell images, conditioning operators may have to be applied to attenuate the effects of noise or to remove regular patterned variations in the background which could produce spurious boundaries. Boundary identification can be performed by iterations of labelling with facet edge detection, thresholding or region growing, interspersed with conditioning iterations. Connected component analysis with region property computation can also be used to differentiate between spurious and legitimate boundaries. Where the boundaries of the objects of interest are combinations of the various kinds of boundaries, the outputs of various edge detection schemes can be combined to yield the desired output.

Algorithms for edge detection in microscopic images

Algorithms and results for edge detection in four different images, from both conventional and confocal microscopes, are presented below. For three of the four images, 'ideal' edge boundaries were identified by an expert. Procedures were designed that produced an edge output that was as close as possible to the 'ideal'. For each image, the features were identified that determined the design of an image analysis procedure. The analysis procedure and the results obtained with it are described below. Lastly, the overall algorithms are presented in a compact mathematical notation. The notation used is derived from that of Joo (1991).

At each sub-step i, G^i or B^i denotes the greylevel or binary image obtained as a result of step i. Step i operates on the output of step $i - 1$. The first step operates on G^0, the input greylevel image. To reiterate, the morphological operators are defined as follows:

- $\oplus$ denotes dilation
- $\ominus$ denotes erosion
- $\bigcirc$ denotes opening
- $\bullet$ denotes closing.

Structuring elements for morphological operations are defined as follows:

1. *disc(r)* denotes a digital disc of radius r with the structuring element centred at the origin.
2. *horizline(l)* denotes a horizontal line of length l with the structuring element origin at (0,0).

Thresholding operators are defined by the symbols $>$ or $\leqslant$ where:

$$B^i = G^{i-1} \overline{\leqslant} t$$

denotes the process of thresholding such that all pixels in G^{i-1} less than the threshold value t are set to a binary 0. Where the thresholding is performed relative to the running row mean, the threshold is expressed as $\bar{x}$, where x times the running row mean is used as a threshold.

1. The inversion of a binary image B^i is denoted by $\bar{B}^i$.
2. The intersection ($\cap$) of two binary images B^i and B^{i-1} is denoted by $B^i \cap B^{i-1}$.
3. The union ($\cup$) of two binary images is denoted by $B^i \cup B^{i-1}$.
4. The set difference operator is denoted by $-$.
5. C^i denotes the connected component image and the associated greylevel and component properties obtained as a result of a connected component and region property computation at step i.
6. The connected component operation on a binary image B^{i-1} is denoted by $C^i = conn(B^{i-1})$.
7. $size(C^i) < t$ denotes the operation of deleting all components from C^i whose size is less than t.
8. $max(C^i)$ denotes the largest connected component in C^i.
9. $mg(C^i) < t$ denotes the operation of deleting all components from C^i whose mean greylevel is less than t.
10. $circul(C^i) \geqslant t$ denotes the operation of deleting all connected components from C^i whose circularity measure is greater than t.
11. Facet edge detection on the image G^i is represented by the function $fedg(G^i,o,s,e,r)$ where o is the order of the facet fit (cubic for example), s is the size of each side of the window of the facet fit, e is the edge contrast threshold and r is the radius threshold for the zero crossing of the second directional derivative edge detector. The resulting edge image has binary 1 pixels at all edge locations.

12 The function *mark*(B^i) denotes the process of marking the boundary pixels of the binary image B^i.

13 The function *rgg*(G^i, B^i, *s*) denotes the process of performing a greylevel based, region growing operation on the image G^i where the regions are constrained to lie within the edges defined by the binary image B^i (with the edge pixels having a binary 1 value). *s* is the significance level of the test for growing regions. The region growing scheme (Haralick & Shapiro, 1991) first performs a top–down, left–right scan where neighbouring regions/pixels are compared for equality of pixel value and region mean using a *t*-statistic test. Regions with sufficiently low *t*-values are merged. Multiple top–down and bottom–up merging scans are also performed. Greylevel properties for each of the regions are also computed. The output of the region grower is denoted by R^i.

14 The function *merge*(R^i) merges all adjacent regions and produces a binary image.

Image 1

The first example image was from a confocal scanning laser microscope. It consists of adult human respiratory mucosa stained with an indirect immuno-fluorescence method to reveal the nerves. The image is shown in Fig. 1. The nerves appear in white. The large object in the centre of the image is a nerve bundle. Above the nerve bundle is a large cavernous blood vessel. In this image all nerves are of interest. The ideal boundaries of the nerves were not available.

The edge contrast is high, and the extraneous objects have a much lower greylevel value than the objects of interest. The boundaries of the objects of interest are of the type 'cliff'. The images have a gradation in the background greylevel which can cause problems if a single threshold value is used for the entire image. The solution to this problem is to use a threshold that depends on the local mean greylevel value. The exact threshold value $t(r)$ for row r of the image is given by the running mean:

$$t(r) = x \times \frac{1}{N_{\text{COLS}} \times 20} \times \sum_{i=r-10}^{r+10} \sum_{j=1}^{N_{\text{COLS}}} I(r,c)$$

where x is a user defined control factor,

  N_{COLS} is the number of pixels per row of the image,
  c is the column number of the pixel and
  $I(r,c)$ is the image greylevel at location (r,c).

The actual value of x used for the image was 2.1 (step 1). The output of the thresholding step is subject to a connected components analysis. All connected components whose size is less than 25 pixels (step 2) (smaller than the smallest nerve) and mean greylevel value less than 110 (darker than the darkest nerve) (step 3) are discarded to yield the final image (step 5).

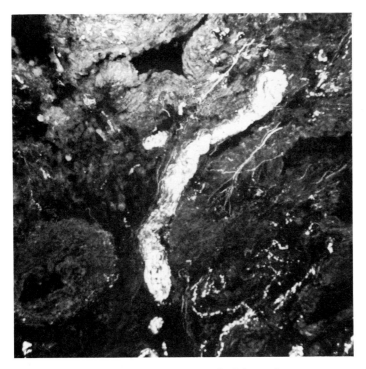

Fig. 1. Image 1. Confocal microscope image of adult respiratory mucosa stained with an indirect immunofluorescence method to reveal the nerves (white).

The overall algorithm is as follows:

1 $B^1 = G^0 < 2.1$
2 $C^2 = conn(B^1)$
3 $C^3 = size(C^2) < 25$
4 $C^4 = mg(C^3) < 110$
5 $B^5 = C^4 \leq 0$

The output of the procedure is shown in Fig. 2.

Image 2

The second example image was obtained from a television camera and is an image of a radial diffusion agarose gel. The objects traced in Fig. 3 are the precipitations of interest. The objects of interest have only their outer outlines marked as being relevant. The image has the following characteristics which have to be taken into account in the image analysis procedure:

1 There is random noise in the image.
2 There is a non-uniform background greylevel.
3 All objects have a bright spot at the centre.

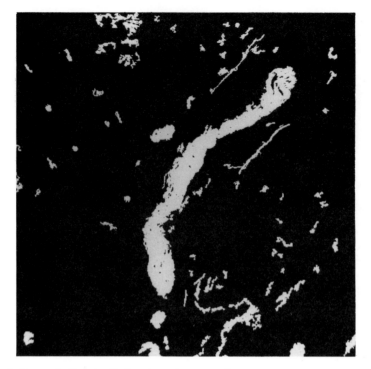

Fig. 2. Image 1. Result of edge detection procedure.

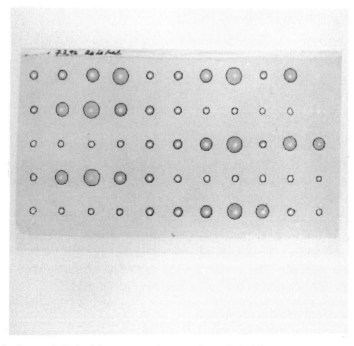

Fig. 3. Image 2. Television camera image of a radial diffusion agarose gel.

4 The only objects of interest are those that have some darkening around the boundary (corresponding to the precipitation of interest).

The precipitation results in a moat region between the bright interior and the bright background. However, since only the outer boundary of the moat is of interest, the moat has first to be converted into a boundary of the type cliff. This is achieved by the first step of conditioning the image, which is to perform a greyscale opening of the image (step 1) with a horizontal line whose extent is slightly larger than the radius of the largest bright spot on the object. The line segment used is of size 15 pixels. The greyscale opening retains all objects with a significant amount of precipitation. However, a few of the objects which have only a small amount of precipitation are merged with the background.

The image obtained from the opening is subject to facet edge detection using a cubic facet with a 5×5 window and an edge contrast threshold of 12.0 (step 2). This produces the boundaries of all the objects which were preserved after the opening. The appropriate algorithm to detect the objects which were missed by the facet edge detector is now applied. The original image is first thresholded with a threshold of 155 (step 3). The threshold is high enough to detect the bright centres of all the objects. All the bright centres that were detected by the facet edge detector now have to be masked out. The image obtained after the initial conditioning by opening is now thresholded at a value (136) such that all objects that have a sufficient contrast (and were hence picked up by the facet edge detector) are detected (step 4). The labelled image from this thresholding is now subject to iterations of conditioning with morpho- logical opening with a disc of radius 3 pixels (to eliminate small additive noise 'blobs' in the foreground) (step 5) and closing with a disc of radius 3 (to reconnect any blobs that were split into two by the opening) (step 6).

The image is then inverted (step 7) and used as a mask on the image (step 8) obtained from step 3 to remove the blobs corresponding to boundaries detected by the facet edge detector. The remaining blobs are dilated by a disc of radius 3 and the boundaries of the dilated blobs are marked (step 9). This yields the boundaries of all the bright objects not detected by the facet edge detector. Only those objects with some precipitation are to be detected. In order to do so, a connected-components analysis is performed on the boundary image (step 10). The means of the greylevels of pixels underlying the boundaries on the original greylevel image were also computed. All boundaries whose mean greylevel values exceed 151 (step 11) were then discarded. This yields the set of all boundaries of interest not detected by the facet edge detector. The two images generated by the facet edge detector and the connected component analysis procedure are then combined (through a logical ⟨OR⟩ operation: step 12) to yield the final edge image which is shown in Fig. 4. It can be seen that some false alarms exist in the final output in terms of spurious boundaries that do not correspond to the boundary of any of the objects of interest and the boundary of the slide on which the precipitations were generated is also detected. However, a post-processing module which analyses the output of the

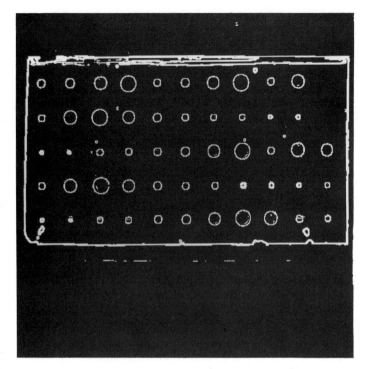

Fig. 4. Image 2. Result of edge detection procedure.

edge detection module could use the knowledge of the relative position of the slide in the frame and the fact that the precipitation centres are located on a square grid on the slide to discard these false alarms. An important aspect of the edge delineation problem was to detect only the outer dark edges of objects corresponding to some precipitation. The algorithm described in this section is able to perform the required edge detection. In mathematical notation the algorithm is as follows:

$\;\;1\;\;G^1 = G^0 \bigcirc horizline(15)$
$\;\;2\;\;B^2 = fedg(G^i, 3, 5, 12.00, 0.7)$
$\;\;3\;\;B^3 = G^0 \leqslant 155$
$\;\;4\;\;B^4 = G^1 \geqslant 136$
$\;\;5\;\;B^5 = B^4 \bigcirc disc(3)$
$\;\;6\;\;B^6 = B^5 \bullet disc(3)$
$\;\;7\;\;B^7 = \bar{B}^6$
$\;\;8\;\;B^8 = B^3 \cup B^7$
$\;\;9\;\;B^9 = mark(B^8 \oplus disc(3))$
$10\;\;C^{10} = conn(B^9)$
$11\;\;C^{11} = mg(C^{10}) > 151$
$12\;\;B^{12} = (C^{11} \leqslant 0) \cup B^2$

The final output of the detection procedure is shown in Fig. 4.

Image 3

The third example image was generated from a light microscope and is an image of adult guineapig lung tissue stained with haematoxylin and eosin. The image is shown in Fig. 5. The boundary of interest is shown traced on the image. The structure traced is an airway. The pulmonary artery is situated to the left of the airway. The structure of interest in the image is fairly well defined in its geometry and is also substantially darker in greylevel than any of the other structures in the image. The boundary structure of interest is clearly a moat because of the characteristics just mentioned. An obvious first step is to start by labelling all pixels whose greylevel value is equal to or less than that of the brightest pixels in the airway of interest (step 1). The threshold value is chosen as 136. This yields a large number of small structures, apart from the airway of interest, which are clutter.

The labelled image now has to be conditioned to eliminate clutter. Once again iterations of morphological operations can be used – first opening with a disc of radius 9 (to remove the small structures) (step 2) and then closing the output of the opening of step 2 with a disc of radius 15 (to reconnect the small segments into which the airway of interest has been broken: step 3). A consequence of the opening iteration is that the airway of interest is now split into two large pieces and a number of relatively small clutter objects remain in

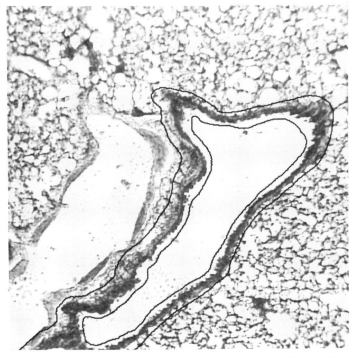

Fig. 5. Image 3. Conventional microscope image of adult guineapig lung tissue stained with haematoxylin and eosin.

the background. Next a connected components analysis is performed on the output of the closing and all but the two largest components are discarded (step 5). The two large components are then joined together by closing with a large disc of radius 25. The single structure is then dilated by a disc of radius 7 (step 6) before obtaining the final boundary (step 7). The boundary is shown in Fig. 6. The dark airway of interest is delineated as needed. The edge detection in this image is more straight forward than for Image 2 because of the distinct geometry and greylevel characteristics of the airway of interest. The overall detection algorithm is as follows:

1 $B^1 = G^0 \geqslant 136$
2 $B^2 = B^1 \bigcirc disc(9)$
3 $B^3 = B^2 \bullet disc(15)$
4 $C^4 = conn(B^3)$
5 $C^5 = max(C^4) \cap max(C^4 - (max(C^4)))$
6 $B^6 = (C^5 \leqslant 0) \oplus disc\ 7$
7 $B^7 = mark(B^6)$

The final output of the edge detector is shown in Fig. 6.

Image 4

The fourth example image was from a light microscope. The section was of adult human respiratory mucosa stained with haematoxylin and eosin. The

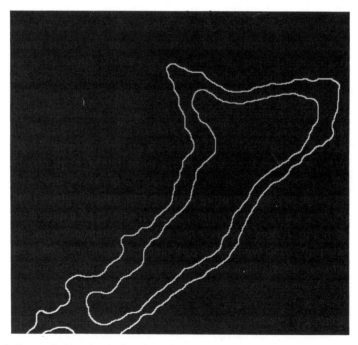

Fig. 6. Image 3. Result of edge detection procedure.

image is shown in Fig. 7, with the boundaries of interest shown traced over the greylevel image. The traced structures are the large cavernous blood vessels. Of the four example images, this one best illustrates the factors an image analysis researcher must cope with in segmenting cell images. The delineated objects of interest and large portions of the background have the same brightness (in terms of greylevel value). The boundaries of the delineated objects (with one exception) have the following characteristics:

1 Portions of the boundaries have a small greylevel contrast with the background – they are cliff boundaries.
2 Other portions of the boundaries have a greylevel 'shadow', i.e. the greylevel value immediately adjacent to the boundary of the object is substantially lower than the greylevel value of either the object or the background adjacent to the boundary – these boundary regions can be considered to be shallow moats.

The one exception is the U-shaped object at the centre of the image in Fig. 7 which has a region at the centre of the object that has greylevel characteristics identical with the boundaries of all the other objects in the scene! This poses problems for the edge detection procedure. In addition, there are extraneous objects in the background that have greylevel characteristics identical with

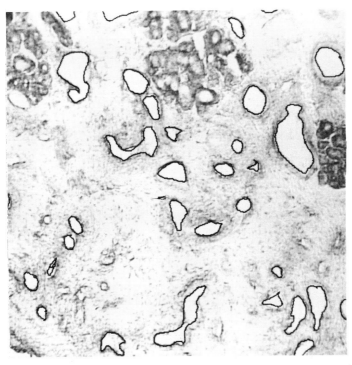

Fig. 7. Image 4. Conventional microscope image of adult human respiratory mucosa stained with haematoxylin and eosin.

those of the objects of interest. The background also has numerous small dark 'pits' which have to eliminated as far as possible in the initial conditioning phase.

As a first step of the algorithm, the image is closed with a disc of radius 5 (step 1). As mentioned in the section on morphology, greylevel closings have the property of being able to fill 'pits'. The output of the closing is subject to facet edge detection (step 2). A cubic facet is used with a 9×9 window and an edge contrast threshold of 10. The edge image obtained is shown in Fig. 8. Clearly, the output of the edge detector has a large number of spurious boundaries in the background of the image. This edge detection strategy, however does a good job of selecting the portions of the boundary corresponding to contrast variations while at the same time preserving the connectivity of the U-shaped object. In order to detect the portions of the boundary that correspond to the 'shadow' regions, another labelling step is performed, thresholding the closed image with a threshold value (of 115) approximately equal to the greylevel value of the 'shadow' regions (step 3). This produces the image of Fig. 9. In order to discard the spurious edge boundaries and to use the greylevel statistics of the objects of interest, a region growing scheme is used (Haralick & Shapiro, 1991) that operates on the greylevel image. The region grower is restricted to growing regions that lie within the boundaries detected by the thresholding and facet edge detection schemes. The output of the region

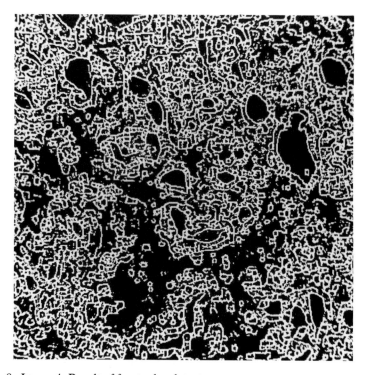

Fig. 8. Image 4. Result of facet edge detector.

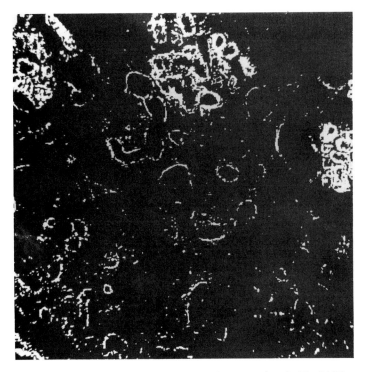

Fig. 9. Image 4. Result of thresholding procedure at a threshold of 115.

grower is subject to connected components analysis and the greylevel properties of the image underlying each of the components are also computed (step
4). All components from the output of the region grower are discarded which
have the following properties:

1 Area less than or equal to 30 pixels (smaller than the smallest object of
   interest – step 5).
2 Area greater than or equal to 3100 pixels (larger than the largest object of
   interest – step 6).
3 Mean greylevel value less than or equal to 198 (greylevel value is less than
   the darkest 'shadow' within the boundaries of any the objects of interest –
   step 7).

   The output of this procedure frequently assigns more than one region to a
single object of interest. So all the regions are merged that are connected and
another iteration performed of labelling by connected components (step 8).
The region properties of the components are also computed. All components
with the following properties are discarded from the output of the connected
components routine:

1 Area less than or equal to 175 pixels (area smaller than the smallest
   object of interest – step 9).

2 Mean greylevel less than or equal to 204 (step 10).

3 Area greater than, less than or equal to 3155 pixels (step 11 – area larger than the largest object of interest).

This iteration eliminates some of the objects of interest that were merged into a large background component. In order to detect these objects, the greylevel image is thresholded at a threshold value of 205 (step 12), conditioned by opening with a disc of radius 3 (step 13), labelled by performing connected components analysis on the output of the opening and the region properties computed for each of the components (step 14). All components are discarded that have a circularity measure higher than a threshold value of 4.4 (step 15) and are smaller than 230 pixels in area (step 16). The outputs of the two procedures are then combined using a logical $\langle \text{OR} \rangle$ operation (step 17). The combined output is conditioned by first closing with a disc of radius 7 and then dilating with a disc of radius 3 (step 18). The boundary pixels of the output of the dilation are shown in Fig. 10 (step 19).

The overall algorithm is described in compact notation as follows:

1 $G^1 = G^0 \bullet disc(5)$
2 $B^2 = fedg(G^1, 3, 9, 10.00, 0.70)$
3 $B^3 = G^0 \geqslant 115$
4 $R^4 = rgg(G^0, (B^2 \cup B^3), 0.001)$
5 $C^5 = size(R^4) \leqslant 30$
6 $C^6 = size(C^5) \geqslant 3100$
7 $C^7 = mg(C^6) \leqslant 198$
8 $C^8 = conn(merge(C^7))$
9 $C^9 = size(C^8) \leqslant 175$
10 $C^{10} = mg(C^9) \leqslant 204$
11 $C^{11} = size(C^{10}) \geqslant 3155$
12 $B^{12} = G^0 \leqslant 205$
13 $B^{13} = B^{12} \bigcirc disc(3)$
14 $C^{14} = conn(B^{13})$
15 $C^{15} = circul(C^{14}) \geqslant 4.4$
16 $C^{16} = size(C^{15}) \leqslant 230$
17 $B^{17} = (C^{16} \leqslant 0) \cup (C^{11} \leqslant 0)$
18 $B^{18} = (B^{17} \bullet disc(7)) \oplus disc(3)$
19 $B^{19} = mark(B^{18})$

Comparing the desired output of the procedure given in Fig. 7 to that obtained by the procedure described above (Fig. 10), the following observations can be made:

1 There are some spurious detections of boundaries where no such boundaries exist on the reference image. The greylevel characteristics of these regions are very similar to those of the objects of interest.

2 The U-shaped object boundary has been detected fairly accurately. How-

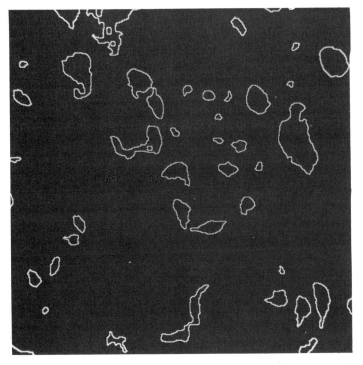

Fig. 10. Image 4. Result of edge detection procedure preserving connectivity.

ever, the region growing algorithm has not defined the boundary of the large object at the top edge of the image well. This is a consequence of our choosing the facet edge detector parameters in order to preserve the connectivity of the two parts of the U-shaped object. If this were not a concern, an alternate procedure could be applied that directly processes the output of a thresholding procedure on the original greylevel image. This is then followed by conditioning using morphology and some connected components analysis to produce the image of Fig. 11. It is apparent that some of the same spurious detections that were present in the more complicated procedure described previously are still present in the thresholding based procedure. However, the boundary of the large object on the top edge is much better defined and the U-shaped object has now become disconnected into two distinct objects. Clearly, the greylevel characteristics of the U-shaped object are not the only factors used by the expert who generated the true delineation of the objects. Using just the greylevel information, it is impossible to preserve simultaneously the fidelity of the boundaries of the U-shaped and the large objects. Clearly, this suggests the need for some higher level knowledge of the nature of the objects of the scene which can then be used to delineate object boundaries. Knowledge about the content of the scene could also be used

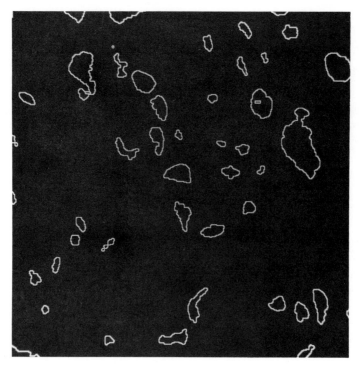

Fig. 11. Image 4. Result of edge detection procedure not preserving connectivity.

to eliminate spurious detections that occur in physically impossible locations.

Conclusions

Edge detection procedures have been applied to four microscope images: one confocal and three conventional images. Three powerful image processing techniques have been used – thresholding, mathematical morphology and facet edge detection. Boundary delineations have been obtained by iterations of conditioning and labelling operations. The boundary delineation procedures combine the output of different edge detection techniques so as to obtain the best possible result relative to the ideal boundary. The trade-offs involved in the design of edge detection procedures have been described. In some instances it is impossible to design an image analysis procedure that uses only greylevel information to perform a boundary detection that is similar to that performed by a human expert. The procedures presented had parameters that depended on the scale and brightness of both the objects of interest and the extraneous objects. This information will have to be supplied by a higher level module that has some *a priori* knowledge of these parameters in a complete system for boundary delineation in cell imagery.

References

Costa, M. (1990). *A Practical Guide to Task-oriented Sequences of Morphological Operations for use in Image Analysis*. Technical Report EE-ISL-90-01, Intelligent Systems Laboratory, Department of Electrical Engineering, University of Washington, Seattle WA.

Garbay, C. (1986). Image structure representation and processing: a discussion of some segmentation methods in cytology. *IEEE Transactions on Pattern Analysis and Machine Intelligence*, **PAMI-8**.

Giardina, C. R. & Dougherty, E. D. (1988). *Morphological Methods in Image and Signal Processing*. Englewood Cliffs, NJ: Prentice Hall.

Haralick, R. M. (1984). Digital step edges from zero crossings of second directional derivatives. *IEEE Transactions on Pattern Analysis and Machine Intelligence*, **PAMI-6**.

Haralick, R. M. & Shapiro, L. G. (1991). *Computer and Robot Vision*. Reading, MA: Addison-Wesley.

Haralick, R. M., Strenberg, S. R. & Zhuang, X. (1987). Image analysis using mathematical morphology. *IEEE Transactions on Pattern Analysis and Machine Intelligence*, **PAMI-9**.

Joo, H. (1991). *Towards the Automatic Generation of Mathematical Morphology Procedures using Predicate Logic*. PhD thesis, University of Washington, Seattle WA.

Lumia, R. L., Shapiro, L. G. & Zuniga, O. (1983). A new connected components algorithm for virtual memory computers. *Computer Vision, Graphics and Image Processing*, **22**.

Prewitt, J. (1970). Object enhancement and extraction. In *Picture Processing and Psychopictorics*, ed. B. Lipkin & A. Rosenfeld. New York: Academic Press.

Rosenfeld, A. & Kak, A. (1982). *Digital Picture Processing*. New York: Academic Press.

15

Image registration

J. R. JAGOE

Introduction and historical perspective

A basic requirement in many image processing applications is the need to compare two or more images, or to compare one image with a chart or atlas. The images may be of one, two, three or more dimensions. The purpose of the comparison may be to detect differences, as in for example, the quantification of changes which occur with time. It may be to enable visualization of structures or events in a higher dimension, as when three-dimensional (3-D) structures can be elucidated from a comparison of two-dimensional (2-D) sequences. It may be to compare images of different modalities, as for example multispectral satellite images where an image in the visual wavelength can be compared with one in the infra-red wavelength.

In the medical sciences, new requirements involving image comparisons are still beyond the limitations of all but the largest and fastest computers and are leading to developments of new software techniques to handle the vast quantities of data. Imaging techniques such as computed tomography (CT), magnetic resonance imaging (MRI), positron emission tomography (PET), digital subtraction angiography (DSA), single photon emission tomography (SPECT), nuclear medicine, ultrasound and thermography, provide a range of different visualization modalities, each producing complementary information. If the images are properly integrated, various advantages accrue, such as improved diagnosis and more accurate surgical planning (Pelizarri et al., 1989; Hill et al., 1991; Woods et al., 1992).

A common theme in all image comparisons is image alignment or registration. Attempts at image alignment have a long history in the biological sciences. This has stemmed from the need to visualize complex 3-D internal structures. A full account of the techniques and problems encountered in this field is given by Gaunt & Gaunt (1978). According to Ware & LoPresti (1975), who give a comprehensive survey of the history of reconstruction in the biological sciences, 'dissection, or semi-ordered sequential destruction has been the rather straightforward method forced upon biologists for seeing inside their chosen material. Assembling information about the structure back together again has been more of a problem'.

The advent of computers has opened the possibilities for easier manipulation and display of 3-D structures. The earliest use of computers was to facilitate the collection and storage of hand-drawn contour data. Typically borders or regions were traced manually on each section using a graphics tablet which controlled a cursor superimposed on the section image, which was displayed on a monitor. In other studies the image has been projected directly onto the surface of the digitizer. Once the section contours have been aligned by eye, the computer can then display the objects with varying degrees of sophistication depending on the characteristics of the display hardware and the software. The development of high speed, high capacity graphics engines, in conjunction with image digitizing hardware has enabled display and manipulation of 3-D objects in real time. Areas where reconstruction has been recently applied are in brain structures (West & Skytte, 1986), neurones (Capowski & Sedivec 1981), heart (Geiser *et al.*, 1980, Wong *et al.*, 1983), vascular network (Ip, 1983), corticotrophs in rat pituitary (Taniguchi & Shiino, 1992) and Ito cells (Tatsumi *et al.*, 1990).

Although computers have greatly facilitated the handling of the image data, the fundamental problem of registration has remained. This is partly because of the algorithmic difficulties of automating the task and partly because of the difficulties arising from distortions introduced by serial sectioning, although Brandle (1989) reported a method for correcting deformations caused by compression or stretching during sectioning. Some image gathering devices avoid the registration problem altogether, as in the case of the optical sections from confocal microscopes or the pre-aligned tomographic slices from CT scanners. However, in most cases it is not possible to circumvent the registration problem, as for example in the alignment of histological sections with autoradiographic images in order to colocalize tissue function and morphology.

Automatic methods of image registration received a great deal of attention with the advent of geosynchronous satellite imaging, which enabled estimation of cloud motion from pairs of earth images taken about 25 minutes apart. Early attempts at visualizing cloud movement were made with the aid of 'loop movies'. Cloud motion was estimated by viewing the loop movies and fixing the positions of the cloud elements at the beginning and end of the picture sequence. This manual process was both tedious and inaccurate because alignment of the images depended on visual matching of the geographical reference points. Automatic methods of determining displacements of the cloud patterns over a finite area in the time interval between two images were reported by Leese *et al.* (1971). They used cross-correlation techniques implemented by computation of the fast Fourier transform (FFT) to match grid squares on a Mercator projection of two ATS images.

Hall *et al.* (1972) also used satellite images to give more precise estimates of cloud motion. They matched the earth's disc to give a global registration. This was followed by a more precise registration using local landmarks which had a high probability of being cloud free, such as Florida, Baja California and the Yucatan peninsula. The first coarse alignment enabled the approximate locations of these landmarks to be estimated. Template matching of small cloud elements was performed by a coarse scan to locate an approximate match, followed by several fine scans from points of near match, which converged to the optimal matching point.

Smith & Phillips (1972) used similar matching techniques to measure accurate displacements of cloud tracers whose rough coordinates were supplied by human operators. Increased accuracy was claimed through more precise alignment of the picture frames. This was because better estimates of the satellite attitude were calculated from multiple pictures rather than from separate calculations on each image. The final matching resolution was estimated to subpixel accuracy by bi-directional quadratic surface fitting in the neighbourhood of the best match.

The techniques for matching cloud patterns depend upon individual matching of small grid squares. For Landsat images it was required to match image data with existing map information for the purpose of comparing with or updating the existing information. This could be done by (a) transforming the picture geometry to that of the map or (b) distorting the map to fit the picture, performing the image interpretation and transferring the results back to the base map by an inverse transform. The latter was more attractive because it was easier to transform graphical data than to warp image data. Steiner & Kirby (1977) explored the problems of using the affine transform to overlay map data on to whole Landsat images.

In 1980 it was decided to develop software to register Landsat images onto the British National Grid. The purpose was to enable comparison of scenes of the same area taken at different times or with different sensors, so that for example, vegetation changes could be monitored, or common points in different scenes of the same area could be located. It also allowed adjacent scenes to be brought into registration so that side-by-side images could be joined. Gordon (1981) reported on the technique which was used to compile manually a library of ground control points for Great Britain using maps and image data. Benny (1981) described a complementary system whereby given the first set of control points which had been mapped to grid coordinates, the control points in repeat images could be located almost entirely automatically after the first pair had been selected manually. This took advantage of the fact that repeat images were similarly scaled and oriented, so that control points could be expected to lie within certain limits from those in previous images. This strategy led to a dramatic reduction in alignment time from 80 hours to perform a visual location, to eight hours for a semi-automatic method and to six minutes for automatic matching of 100 ground control points in an image.

Registration overview

Registration requires that one image be changed or warped to match another image as closely as possible. The limitations of the allowable change are determined by the equations that transform the position of a point in one image to a corresponding point in the matched image. It is possible to specify that only the simplest changes can be made such as translation in the x and y directions for a 2-D image. It is possible to include rotational and scale changes, or to allow rotational but not scale change. Many medical images can be aligned using these transformations alone, but more complicated warping can be carried out, such as shear distortion, perspective change and non-linear distortion (Fig. 1). Whereas the more complicated warping models can accommodate the simpler transformations, it is important to decide in advance on the maximum distortion model required, as this will influence the course of the automatic (or semi-automatic) method used. It is also advisable not to use a model that could allow unwanted image distortions, but to constrain the changes to the minimum required.

Given that the transformation model has been decided upon, the particular parameters of the model are frequently calculated from a set of points in one image whose correspondences in the other image are known. These are generally referred to as control points (or sometimes fiducial or registration points). The required number of control points depends on the model used. A commonly used technique is the affine transformation. This is a linear matching of one image to another which can allow for translation, rotation, independent scale changes in each axis and shear transformation. Fig. 1 shows examples of warping a unit square using the affine transformation. Parallel lines remain parallel under this transformation. It is equivalent to the first order polynomial transformation which can be expressed as:

$$x' = a_0 + a_1x + a_2y$$
$$y' = b_0 + b_1x + b_2y,$$

where (x',y') is a coordinate point in the warped (output) image corresponding to (x,y) in the original (input) image, and the coefficients are $a_0 \ldots a_2$ and $b_0 \ldots b_2$.

A minimum of three control points are required to calculate the coefficients of the transformation. The six coefficients can be calculated from three (x,y) pairs, although this leaves no room for error. More accurate matching is achieved by finding more than three control points and calculating the coefficients which give a minimum residual error between the calculated output points and the coordinates in the output image. The residual error is usually calculated as the sum of the squared distances between the calculated points and the output control point coordinates.

Higher order polynomial transformations can be used for non-linear image

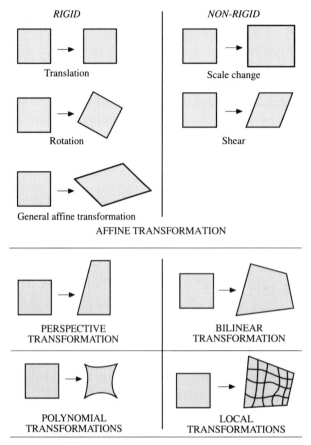

RIGID

Translation

Rotation

General affine transformation

NON-RIGID

Scale change

Shear

AFFINE TRANSFORMATION

PERSPECTIVE
TRANSFORMATION

BILINEAR
TRANSFORMATION

POLYNOMIAL
TRANSFORMATIONS

LOCAL
TRANSFORMATIONS

Fig. 1. Some image transformations. An affine translation preserves parallel lines. A subset is a rigid translation which preserves scale.

warping. One which is useful is sometimes referred to as the bi-linear transformation:

$$x' = a_0 + a_1x + a_2y + a_3xy$$
$$y' = b_0 + b_1x + b_2y + b_3xy$$

This can give rise to a type of warping, an example of which is shown in Fig. 1. These equations with eight unknown coefficients require a minimum of four control points to solve. This family of transformations has been investigated by Fitzpatrick & Leuze (1987).

Second order polynomial transformations have also been used to match satellite images:

$$x' = a_0 + a_1x + a_2y + a_3xy + a_4x^2 + a_5y^2$$
$$y' = b_0 + b_1x + b_2y + b_3xy + b_4x^2 + b_5y^2$$

Six control points are required to calculate the 12 coefficients, but in practice, many more carefully selected control points are required to constrain the transformation from going badly wrong in regions not close to a control point.

It may be that a rigid transformation is required, i.e. one requiring translation or rotation but specifically excluding scale change or any other form of warp. In theory this requires only two control points. A least squares analytical solution to this problem based on quaternions was first published by Faugeras & Herbert (1986). Arun *et al.* (1987) proposed an alternative analytical solution based on the singular value decomposition of a matrix.

Having decided on a suitable mapping function, an appropriate set of control points needs to be located. These points are then used to estimate the coefficients in the transformation equations. The final step is to transform all the points in the input image to their corresponding positions in the output image. In summary the basic steps in image registration are:

1 Choose a suitable mapping function.
2 Find an appropriate set of matching control points in the input and output images.
3 Calculate the coefficients of the chosen transformation.
4 Generate the output image point by point.

Intermediate steps may be required in some schemes as will be seen below.

Location of control points

Control points in the input and output images may be selected manually, semi-automatically or totally automatically. In manual methods, an operator marks the control points. Semi-automatic selection of control points is the process where a human operator indicates approximate matching regions, and the computer then calculates the best matching position in the region of the indicated spot. This sort of semi-automatic matching was commonly used in cloud motion studies (Smith & Phillips, 1972). In totally automatic methods, there are basically two lines of approach. In the first, a template from one image is matched in the other image and the coordinates of the centre of the template and of its optimal matching position are taken as a pair of corresponding points. In the second method, distinctive features of each image are found. These may be objects such as corners, lines, edges, intersections or higher level objects segmented from the scene with specific characteristics, such as 'blobs' within preset bounds of size and/or shape, or regions of specific greylevel or texture. In this latter case, objects from each image may be picked out separately with no reference to the other image. A further step is then required to find the correspondences between the objects in each image.

Template matching

Template matching is the process of determining the position of a subimage inside a larger image. The subimage is called the template and the larger image is called the search area (Fig. 2). The template matching process involves shifting the template over the search area and computing the similarity between the template and a corresponding window in the search area. The centre of the window that yields maximum similarity in the search area defines the location of correspondence. By selecting a set of templates from one image and matching them in the other image, a set of matching control points can be accumulated, from which the transformation parameters can be calculated. The exact position of the optimum template match and the speed at which this can be computed depends (a) on the method used to estimate the similarity between the template and the window in the search area and (b) on the search strategy used to locate the optimum correspondence.

Template matching is usually only applicable when the images are of similar scale. Most matching methods also rely on similar orientation, although rotation invariant techniques have been described. When template matching is used as a method to locate control points, it may be useful to ensure that the template and window regions contain features which provide a good matching key. For example, it is no use trying to match templates in flat featureless regions of the images. Strong dominant linear structures can be dangerous, because a match can occur equally well anywhere along the length of the structure. Corners and intersections provide good keys and it may be worthwhile making a preliminary pass over the image to locate regions where good

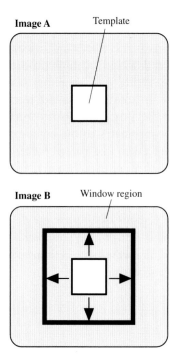

Fig. 2. Template matching by translation. The template T in image A is compared to all sub-windows of the same size in a window region of image B.

matches are likely to occur. Unfortunately, this process can be even more time consuming than the matching process itself.

Similarity estimators

Similarity estimators are used to quantify the similarity of two images. A number of techniques exist.

Cross-correlation coefficients

A commonly used similarity estimator is the cross-correlation or normalized cross-correlation coefficient (Fig. 3). This is simply the correlation coefficient between the greylevel of every pixel in the template and the corresponding pixel in the window. The normalized coefficient has a maximum value of 1.0 for a perfect match with values close to zero for no matching. It has the advantage that it is little affected by the relative brightness of the two images, so that if one image is intensity rescaled, the correlation coefficient is not in theory affected. It has the disadvantage that it involves lengthy computation: n^2 correlations are required for each shift position, where n is the template size. This can, however, be speeded up enormously by use of the FFT to compute the coefficients. A transform of two image regions, multiplied together and followed by an inverse transform will give the coefficients, which merely have to be searched for a maximum value. However, because of its

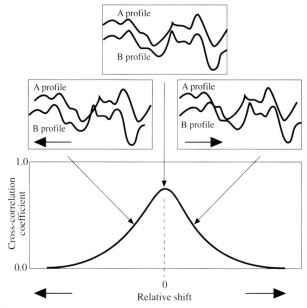

Fig. 3. Schematic illustration of the cross correlation technique using 1-D curves. The correlation coefficient is maximum when the two profiles A and B coincide. This falls off as they are shifted relative to each other.

heavy dependence on outlying values, the cross correlation is not suitable for some types of image matching.

Sum of differences

This method calculates the sum of the absolute differences between pixels in the template and the window. Alternatively, the sum of the squared differences can be used. This latter variation is called the distance measurement. These estimators have the advantage that they are many times faster than the cross-correlation method. They are, however, affected by changes in image intensity in a way which the correlation coefficients are not. In a comparison of two windows, if the pixel values of the first window are halved while the second remains constant, then the correlation coefficient remains unchanged, but the difference measurements will be drastically altered. It is most effective when the images to be compared are of about equal brightness. This can sometimes be arranged using pre-processing techniques such as histogram equalisation.

In a comparison of similarity estimators, Svedlow *et al.* (1976) found that the correlation coefficient method was more reliable than the sum of differences, especially when the images were pre-processed by a gradient operator.

Sequential similarity detection algorithm

The sequential similarity detection algorithm (SSDA) was proposed by Barnea & Silverman (1972) and is similar to the absolute differences method. However, there are several important modifications. First, the local mean value of the template and search region can be taken into account. Thus if T_m and S_m are the local mean values of the template and window, then the difference between corresponding pixels i with greylevels T_i and S_i is expressed as:

$$D_i = |T_i - T_m| - |S_i - S_m|,$$

and the total difference between template and window with n pixels is:

$$D = \sum D_i.$$

This overcomes to some extent the difficulty with differences in image intensity, but involves an additional computational overhead for the recalculation of the mean sub-window value for every shift position.

The second modification can offset this computational overhead. Not all corresponding pixels in the template need to be compared. This is because in non-matching regions, the cumulative difference between corresponding pixels will grow rapidly. If a difference threshold value is set, then this will be exceeded after only a few comparisons, after which the comparisons can be abandoned. In contrast, in similar regions, the differences will be small and the threshold value will be reached, if at all, after many comparisons. Therefore, the number of pixel comparisons made to reach the threshold difference is a measure of similarity. The matching process will quickly pass over obviously non-matching regions. It is also possible to set a dynamic threshold value. The growth curve of the cumulative differences is a monotonically increasing function. So the average slope of the growth curve can be used in the determination of the threshold. In other words, a constant threshold value can be replaced by a threshold that is dependent on the number of comparisons already made. These strategies are illustrated schematically in Fig. 4. A third improvement to template comparison is selection of pixel pairs in random order, so that on average, regional information is sampled more quickly than in an ordered comparison. A variant of this technique was used by Peli *et al.* (1987) who chose random window pairs from regions which had been segmented, thus showing structure. It was argued that pixels from these regions were more likely to show differences and therefore reach the threshold value more quickly.

The problem with adding more refinements to this technique is that the speed advantages are reduced. There is considerable overhead in keeping a running average of the sub-window greylevels, so that efficient programming techniques play an important part in the overall computation time.

Similarity criteria

Stochastic and deterministic similarity criteria (SSC and DSC) are a class of similarity measures proposed by Venot *et al.* (1984). They differ from the previous ones mainly because the pixel values are not directly involved in the calculation. The SSC criterion is used for images where the noise level in the images is greater than the precision of digitization as happens with nuclear

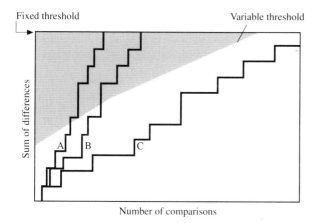

Fig. 4. Cumulative absolute differences between template and window pixels as used in the SSDA algorithm. For A and B, the differences soon reach the threshold value, after which no more comparisons are made. For C, the differences rise more slowly, indicating that there may be a match.

medicine images, while the DSC method is used for images where the noise level can be neglected.

Suppose two images differ only because of the noise component. The difference image will exhibit random fluctuations about zero, and there will be frequent sign changes along rows or columns of the difference image. However, if the images are different, the difference image will be more structured and exhibit fewer random sign change fluctuations. Therefore a count of the sign changes is an indication of similarity.

The idea for the DSC criteria is similar except that a periodic pattern is added to one image before subtraction. The pattern is of the form:

$$
\begin{array}{cccccc}
+q & -q & +q & -q & \cdot & \cdot \\
-q & +q & -q & +q & \cdot & \cdot \\
+q & -q & +q & -q & \cdot & \cdot \\
-q & +q & -q & +q & \cdot & \cdot \\
\cdot & \cdot & \cdot & \cdot & \cdot & \cdot
\end{array}
$$

where q is a small positive integer. This has the effect of compensating for the absence of noise.

Venot *et al.* (1984) showed that these similarity measures behaved as well as the correlation and absolute difference methods on similar images, but were more robust and more accurate on images which were highly dissimilar. They located accurate templates in regions where the correlation technique showed no optimum value.

Invariant moments

As two images are rotated with respect to each other, the above matching techniques become more inaccurate and difficult to use. Even though the centres of the windows correspond, other points do not. In addition, it is impossible to match two rectangular windows in rotated images. Matching by invariant moments was first described by Hu (1962). The 2-D $(p + q)$th order moment of a digital image $g(x,y)$ about its centre of gravity (x_c,y_c) is calculated as:

$$
M_{pq} = \sum\sum g(x,y) * (x - x_c)p * (y - y_c)q.
$$

Hu showed that there are seven second- and third-order invariant moments with respect to translation and rotation of the image which can be derived from combinations of the M_{pq} $(0 \leqslant p,\ q < 3)$. Wong & Hall (1978) used the correlation of the logarithm of the moments to estimate similarity between two windows. However as pointed out by Goshtasby (1985), this method requires that the feature elements of the moment vectors be of the same scale, which they are not, and this is not solved by taking logarithms. Garret *et al.* (1976) proposed quantifying the features into the same number of discrete levels, but this has the effect of causing information loss. Goshtasby (1985) overcame the problem by using circular templates and search regions, and normalizing all moments to have the same scale. Because moment computation is lengthy, he speeded up the process by a two-stage matching process. In the first stage, the zeroth moment was used to estimate likely matching template positions. In the second slower stage, the seven second- and third-order moments were used to select the best match from among the candidates.

Template search strategies

The method of location of the optimal template is clearly an important computational consideration. In the SSDA algorithm, there is no guideline as to how threshold values can be set in advance. If too high a threshold is set, the efficiency of the algorithm is reduced, whereas if too low a value is set, the optimal matching position may be missed. Onoe & Saito (1976) described an algorithm that requires no *a priori* knowledge of the image statistics for monotonically decreasing the threshold value. The first threshold is set to the difference value obtained by a complete summation over the template. After that, whenever each summation is carried out to the end without reaching the threshold, the resultant sum is used as a new threshold. This method is guaranteed to locate the minimum. They also described a modification to the variable threshold technique of Barnea & Silverman (1972).

Rosenfeld & Vanderberg (1977) demonstrated efficiency improvements in template matching by using a two stage coarse–fine template matching procedure. This method used a reduced resolution template and window for the initial screening. The reduced resolution was achieved by averaging over square groups of pixels. This enables the gross structure to be checked which permits rapid rejection of mismatched positions. The increase in speed depends both on the degree of coarsening and the image differences.

Goshtasby *et al.* (1984) used a two stage matching process that is applicable to the cross-correlation technique. By taking a sub-template consisting of a random set of pixels from the template, a set of coefficients, which are estimates of the true coefficients, can be calculated. From these, a correlation coefficient threshold was computed. All template positions where the sampled coefficient was above this threshold were examined using all template pixels. Using a window of 32×32 pixels, a template of 16×16 and a sample of 16 points, they showed that this method was faster than equivalent methods using the FFT. A further advantage was that it was considerably more flexible.

Location of independent control points

Outstanding features in the images, such as lines, corners, spots or blobs, which can be automatically detected by a combination of filtering, thresholding and binary operations, can be used as control points. The location of these features is determined independently in each image. Not only are the correspondences between features unknown, but the number of detected features will be, in general, different in both images. An added difficulty is that the positional correspondences of the matching subset will not be exact. The positions of the features are likely to be perturbed by real differences between the images and by noise effects in the thresholding and binary processing. An example of two point sets with a common matching subset is shown in Fig. 5. It is important that the matching points be well distributed throughout the image. Matching points near the periphery will be the most important in a least squares solution as regards accurate estimates of the registration parameters. Associated with each point may be measurements of other attributes, such as gradient strength, corner angles etc., which can be used for additional matching evidence. The problem of identifying the matching subset is called the point pattern matching problem. It has received considerable attention recently due to its relevance to robot navigation and to the monitoring of dynamic industrial processes. Motion correspondence requires that a set of points in a time series of image frames be mapped from one frame to the next in a consistent manner (Rangarajan & Shah, 1991). The problem can be divided into two parts. First establish the correspondence of object features and then solve the translational and rotational parameters that relate the corresponding features given known constraints. The first problem, also known as the correspondence problem is the most important one and has been approached in a number of ways. Matching of point sets is a subset of the general problem.

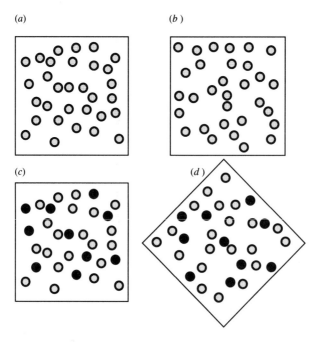

Fig. 5. The two images in (a) and (b) have a subset of 10 matching points as shown in (c) and (d) where they are marked in black and one image is rotated.

Point-pattern matching

Early work on the point-pattern-matching problem was done by Zahn (1974) who pointed out that the problem can be solved by the brute force method. If there are m points in one set and n points in the other, then each point pair in the first set can be matched to each point pair in the second set to generate a translation, rotation and scaling transformation. The number of other points which match or nearly match under each transformation can be counted. The transformation which gives the maximum number of matches is chosen. Unfortunately this method requires $nm(n-1)(m-1)$ template matches which, for a reasonable size point set was not computationally practical at that time. Instead, Zahn implemented a more efficient algorithm that located local structural similarity in the minimum spanning trees (MSTs) of the two sets. The nodes of the MSTs are matched for degree, minimum angle and length ratio of the sides subtending the minimum angle. Only when a degree of local similarity occurred was the template matching tested. The algorithm was tested on computer-generated point sets with constrained random noise added. A 91% success rate was reported. It is, however sensitive to point additions and deletions that change the structure of the trees.

Ranade & Rosenfeld (1980) discuss an iterative point-pattern-matching algorithm for two point sets having translational differences, although it should still work under small rotational displacements. For a point P_i in set P and a point Q_j in set Q, a figure of merit is assigned to each pair (P_i, Q_j) according to how closely other pairs match when P_i is mapped to Q_j. This figure can then be recomputed, giving weights to the other point pairs based on their own scores. This iterative method was extended by Wang *et al.* (1983) to point sets consisting of corner points with a known orientation having rotational displacements.

Stockman *et al.* (1982) described a clustering approach to matching two point sets differing by translation, rotation and scaling. Each point pair in one set was matched with each point pair in the other set. This defines the four parameters required to match these two lines exactly. The corresponding location in 4-D parameter space was marked. After all point pairs have been compared, there should be a cluster in the parameter space that corresponds to the optimum transformation coefficients.

Goshtasby & Stockman (1985) described a technique of point-pattern matching using only a subset of the points. The subset chosen was the convex hull of the point set. This subset has the dual advantage of reducing the computation and using those points that give the most robust transformation estimators. For each point pair in this subset, they computed the transformation parameters as described by Stockman *et al.* (1982) but instead of building a cluster in parameter space, the transformation was made and the number of other points that matched within a threshold distance counted. The transformation that gave rise to the highest count was selected as the approximate transformation.

This was then optimized using the matched points to give a least squares solution. This technique relies on having a sufficient number of corresponding points in the convex hull subset, which cannot always be guaranteed.

The technique of using a subset of points to estimate the matching parameters and then finding how many other points match given those parameters, is a variant of the random sample consensus technique introduced by Fischler & Bolles (1981). They showed that estimation of the parameters of a model in the presence of even a single gross error (a 'poisoned point') mixed with good data may not work using the classical technique of least squares fitting followed by rejection of outliers with high residuals. Rather than using as much of the data as possible to obtain an initial solution and then attempting to eliminate invalid points, the random sample consensus technique selects a random subsample of those points, estimates the parameters and if a sufficient number of other points match the model, selects those parameters.

Hong & Tan (1988) introduced a method of comparing two point sets by transforming each point set to a canonical form under affine transformation and then comparing their canonical forms. If there is a one to one correspondence between the point sets, the same is true between their canonical forms. A point set is in canonical form if:

1 The centre of gravity is at the origin.
2 The moment curve is a circle.
3 The longest distance from any point to the origin is 1.

Their technique is efficient, but is only applicable to point sets with equal numbers in each set.

Chen & Huang (1988) considered the problem of matching 3-D point features of objects observed at two different times. This is a problem which is encountered in mobile robot navigation where the task is to segment those objects that move relative to each other and to identify the corresponding points for each object. They used local rigidity constraints to prune the systematic search for matching points. The algorithm begins with an initial partial match and grows the match by pairing points so that the structures of the two matched point sets are congruent. Geometric relationships used between the point sets are distance and angle measurements. The initial match is a pairing of a triplet of non-colinear points in the two images. A match growing procedure is implemented in which an additional point is added to the triplet in one image and a corresponding congruent tetrahedron is searched for in the other image. The growing is continued until no more points can be added, at which stage the next triplet of matching points, not already matched in the previous set, is grown to completion in a similar way. Thus, points belonging to the same object will match in different scenes independently of any relative movement of neighbouring objects. Matching of an additional point to the existing structure is done by distance relationships with a pre-set tolerance on the allowable error in point to point distances. Jagoe *et al.* (1990)

matched point sets in retinal images using a triangular matching procedure. The points were derived from vessel corners and by use of corner attributes such as direction, the combinatorial problem arising from considering all possible comparisons could be contained.

Line matching

Straight-line matching is more likely to be useful when matching scenes from man made environments. Medioni & Nevatia (1984) used an iterative technique to register images that differed only in translation, by using line orientation similarity. Price (1984) matched closed contours, where the contours were composed of straight-line segments. The constraints imposed by neighbouring segments, such as the angles between them, must be consistent between matching contours. McIntosh & Mutch (1988) estimated similarity between line pairs by using a set of eight descriptive features for each line. These included position, length, orientation, width, contrast etc. Matched lines were identified from a 2-D array of between line similarities, provided the matching was above a threshold value. Linking broken-line segments is a required pre-processing step to prevent matching confusion.

Matching bits of the same line that are broken or occluded by relatively large distances can be done using the Hough transform (Rosenfeld, 1969). In this technique, each edge point in an image can be considered as part of a straight line whose parameters (p,q) (perpendicular distance from the origin, and angle) can be estimated. Each edge point can increment a location in the (p,q) space, which is subsequently examined for clusters. Thus all the elements of a broken straight line no matter how far apart, will be located in the same cluster and therefore be detected as belonging to the same line. Cheng & Huang (1984) described a scheme for matching significant edge elements using relational structures. They include symbolic relationships between edge elements such as the concepts parallel and anti-parallel as well as numeric attributes such as distance between line pairs and angles between them.

Shape matching

There is a profusion of literature on the techniques used in shape analysis and shape matching. A review of these techniques can be found in Pavlides (1978). Some more recent techniques of shape matching are mentioned below.

Mitchie & Aggarwal (1983) described a method for registering planar figures using shape-specific points. They demonstrated this by using the centroid- and radius-weighted mean of two planar figures which were transformed with respect to each other by translation, rotation and scaling. The two points in each shape were sufficient to calculate the transformation coefficients. The method, however, is not robust in that it cannot cope with missing boundary segments.

Bhanu & Faugeras (1984) solved the segment-matching problem, which is defined as the recognition of a piece of a shape as an approximate match to a part of a larger shape. They did this using a stochastic labelling technique. Suppose the two shapes to be matched are represented by polygonal approximations. Let $A = (A_1, A_2, \ldots, A_n)$ and $B = (B_1, B_2, \ldots, B_m)$ be the polygonal representations of two shapes with n and m line segments respectfully. In general n is not equal to m. Each segment A_i can be matched with each segment B_j, so that initially each A_i can have m labels. The matching is done on the basis of segment feature values, such as its length and the angles with its neighbours. The initial ambiguous labelling is then updated by comparing the local structure of neighbouring segments and their compatibilities.

Distance measurements have been used to match parts of a boundary to a complete one, or to match two boundaries of approximately the same shape. Given one boundary, the nearest distance from every image pixel to the boundary can be computed. Using the distance image, the second boundary or boundary template, can be overlaid on the distance map such that the sum of the distance measurements along the length of the second boundary is minimum. The problem with this technique is the efficient and accurate computation of the distance map, as calculation of the Euclidean distances is prohibitively expensive. Borgefors (1988) described edge matching using chamfer distance estimators, which can be computed in two passes through the binary feature image. The error difference between the chamfer distances and the true Euclidean distances is acceptably small.

The Hough transform technique for matching straight lines has been extended to find circles (Kimme *et al.*, 1975), ellipses and arbitrary shapes (Ballard, 1981). Lee & Quek (1988) described a further extension of the technique to matching shapes which is both invariant of scale and orientation. It depends on a representation of the boundary using two properties that are both scale and orientation invariant. The first is the angle between two straight lines, the other is the ratio of arc to chord length. Each boundary point on the reference shape is coded by the angle β (Fig. 6) which the tangent at that point makes with a specific chord. The chord is such that it connects the boundary point to the nearest boundary point (in a given direction of traversal) where the ratio of arc length to chord length is equal to a pre-determined value. The angle ϕ which this chord makes to a reference line such as the x-axis is computed. An additional independent angle α between the tangents at the two points is also calculated. A table is then constructed which records for each value of the angle β, the associated pair of angles (α, ϕ). On the input shape, the values of β', α', and ϕ' are computed for each boundary point. For each β' value, the set of (α, ϕ) angle pairs which are found in the table from the reference shape, are compared with the (α', ϕ') angle pair in the input shape. If the angle difference between tangents $|\alpha - \alpha'|$ is less than a pre-defined tolerance, then candidate matching points on the boundaries exist, and the difference between the reference angles $\alpha - \alpha'$ is the possible orientation

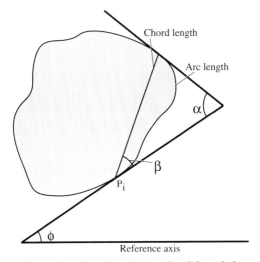

Fig. 6. The ratio of arc length to chord length between two corresponding points on similar shape boundaries is scale and orientation invariant. Given a fixed ratio, for every point p_i on the boundary, the angle β between the chord and the tangent at that point is computed. Additional information such as the angle α between the two tangents enables matching of similar shapes. The angle ϕ which the chord makes with a reference line enables relative orientation of the shapes to be calculated.

difference between the shapes. The most commonly occurring orientation difference found by examining all points on the boundary is obtained and this is the relative orientation between the shapes. This technique is unfortunately sensitive to boundary noise.

Locating a specific shape in a cluster of overlapping known shapes is a task in robotic vision which is frequently encountered in industrial inspection systems. Hong & Wolfson (1988) described a technique which uses local shape signatures (called footprints) that enable comparison between short segments of boundary curves. All the known shapes are scanned and footprints based on the arc length versus turning angle are generated at equally spaced points along the boundary. Each footprint is used as a key to a table where the object and position of the footprint in the object are recorded. In the recognition stage, the boundary curve of the composite scene is scanned and footprints are again calculated at equally spaced points. The table that has been built up from the individually scanned objects is consulted and each object position corresponding to a footprint from the composite image is given an incremental vote. At the end of the process, those object segments that receive most votes are selected and the start and end points of matches between the footprint string of the composite scene and the footprint string of the object are located. The object that has the longest matching sub-curve with the composite image is thus found. The matching part is eliminated from the composite boundary and the process is then repeated for the remaining partial curve in the composite boundary.

Cootes *et al.* (1992) derived a model of a flexible shape from a set of learned examples. By characterizing a typical member of a class of object shapes using boundary landmarks, a mean shape can be derived. Also the modes of variation can be described with a small number of independent parameters. Using this flexible model, an example of the class can be accurately located in the scene given a reasonable initial estimate.

Region based matching

A registration procedure based on features extracted from segmentation has been described by Goshtasby *et al.* (1986). In this method, the centres of gravity of segmented regions are first used as potential control points. Correspondences between these points is then determined by a point-pattern-matching procedure. The regions around corresponding points are then examined and the segmentation procedure for each region is refined until the shapes of the extracted features are optimally matched. Updated centres of gravity can then be measured and these are used to estimate the parameters of the least-squares transformation in the normal manner.

Image re-mapping

Given that a set of corresponding control points have been located and are well spread in the image, the next step is the calculation of the coefficients that enable the registration of any point in one image given its corresponding position in the other. Knowing the required transformation, this is usually done by solving the least squares equations, i.e. minimizing the squared differences between the calculated positions of the transformed control points and their measured positions. The image to be warped is the input image and the resultant image the output image. Calculating the parameters such that every point on the input image is mapped to a new position in the output image will give rise to problems. These arise from the non-integral nature of the resultant points, which must be assigned to integral image positions. Thus two input points may map to a single output point, or an output position may remain unfilled (Fig. 7). The easiest way to overcome this difficulty is to calculate the reverse mapping, that is, for every output image position, calculate the non-integral input image position. The greylevel value of this point, will in general fall between pixels, and can be estimated by various interpolation schemes.

Estimation of the polynomial coefficients

Suppose the transformation is to be done via a pair of polynomials of the form:

$$x' = a_0 + a_1x + a_2y + a_3xy + a_4x^2 + a_5y^2$$

(*a*) Input to output mapping

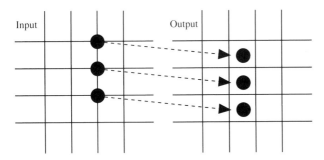

(*b*) Output to input mapping

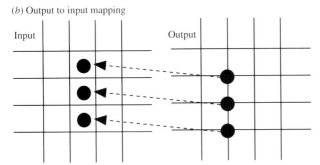

Fig. 7. In (*a*) the pixel positions in the input image are mapped to coordinates in the output image which, in general, will not coincide with output image pixel points. In this case, they could be assigned to the nearest pixel, but this can lead to some output pixels not being filled. A better approach is to map the output pixel positions to input image coordinates as in (*b*). The greylevel of the input coordinates can then be interpolated from the surrounding pixel values.

$$y' = b_0 + b_1 x + b_2 y + b_3 xy + b_4 x^2 + b_5 y^2$$

where (x', y') are the reference image coordinates corresponding to the input image pair (x, y). Given a minimum of six matching pairs, the coefficients a_0 ... a_5 and b_0 ... b_5 can be calculated such that the sum of squares of the distances between mapped input points and their corresponding reference points is minimum. If:

$$X = [x_1, x_2, \ldots, x_n]^T \text{ and } Y = [y_1, y_2, \ldots, y_n]^T$$

are the vectors of input column and row coordinates and M is the matrix of polynomial terms formed from the reference image coordinates as in:

$$M = \begin{bmatrix} 1 & x'_1 & y'_1 & x'_1 y'_1 x'^2_1 & y'^2_1 \\ 1 & x'_2 & y'_2 & x'_2 y'_2 x'_{22} & y'_{22} \\ 1 & x'_3 & y'_3 & x'_3 y'_3 x'_{32} & y'_{32} \\ & \cdots & & & \cdots \\ 1 & x'_n & y'_n & x'_n y'_n x'^2_n & y'^2_n \end{bmatrix}$$

then the coefficients $A = [a_0, a_1, \ldots, a_5]^T$ and $B = [b_0, b_1, \ldots, b_5]^T$ are given by:

$$A = (M^T M)^{-1} M^T X$$
$$B = (M^T M)^{-1} M^T Y$$

Given A and B, each control point in the input image can be mapped to its corresponding point in the reference image. The Euclidean distance between a mapped point and its corresponding reference point is called the residual. The mean value of the residuals is an estimation of the goodness of fit. Sometimes one or two residuals may be significantly larger than the rest. A common strategy is to remove point pairs with high residuals and recalculate the coefficients from the remaining pairs. This can be repeated iteratively until all residuals fall below a threshold distance.

Image resampling

The easiest and quickest way to map output coordinates to non-integer input positions is to select the greylevel of the nearest neighbour. This is not a very satisfactory solution in practice. A more acceptable method is to estimate its value by bi-linear interpolation, using the pixel values of the four nearest neighbours. At the price of further computation, more sophisticated re-sampling schemes can be used. These have higher theoretical accuracy and will preserve the original resolution better. One such method is cubic convolution, which uses two cubic polynomials to define the weights given to the surrounding points. Using 16 surrounding pixel values, good results can be achieved (Shlien, 1979).

Local registration methods

Sometimes the above matching schemes are not appropriate, because the distortions between the images are of a more local nature. The least squares method with a global transformation function registers images by minimizing a global measure and does not have any local control over the registration process. One approach to this problem is to to use polynomials which are defined locally. A set of coefficients are computed at each grid point using a weighted least squares fit to the neighbouring control points, giving more weight to the nearest neighbours. The computation is similar to the calculation of the coefficients given above with the addition of a weighting matrix, which weights a control point according to its inverse distance to the grid point, making sure that very close points do not have weights approaching infinity. The computational overhead is considerable, but good results can be obtained by this method. A variant of this gives zero weights to points which are farther than a threshold value from the local grid point.

Surface splines can be used to model local 'rubber sheet' deformations more accurately than polynomials (Goshtasby, 1988). Goshtasby (1986) described a scheme for piecewise linear mapping of triangular areas in two images. The corresponding control points were used to generate triangular regions in both images. Corresponding triangles were then used to calculate the local trans-formation parameters within each triangle. Registration parameters at a point were determined from a linear interpolation of registration parameters at its three nearest control points.

Accuracy of registration

The accuracy of registration procedures that use control points can sometimes be roughly assessed by how far the registered control points are mapped from the real points. However this is not a good way of measuring accuracy because the residual errors can be made as small as desired by choosing a suitable mapping function. Corresponding point pairs in the images, other than those used to generate the transformation, need to be compared. A visual check can be made by displaying the difference image. Fig. 8 shows the difference image of two circular discs misregistered by half a pixel in the x and y directions.

The accuracy of registration of two images may be assessed on a statistical basis by locating several corresponding point pairs in several small regions throughout the image (Niblack, 1986). If the observed error in a correspond-ence is assumed to be the sum of the registration error plus the measurement error, and these are assumed to be uncorrelated, then using the statistical

Fig. 8. The difference image obtained by subtracting the images of two disks which are misregistered by half a pixel in the x and y directions.

technique of analysis of variance, it is possible to make estimates for the registration error. This makes the reasonable assumption that the registration error will be constant within each of the small regions.

Conclusion

Despite the volume of work published on registration of images, there is as yet no universal method which can be applied in all circumstances. Where automatic methods can be applied, they are usually more accurate than manually assisted methods. Nevertheless, in many cases, the registration must be done in a manual or semi-interactive way, with the user supplying the control points either directly or at least indirectly by indicating the neighbourhood of an optimum match. Under these circumstances, it is essential that the computer interface provides the best possible environment to the user allowing the flexibility to edit out existing pairs or add new ones after inspection and evaluation of the results.

References

Arun, K. S., Huang, T. S. & Blostein, S. D. (1987). Least squares fitting of two 3-D point sets. *IEEE Transactions on Pattern Analysis and Machine Intelligence*, **PAMI-9**, 698–700.

Ballard, D. H. (1981). Generalizing the Hough transform to detect arbitrary shapes. *Pattern Recognition*, **13**, 111–12.

Barnea, D. I. & Silverman, H. F. (1972). A class of algorithms for fast digital image registration. *IEEE Transactions on Computers*, **C-21**, 179–86.

Benny, A. H. (1981). Automatic relocation of ground control points in Landsat imagery. In *Proceedings of the 9th Annual Conference of the Remote Sensing Society on Matching remote sensing technologies and their applications*. London: Remote Sensing Society.

Bhanu, B., & Faugeras, O. D. (1984). Shape matching of two-dimensional objects. *IEEE Transactions on Pattern Analysis and Machine Intelligence*, **PAMI-6**, 137–56.

Borgefors, G. (1988). Hierarchical chamfer matching: a parametric edge matching algorithm. *IEEE Transactions on Pattern Analysis and Machine Intelligence*, **PAMI-10**, 849–65.

Brandle, K. (1989). A new method for aligning histological serial sections for three-dimensional reconstruction. *Computers and Biomedical Research*, **22**, 52–62.

Capowski, J. J. & Sedivec, M. J. (1981). Accurate computer reconstruction and graphics display of complex neurones utilizing state-of-the-art interactive techniques. *Computers and Biomedical Research*, **14**, 518–32.

Chen, H. H. & Huang, T. S. (1988). Maximal matching of 3-D points for multiple-object motion estimation. *Pattern Recognition*, **21**, 75–90.

Cheng, J. K. & Huang, T. S. (1984). Image registration by matching relational structures. *Pattern Recognition*, **17**, 149–59.

Cootes, T. F., Taylor, C. J., Cooper, D. H., Graham, J. (1992). Training models of shape from sets of examples. *Proceedings of British Machine Vision Conference*, **92** (in the press).

Faugeras, O. D. & Herbert, M. (1986). The representation, recognition and location of 3-D objects. *International Journal of Robotics Research*, **5**, 27–52.

Fischler, M. A. & Bolles, R. C. (1981). Random sample consensus: A paradigm for model fitting with with application to image analysis and automated cartography. *Communications of the ACM*, **24**, 381–95.

Fitzpatrick, J. M. & Leuze, M. R. (1987). A class of one-to-one two-dimensional transformations. *Computer Vision, Graphics and Image Processing*, **39**, 369–82.

Garret, G. S., Reagh, E. L. & Hibbs, E. B. (1976). Detection threshold estimation for digital area correlation. *IEEE Transactions on Systems Man and Cybernetics*, **SMC-1**, 65–70.

Gaunt, P. M. & Gaunt, W. A. (1978). *Three-Dimensional Reconstruction in Biology*. Tunbridge Wells, Kent: Pitman Medical Publishing.

Geiser, E. A., Lupkiewicz, S. M., Christie, L. G., Ariet, M., Conetta, D. A. & Conti, C. R. (1980). A framework for three-dimensional time-varying reconstruction of human left ventricle: sources of error and estimation of their magnitude. *Computers and Biomedical Research*, **13**, 225–41.

Gordon, M. R. (1981). Ground control pointing of the UK. In *Proceedings of the 9th Annual Conference of the Remote Sensing Society on Matching remote sensing technologies and their applications*. London: Remote Sensing Society.

Goshtasby A. (1985). Template matching in rotated images. *IEEE Transactions on Pattern Analysis and Machine Intelligence*, **PAMI-7**, 338–44.

Goshtasby, A. (1986). Piecewise linear mapping functions for image registration. *Pattern Recognition*, **19**, 459–66.

Goshtasby A. (1988). Image registration by local approximation methods. *Image and Vision Computing*, **6**, 255–61.

Goshtasby, A., Gage, S. H. & Bartholic, J. F. (1984). A two-stage cross correlation approach to template matching. *IEEE Transactions on Pattern Analysis and Machine Intelligence*, **PAMI-6**, 374–8.

Goshtasby, A. & Stockman, G. C. (1985). Point pattern matching using convex hull edges. *IEEE Transactions on Systems, Man and Cybernetics*, **SMC-15**, 631–7.

Goshtasby, A., Stockman, G. C. & Page, C. V. (1986). A region-based approach to digital image registration with subpixel accuracy. *IEEE Transactions on Geoscience and Remote Sensing*, **GE-24**, 390–9.

Hall, D. J., Endlich, R. M., Wolf, D. E. & Brain, A. E. (1972). Objective methods for registering landmarks and determining cloud motions from satellite data. *IEEE Transactions on Computers*, **C-21**, 768–76.

Hill, D. G. L., Hawkes, D. J., Crossman, J. E., Gleeson, M. J., Cox, T. C. S., Bracey, E. E. C. M. L., Strong, A. J., & Graves, P. (1991). Registration of MR and CT images for skull base surgery using point-like anatomical features. *British Journal of Radiology*, **64**, 1030–5.

Hong, J. & Tan, X. (1988). A new approach to point pattern matching. In *Proceedings IEEE International Conference on Pattern Recognition*, pp. 82–4.

Hong, J. & Wolfson, H. J. (1988). An improved model-based matching method using footprints. In *Proceedings IEEE International Conference on Pattern Recognition*, pp. 72–8.

Hu, M-K. (1962). Visual pattern recognition by moment invariants. *IRE Transactions on Information Theory*, **IT-8**, 179–87.

Ip, H. H-S. (1983). Detection and three-dimensional reconstruction of a vascular network from serial sections. *Pattern Recognition Letters*, **1**, 497–505.

Jagoe, R., Blauth C. I., Smith P. L., Arnold, J. V., Taylor, K. & Wootton R. (1990). Automatic geometrical registration of fluorescein retinal angiograms. *Computers and Biomedical Research*, **23**, 403–9.

Kimme, C., Ballard, D. & Sklansky, J. (1975). Finding circles by an array of accumulators. *Communications of the ACM*, **18**, 120–2.

Lee, C-H. & Quek, G. P. (1988). Partial matching of two-dimensional shapes using random coding. In *Proceedings IEEE International Conference on Pattern Recognition*, pp. 64–8.

Leese, J. A., Novak, C. S. & Clark, B. B. (1971). An automated technique for obtaining cloud motion from geosynchronous satellite data using cross correlation. *Journal of Applied Meteorology*, **10**, 18–132.

McIntosh, J. H. & Mutch, K. M. (1988). Matching straight lines. *Computer Vision, Graphics and Image Processing*, **43**, 386–408.

Medioni, G. & Nevatia, R. (1984). Matching images using linear features. *IEEE Transactions on Pattern Analysis and Machine Intelligence*, **PAMI-6**, 675–85.

Mitchie, A & Aggarwal, J. K. (1983). Contour registration by shape-specific points for shape matching. *Computer Vision, Graphics and Image Processing*, **22**, 296–408.

Niblack, W. (1986). *An Introduction to Digital Image Processing*. London: Prentice-Hall International.

Onoe, M. & Saito, M. (1976). Automatic threshold setting for the sequential similarity detection algorithm. *IEEE Transactions on Computers*, C-25, **10**, 1052–3.

Pavlides, T. (1978). A review of algorithms for shape analysis. *Computer Graphics and Image Processing*, **7**, 243–58.

Peli, E., Augliere, R. A. & Timberlake, G. T. (1987). A feature-based registration of retinal images. *IEEE Transactions on Medical Imaging*, **MI-6**, 272–8.

Pelizarri, C. A., Spelbring, D. R., Weichselbaum, R. R., Chen, G. T. Y. & Chen, C. T. (1989). Accurate 3-dimensional registration of CT, PET or MR images of the brain. *Journal of Computer Assisted Tomography*, **13**, 20–6.

Price, K. E. (1984). Matching closed contours. In *Proceedings 7th International Conference on Pattern Recognition*, Montreal, IEEE Computer Society Press, pp. 990–2.

Ranade, S. & Rosenfeld, A. (1980). Point pattern matching by relaxation. *Pattern Recognition*, **12**, 269–75.

Rangarajan, K. & Shah, M. (1991). Establishing motion correspondence. *Computer Vision, Graphics and Image Processing: Image Understanding*, **54**, 56–73.

Rosenfeld, A. (1969). *Picture Processing by Computer*. New York: Academic Press.

Rosenfeld, A. & Vanderberg, G. J. (1977). Coarse-fine template matching. *IEEE Transactions on Systems, Man and Cybernetics*, **SMC-7**, 104–7.

Shlien, S. (1979). Geometric correction, registration and resampling of Landsat imagery. *Canadian Journal of Remote Sensing*, **5**, 74–88.

Smith, E. A. & Phillips, D. R. (1972). Automated cloud tracking using precisely aligned digital ATS pictures. *IEEE Transactions on Computers*, **C-21**, 715–29.

Steiner, D. & Kirby, M. E. (1977). Geometrical referencing of Landsat images by affine transformation and overlaying of map data. *Photogrammetria*, **33**, 41–75.

Stockman, G. C., Kopstein, S. & Benett, S. (1982). Matching images to models for registration and object detection via clustering. *IEEE Transactions on Pattern Analysis and Machine Intelligence*, **PAMI-4**, 229–41.

Svedlow, M., McGillem, C. D. & Anuta, P. E. (1976). Experimental examination of similarity measures and preprocessing methods used for image registration. *Symposium on Machine Processing of Remotely Sensed Data*, **4A**, 9–17.

Taniguchi, Y. & Shiino, M. (1992). Three-dimensional and quantitative observation of the hypertrophy of rat corticotrophs following adrenalectomy. *Cell and Tissue Research*, **267**, 519–23.

Tatsumi, H., Takaoki, E., Omura, K. & Fujita, H. (1990). A new method for three-dimensional reconstruction from serial sections by computer graphics using 'meta-balls': reconstruction of 'hepato skeletal system' formed by Ito cells in the cod liver. *Computers and Biomedical Research*, **23**, 37–45.

Venot, A. Lebruchec, J. F. & Roucayrol, J. C. (1984). A new class of similarity measures for robust image registration. *Computer Vision, Graphics and Image Processing*, **28**, 176–84.

Wang, C-Y., Sun, H., Yada, S. & Rosenfeld, A. (1983). Some experiments in relaxation image matching using corner features. *Pattern Recognition*, **16**, 167–82.

Ware, R. W. & LoPresti, V. (1975). Three-dimensional reconstruction from serial sections. *International Reviews of Cytology*, **40**, 325–440.

West, M. J., & Skytte J. (1986). Anatomical modeling with computer aided design. *Computers and Biomedical Research*, **19**, 535–42.

Wong, R. L. & Hall, E. L. (1978). Image transformations. In *Proceedings 4th International Joint Conference on Pattern Recognition*, Kyoto, pp. 939–942.

Wong, Y. M., Thomson, R. P., Cobb, L. & Fitzharris, T. P. (1983). Computer reconstructions of serial sections. *Computers and Biomedical Research*, **16**, 580–6.

Woods, R. P., Cherry, S. R. & Mazziotta, J. C. (1992). Rapid automated algorithm for aligning and reslicing PET images. *Journal of Computer Assisted Tomography*, **16**, 620–33.

Zahn, C. T. (1974). An algorithm for noisy template matching. In *Information Processing 74*, pp. 698–701, IFIP Congress, Stockholm, Elsevier Science Publishers.

16

Computational haze removal

N . F . CLINCH and V . A . MOSS

Image enhancement and image reconstruction

The familiar techniques of image enhancement take advantage of the psycho-physics of the human visual system to enhance perception of features of interest in an image. For example, the use of pseudocolour and contrast enhancement may make greyscale discrimination easier, and edge detection filters can help visualize discontinuities. Restoration techniques, on the other hand, attempt to make use of knowledge of the physical basis of image degradation to invert the process and restore the original, true image. The image degradation process can be represented as shown in Fig. 1. Mathematic-ally, the observed image, $g(x,y)$, is given by:

$$g(x,y) = \mathbf{H}.f(x,y) + \mathbf{R}(x,y),$$

where $\mathbf{H}$ is a degradation operator,
$\qquad f(x,y)$ is the ideal image and
$\qquad \mathbf{R}(x,y)$ is unwanted noise, for example from the camera.

The point spread function

In order for a reconstruction technique to be successful, a precise description of the image degradation process must be available. This is obtained from the response of $\mathbf{H}$ to the impulse input given by a single point of light in the focal plane: the point spread function, or PSF, denoted by $s(x,y)$. Using this, and assuming the noise factor to be negligible, the observed image is:

$$g(x,y) = f(x,y) * s(x,y),$$

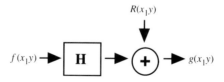

Fig. 1. A model of the image degradation process, after Gonzales & Wintz (1987).

where * represents the convolution operator. The PSF can be measured empirically, or it can be computed from the principles of optics (Gibson & Lanni, 1990; Sheppard & Gu, 1991). Several different methods can then be used to perform the deconvolution which extracts $f(x,y)$ from the observed image $g(x,y)$. All of the practical methods assume that **H** is position invariant in the $x-y$ plane (see, for example, Gonzales & Wintz, 1987; Inoue, 1989).

In-focus point spread

In classical, thin section histology, the microscopic specimen may be thinner than the depth of field of the objective lens (less than 0.5 μm for a high numerical aperture (NA) oil immersion lens, and about 2 μm for a 0.7 NA dry lens). In this case there is no contamination of the image from out-of-focus regions of the specimen, but the optical properties of the microscope still impose constraints on the quality of the final image. In particular, the NAs of the objective lens and condenser determine the highest spatial frequencies which can be transmitted. Fig. 2 shows the way in which transverse resolving power is determined by the NA of the objective. For a general discussion of the use of the PSF to improve the quality of 2-D images see Gonzales & Wintz (1987) and for a discussion of the possibilities of using the computer to overcome the diffraction limits and produce a super-resolving microscope, see Young *et al.*, 1992). Until now however, the use of deconvolution techniques in cell biology and histology has been directed at removing out-of-focus haze in thick section microscopy (Agard, 1984; Agard, Yasushi & Sedat, 1989; Agard & Sedat, 1983; Carrington *et al.*, 1989; Fay, Carrington & Fogarty, 1989;

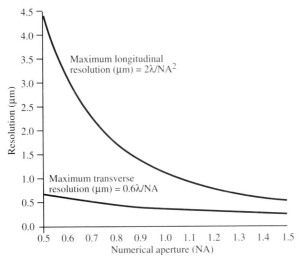

Fig. 2. Relationships between transverse and longitudinal resolving power and numerical aperture. Curves based on equations developed by Born & Wolf (1980).

Carrington, Fogarty & Fay, 1990; Kam *et al.*, 1991; Monck *et al.*, 1991; Paddy & Chelsky, 1991; Waybill *et al.*, 1991; Clinch *et al.*, 1992; Monck *et al.*, 1992).

Out-of-focus point spread

If a thick, say 2 to 50 μm, specimen is set up on the stage of a conventional wide field microscope and the focusing mechanism is stepped along the longitudinal (z) axis, a series of video images can be obtained. These can be used to create 3-D images (see below), but the result will almost always be disappointing. Especially when viewed from the side, the volume dataset will appear very blurred and may display little detail. This is because light that enters the aperture of the objective lens comes from throughout the whole thickness of the specimen; almost all the light arriving at the image plane comes from levels above and below the focal plane of the objective. Hence any individual slice image will always be heavily contaminated with information from neighbouring focal planes. While reducing this signal-to-noise problem is the main function of the confocal microscope (Sheppard, 1987), similar results can be obtained by performing a 3-D deconvolution.

The simplest of the purely computational strategies for out-of-focus haze removal is the Nearest Neighbour Algorithm (NNA) introduced by Castleman (1979: see also Agard & Sedat, 1983; Agard, 1984; Agard *et al.*, 1989; Yelamarty *et al.*, 1990). Castleman pointed out that neglecting the contribution of all the data slices except those on either side of the image in question simplifies the deconvolution calculation without a significant loss in the quality of the final reconstructed image. Otherwise the process is made computationally expensive by the complexity of the 3-D PSF. To quote Agard (1984), discussing the different approaches to solving the deconvolution problem, 'It is important to note that even the simplest of the methods (the NNA) produces a substantial improvement and is suitable for all but the most demanding applications, with results roughly comparable to the MRC Lasersharp confocal microscope'.

This discussion is restricted to the NNA, since the algorithm is now available in a convenient commercial package, MicroTome, for use in desktop computers or in Unix workstations. MicroTome is designed to make use of an array processor board in an IBM standard personal computer. The software is capable of processing three 512×512 images to produce a single reconstructed image in five seconds. It can accept the user's measured PSF or can compute one based on the assumption of an aberation-free objective.

The process which is used to reduce out-of-focus blur can be summarized as follows:

$$f_j = g_j - k\{g_{j-1} \oplus s_{j-1} + g_{j+1} \oplus s_{j+1}\},$$

where f and g have the same meaning as before,

    k is the haze removal factor,

⊕ represents the process of convolution,

s represents a 2-D PSF abstracted from the overall 3-D PSF and the subscripts refer to the three individual images.

The haze removal factor, k, can be adjusted interactively by the user to any value in the range 0–1. It has been called the virtual pinhole as it acts in a way analogous to the pinhole aperture of the CSLM. Increasing the value of k is like reducing the pinhole diameter and improves resolution in the final image while decreasing its dynamic range (brightness). A feature of the MicroTome package is that the user can interactively amplify the incoming images before the deconvolution, so as to compensate for loss in brightness of the final image (Kesterson & Richardson, 1991).

Out-of-focus blur removal using the NNA

The NNA is most often used in wide field fluorescence microscopy, but as shown in Fig. 3 it can often be usefully applied to conventional transmission microscopy as well. Use of the NNA requires that at least three equally spaced images are acquired along the optical axis of the microscope. Fig. 3 and Plates 5 and 6 show examples of the improvement in image quality given by NNA

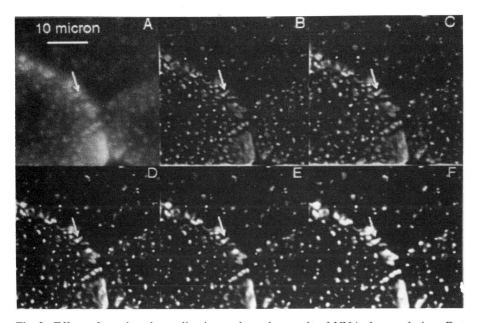

Fig. 3. Effect of varying the z-slice interval on the result of NNA deconvolution. Rat cerebral cortex with mitochondrial stain. Approximately 25 μm section. Transmitted light. Inverted greyscale images. NA 1.2, calibration bar shows 10 μm. (A) original image, (B)–(F) same image deconvolved with two neighbours at 0.5, 1, 2, 3 and 4 μm z-interval respectively. Note excessive contrast and loss of fine detail beginning at dz 3 μm. (Data courtesy of Dr N. Spurway, Glasgow University).

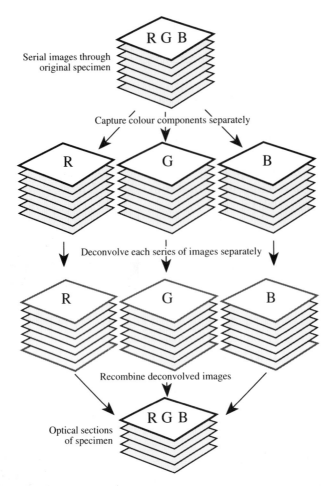

Fig. 4. Deconvolution of colour images using separate series for each of the colour components. Note that the NNA algorithm uses the sections above and below the section being deconvolved, so the final reconstruction contains two fewer sections than the original series.

deconvolution. In every case, the image on the right is computed from three video images, of which the centre one is shown at the left of the Figure. Fig. 3 shows the effect of changing the inter-slice spacing, which must be chosen with reference to the NA of the objective lens. It is important in practice that the spacing should not be too great. If the slice separation is much greater than the axial resolving power (shown in Fig. 2), the quality of the reconstructed image will often not be satisfactory and it may be preferable to use image enhancement techniques to improve image contrast (see, for example, Kam *et al.*, 1991). Oversampling, on the other hand, has little effect on the final image. A slice interval of half the axial resolution is optimum in most cases. For a useful discussion of slice spacing in volume microscopy, see Wilson & Sheppard (1984).

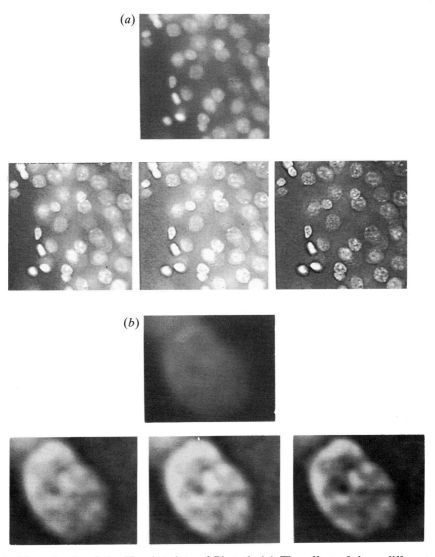

Fig. 5. More details of the Hoechst data of Plate 6. (*a*) The effect of three different settings of the haze removal factor; (*b*) the same thing after zooming to a single nucleus at the top left of (*a*).

Deconvolution in true colour

Colour is an essential feature of much of light microscopy. The original confocal microscope with a spinning Nipkow disc (Boyd, 1985; Petran *et al.*, 1985) can be used directly to visualize and record colour optical sections. Providing the disc contains a sufficient number of holes, adequate spatial resolution can be obtained. Whilst early models of the tandem scanning confocal microscope used a mercury arc light source, which produced poor colour balance, a xenon arc is now used, which gives good colour rendering.

Laser scanning microscopes can be fitted with two or three separate lasers for the colour components (Cogswell *et al.*, 1992). However these systems present formidable technical difficulties in operation and require great skill to align the components of the image. Deconvolution can be applied to colour images, by separately processing the colour components of the video signal (Moss, 1992). This is most easily done by capturing the images using a microscope fitted with a good quality, three chip CCD camera to generate separate red, green and blue images. Instead of a single series of images through the specimen, three separate series of images are captured for each component colour and each series is deconvolved separately. Recombining the resultant images gives full colour optical sections. Plate 5 shows this method applied to a Masson-stained kidney glomerulus.

Often a histochemical specimen has specific wavelengths which can be recorded separately using interference filters. In principle it is possible to use more than three images to capture the component colours of a histological specimen. For transmitted light, colour images can be captured by using interference filters or a wedge interference filter to give approximately mono-chromatic light at the condenser, then recording the image with a standard monochrome camera. Gelatin dye filters do not normally provide sufficient colour separation. Although using a monochrome camera increases light sensitivity and is cheaper, it is difficult to ensure that the colours are correctly aligned and adjusted for the relative brightness of the different components (colour balance). Image capture may be a particular problem when recording colour images from a dual emission fluorescent image since the images are often of low intensity and a colour camera is much less sensitive than a monochrome camera. Separate images can be recorded using a monochrome CCD camera with filters. Interference filters can be matched to the emission wavelengths and put adjacent to the camera, providing the alignment of the images is not compromised. Plate 6 shows the result of applying this technique to mouse hippocampus labelled with Hoescht stain (blue) and ethidium bro-mide (red).

Deconvolution and 3-D volumetric rendering

It is now becoming possible for biologists to use computers to construct successful images of 3-D microscopical objects. In most situations, this means using software that can create a 3-D display directly from a series of 2-D video images (arrays of colour or brightness values). For the highly complex, cloudy, ill-defined or reticulated structures which are routinely encountered in living cells, it is appropriate to use a method such as the back-to-front alpha blending method described by Drebin and others (Drebin, 1988; Richardson, 1990; Argiro & Van Zandt, 1992). In this method, a series of registered 2-D images, taken at equal intervals along the longitudinal (z) axis of the microscope, is blended according to a table of weighting factors, or alpha values, chosen by the user to define the relative opacities of the different possible intensity values in the original images. As long as an RGB analogue display device is used, the final pseudocoloured image has a possible range of over 16 million colours. 'Alpha renderers' now run on the entire range of computing hardware from the most sophisticated graphics workstations to standard IBM AT and MacIntosh personal computers. The available implementations differ in price, rendering speed, and the sophistication of the user interface. All allow the viewer to control transparency, to select arbitrary rotations of the object and to make movie loops or animations. At the high performance end of the spectrum, the major limitation of alpha blenders is imposed by the bandwidth of the graphics hardware. But alpha blending is not the only way to composite directly video images in order to visualize a 3-D object: several simpler methods are available which are highly effective for some types of data. Examples are the maximum point projection which simply displays the brightest points along the paths of rays cast through the volume from the viewing plane. Another type of ray tracing method is the front-to-back technique in which rays are projected into the object from the viewing plane until a pre-set voxel value is encountered. This method has the advantage of being able to return a z coordinate for each point in the $x-y$ viewing plane, but is little used in microscopy because it is almost useless for rendering images of transparent, particulate, or cloudy objects.

Surface rendering treats the object as set of geometrically describable surfaces, and is useful when the boundaries of the features of interest are clearly defined. Very satisfactory results can sometimes be obtained with complex structures by extracting data from the individual 2-D images (either manually with a graphics tablet or automatically by boundary tracing in a digital image) and then using this 'extracted geometry' to construct 3-D projections of the surfaces of the measured objects. Individual parts can be selected and shown in appropriate plotting modes so that internal detail is not obscured. As a typical example, Plate 7 shows a reconstruction of the spread of orf virus down a hair follicle, digitized automatically from binary images. To avoid obscuring detail the orf virus antigen is shown partially cut away and the hair follicle is plotted in outline. This method takes advantage of the ability of the human nervous system to extract significant structure from what may otherwise be a mass of bewildering detail, for example in tracing the dendrites of a single neuron among its many neighbours.

Deconvolution and the confocal microscope

Out-of-focus blur in thick specimens can be removed by the special optics of the confocal microscope, or by numerical deconvolution as outlined above. The following questions are relevant:

1 How do the results of wide field deconvolution compare with CSLM images?

(*a*)

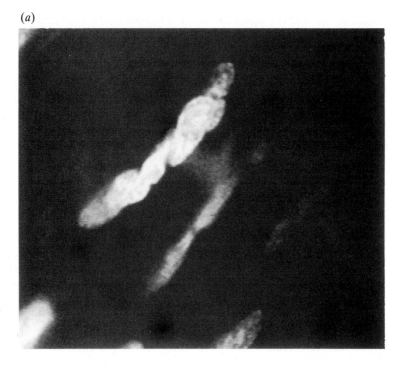

(*b*)

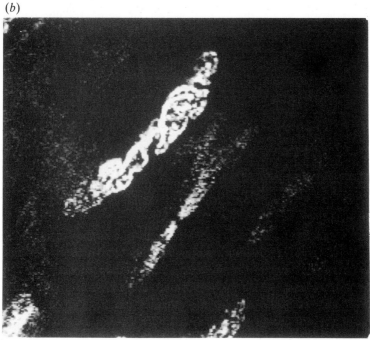

Fig. 6. Nearest neighbour deconvolution of images from a confocal microscope (Noran). The large bright object is a nucleus of an arteriolar smooth muscle cell in rat mesentery, labelled with dihydroethidium. Oil immersion objective (× 60, NA 1.4), *z*-slice interval 0.5 μm. (*a*) Before, and (*b*) after NNA deconvolution.

2 Can confocal images be further improved by subsequent PSF deconvolution?

Several authors have addressed the first question (see Agard, 1984; Carrington *et al.*, 1989; Carrington *et al.*, 1990). All agree that deconvolution is capable of giving results equivalent to, and in some cases superior to, the confocal microscope. According to Ghislain & Webb (1991), the improvement in effective transverse resolution given by the NNA approaches that of the BioRad CSLM. Shaw & Rawlins (1991) found that optimum results were given by a constrained iterative deconvolution operating on data provided by a low noise, cooled CCD camera. In this case, more significant detail could be seen in their chromosome images than in confocal images of the same specimen under similar conditions. Shaw & Rawlins went further and applied their deconvolution method to the confocal images themselves, using the measured PSF of the CSLM, and found that a further improvement in image quality was obtained. A greater improvement followed deconvolution of wide pinhole data than could be achieved by simply closing down the pinhole alone. The result of applying the NNA to confocal data is illustrated in Fig. 6, which shows in (*a*) one of a series of confocal optical slices through a smooth muscle nucleus made with the Noran LSM, and in (*b*) the same slice after deconvolution. It is clear that deconvolution can be usefully applied to enhance image quality, just as in wide field microscopy, as long as the slice interval is kept below the 'optical thickness' of the confocal sections.

Choice of deconvolution technique

'The NNA is quick, robust, and can give a substantial improvement in image quality. Just as with the confocal microscope, PSF deconvolution is powerless to cope with phase effects due to refractive index differences in the specimen. On the other hand, the much slower constrained iterative method is sometimes capable of producing even better results, provided that an experimentally measured PSF is available and that a suitable camera is used. Current developments focus on improving image aquisition through the use of low noise, calibrated CCD cameras, and improved z-axis driver mechanisms to obtain more accurately sampled data, and on the development of appropriate techniques for obtaining reliable point spread functions. At present the high speed and reliability of the NNA continue to ensure that this method is the most widely used for routine computational out-of-focus haze removal.

References

Agard, D. (1984). Optical sectioning microscopy: cellular architecture in three dimensions. *Annual Reviews in Biophysics and Bioengeering*, **13**, 191–219.
Agard, D. & Sedat, J. W. (1983). Three-dimensional architecture of a polytene nucleus. *Nature*, **302**, 676–81.

Agard, D., Yasushi, H. & Sedat, J. (1989). Three-dimensional microscopy: image processing for high resolution subcellular imaging. In *New Methods in Microscopy and Low Light Imaging*, ed. J. Wampler, pp. 24–30, Proceedings of SPIE.

Argiro, V. & van Zandt, W. (1992). Voxel rendering. *Byte*, **17**, 177–82.

Born, A. M. & Wolf, R. (1980). *Principles of Optics*. New York: Pergamon Press.

Boyd, A. (1985). The tandem-scanning reflected light microscope. *Proceedings of the Royal Microscopical Society*, **20**, 130–9.

Castleman, K. R. (1979). *Digital Image Processing*, pp. 347–79. Englewood Cliffs, NJ: Prentice-Hall.

Carrington, W. A., Fogarty, K. E., Lifschitz, L. & Fay, F. S. (1989). Three-dimensional imaging on confocal and wide-field microscopes. In *The Handbook of Biological Confocal Microscopy*, ed. J. Pawley, pp. 137–46. Madison: IMR Press.

Carrington, W. A., Fogarty, K. E. & Fay, F. S. (1990). 3D fluorescence imaging of single cells using image restoration. In *Noninvasive Techniques in Cell Biology*, pp. 53–72. New York: Wiley-Liss Inc.

Clinch, N. F., Daly, C. J., Gordon, J. F., Moss, V. A. & Spurway, N. C. (1992). Wide-field volume visualisation of thick microscope sections by computed nearest neighbour deconvolutions. *Journal of Physiology (London)*, **3P**, 452.

Cogswell, C. J., Hamilton, D. K. & Sheppard, C. J. R. (1992). Colour confocal reflection microscopy using red, green and blue lasers. *Journal of Microscopy*, **165**, 103–17.

Drebin, A. (1988). 3D volume rendering. *Computer Graphics* (Proc. SIGGRAPH '88) **22**, 65–74.

Fay, F. S., Carrington, W. & Fogarty, K. E. (1989). Three-dimensional molecular distribution in single cells analysed using the digital imaging microscope. *Journal of Microscopy*, **153**, 133–49.

Gibson, S. F. & Lanni, F. (1990). Measured and analytical point-spread functions of the optical microscope for use in 3D optical sectioning microscopy. In *Optical Microscopy for Biology*, ed. B. Herman & K. Jackobson, pp. 109–19. New York: Wiley.

Ghislain, L. P. & Webb, W. W. (1991). Comparison of optical sectioning by confocal microscopy (LSCM) and widefield image processing. (abstr) *Biophysics Journal*, **60**.

Gonzalez, R. C. & Wintz, P. (1987). *Digital Image Processing*. Reading, MA: Addison-Wesley.

Inoue, S. (1989). *Video Microscopy*. New York: Plenum.

Kam, Z., Minden, J. S., Agard, D. A., Sedat, J. W. & Leptin, M. (1991). Drosophila gastrulation:analysis of cell shape changes in living embryos by three-dimensional flourescence microscopy. *Development*, **112**, 365–70.

Kesterson, J. & Richardson, M. (1991). Confocal microscope capability with desktop affordability. *Advanced Imaging*, **6**, 23–8.

Monck, A., Oberhauser, T., Keating, J. & Fernandez, J. M. (1991). Confocal ratiometric calcium images measured using fura-2 and a conventional epifluorescence microscope. *Biophysical Journal*, **59**, 378–85.

Monck, A., Oberhauser, T. Keating, J. & Fernandez, J. M. (1992). Thin-section ratiometric Ca^{2+} images obtained by optical sectioning of fura-2 loaded mast cells. *Journal of Cell Biology*, **116**, 745–69.

Moss, V. A. (1992). Digital deconvolution of colour images. *Proceedings of the 4th Amsterdam Confocal Microscopy Conference*, March 1992.

Paddy, M. R. & Chelsky, D. (1991). Spoke: a 120-kD protein associated with a novel filament structure on or near kinetochore microtubules in the mitotic spindle. *Journal of Cell Biology*, **113**, 161–71.

Petran, M., Hadravsky, M., Benes, J. & Kucera, R. (1985). The tandem scanning reflected light microscope. *Proceedings of the Royal Microscopical Society*, **20**, 120–9.

Richardson, M. (1990). Confocal microscopy and 3D visualisation. *American Laboratory*, **35**, 19–24.

Shaw, P. J. & Rawlins, D. J. (1991). The point-spread function of a confocal microscope: its measurement and use in deconvolution of 3D data. *Journal of Microscopy*, **163**, 151–65.

Sheppard, C. J. R. (1987). Scanning optical microscopy. *Advances in Optical and Electron Microscopy*, Vol. 10. ed. R. Barer & V. E. Cosslett, pp. 1–98. London: Academic Press.

Sheppard, C. J. R. & Gu, M. (1991). Approximation to the 3D optical transfer function. *Journal of the Optical Society of America*, **6**, 692–4.

Waybill, M. M., Yelamarty, R. V., Zhang, Y., Scaduto, R. C., LaNoue, K. F., Hsu, C-J., Smith, B. C., Tillotson, D. L., & Cheung, J. Y. (1991). Nuclear calcium gradients in cultured rat hepatocytes. *American Journal of Physiology*, **261**, E49–E57.

Wilson, T. & Sheppard, C. J. R. (1984). *Theory and Practice of Scanning Optical Microscopy*. New York: Academic Press.

Yelamarty, R. V., Miller, B. A., Scaduto, R. C., Yu, F., Tillotson, D. L. & Cheung, J. Y. (1990). Three dimensional intracellular calcium gradients in single human burst-forming units-erythroid-derived erythroblasts induced by erythropoietin. *Journal of Clinical Investigation*, **85**, 1799–1809.

Young, M. R., Jiang, S. H., Davies, R. E., Walker, J. G., Pike, E. R. & Bertero, M. (1992). Experimental confirmation of super-resolution in coherent confocal scanning microscopy using optical masks. *Journal of Microscopy*, **165**, 131–8.

17

Computer based 3-D models of biological structures

M. J. COOKSON and W. F. WHIMSTER

Introduction

The advent of computerized systems for capture of images from a wide variety of detection systems has lead to an explosion in the multidimensional structural and functional information now available. The data used as a basis for 3-D modelling may be physical, actual slices of an organ viewed with the naked eye, for example. It may be digitized sequences of 2-D image datasets obtained by computerized tomography (CT) scanning, positron emission tomography (PET), or magnetic resonance imaging (MRI). The data may be microscopic structures visualized by conventional or electron microscopy captured as photographs or drawings or derived in digital form directly from the machines. The development of confocal scanning laser microscopy (CSLM) has provided a rich source of 3-D datasets.

Given the enormous amount of such information there is a need to identify the methods by which it can be most easily and effectively processed, summarized and displayed. In this chapter, we describe the process of constructing 3-D models of biological objects from serial section data of various kinds. Numerous pitfalls make the creation of such models difficult. These problems arise at all stages of the process and so it is necessary to examine all aspects of model creation from the production of sections to the final construction of a 3-D representation.

The complexities of display techniques for 3-D models are dealt with in Chapter 18.

Types of models of biological structures

There are different types of models which can be created from serial sets of 2-D data forming 3-D datasets. Physical models were popular in the 19th century and in the early part of this century. Such models have proved useful even in recent years (Werner & Morganstern, 1980; Augustine, 1981). They are, however, very time consuming to prepare and difficult to create and amend. Two types of general models based on serial section data are possible:

surface models and volume models. Surface models create a surface which covers sampled data points. Volume models consist of representations of the volume of material between adjacent slices. For physical models both methods have significant problems. Volume models allow very limited visualization of internal structures, and surface models, based for example on drawn outlines, are often extremely confusing. A summary of methods available largely in the pre-computer era is given by Gaunt & Gaunt (1978).

Serial section production

The successful creation of 3-D models of biological structures from serial section data is critically dependent on the quality of serial sections produced. It is at this stage that many 3-D modelling projects fail. Most workers producing 2-D sections concentrate on the fidelity of 2-D images. It is only when 3-D relationships between stacked adjacent sections are studied that limitations of sectioning technologies and the technical skills of section producers become apparent.

Problems of physical sectioning

The process of physically sectioning objects creates several potential sources of error that non-destructive sectioning (using scanning systems) avoids. Unfortunately the production of the appropriately sectioned biological material to be reconstructed generally remains a slow, laborious process.

In a whole organ, serial slicing may readily reveal the structure and allow reconstruction without difficulty. However, if the structure has to be found and removed from within an organ, identifying the correct orientation and slicing procedure may be difficult. Section cutting technology imposes size limitations and it may be particularly difficult to ensure that the whole of the structure is within the tissue sample.

An important decision is in choosing the plane in which sections are to be made. If physical sectioning is to be the basis for the reconstruction, the plane is generally chosen which is likely to give the most sections. This choice may, however, be inappropriate if the orientation chosen increases the difficulties of constructing the 3-D model. This can occur where reconstruction of the image in one plane is a more complex task than in another. To reconstruct a structure consisting of a sequence of simple closed outlines is easier than unifying multiple discrete structures into a single one.

With techniques such as CT scanning, where sectioning is non-destructive, sections in different orientations can be produced to assess the best orientation for serial section production. A further factor which may affect the choice of orientation for the serial sections is the sampling resolution achievable. In all the sectioning methodologies discussed, the overall sampling frequency is generally limited by the section thickness, i.e. the sampling frequency along the *z* axis. Ideally the sampling frequency should be the same in all directions. In reality, the sampling frequency attainable in the *x*–*y* plane is usually greater than in the *z*-plane. In this case consideration of the resolution achievable may affect the choice of orientation of the specimen prior to sectioning.

Alignment of slices

To produce a 3-D model it is essential to align the 2-D slices to form a 3-D dataset so that their components have exactly the same relationships they had before slicing took place. Translational misalignment, in the *x* or *y* axes, and rotational misalignment, around the *z* axis, may occur between adjacent slices therefore causing cumulative errors. Intuitive corrections of misalignment (using the eye of the reconstructor) may also lead to errors, for example, reconstructing a tubular structure to be straight and cylindrical by injudicious corrections when it is really oblique and irregular.

To overcome these alignment difficulties registration points of various kinds have been proposed, such as holes drilled in the wax or resin (Gough, 1967), possibly using a laser beam (Spacek, 1971), inserted nerve fibres, endogenous structures such as blood vessels (Burston & Thurley, 1957), or cactus spines of the genus Mammillaria (Deverell & Whimster, 1989). For hard tissues, such as teeth or bone, for example, alignment can be ensured by milling parallel v-shaped grooves into the block within which the subject of the investigation is embedded (Kimura *et al.*, 1977).

With the increasing use of electronic image capture in electron microscopy an integrated approach to the generation of 3-D datasets is possible. Bron *et al.* (1990*a*,*b*) have demonstrated the digital processing of electron microscopic images from serial sections that contain laser-created alignment markers. This permits 3-D reconstruction at a depth resolution of 30–40 nm of entire cells for both transmission electron microscopy and scanning transmission electron microscopy. Bron *et al.* (1990*a*,*b*) used computer programs to correct artefacts arising both from the use of scanning transmission electron microscopy (STEM) and from the serial sectioning process to reconstruct automatically the third dimension of the cells. They used a minimum of three reference markers per section using an excimer laser. Their results show that digital processing of electron microscopy (EM) images combined with the laser-created fiducial markers is a powerful tool which will eventually be useable for the routine generation of 3-D EM reconstructions. The results of Hamilton (personal communication) on histological sections and Bron *et al.* (1990*a*,*b*) on EM sections suggest that laser-produced markers will in future play an important role in the generation of accurate 3-D datasets.

For specimens that do not have external markers, internal structures that show little variation in position in adjacent sections may be used. This can be successful if the slices are thin enough that there is a high degree of 'coherence' between adjacent sections. For electron microscopy based reconstruction using thin slices, this may be useful. Equally, where a structure of known shape or little variation is present (e.g. the shaft of femur in a leg reconstruction), this can be used as an alignment guide.

If the sections to be aligned are stored in digital form on the computer it may be possible to align them by using correlation methods or boundary matching, by algorithms that move adjacent sections relative to each other until some acceptability criterion is satisfied. Hibbard & Hawkins (1988) have evaluated two image processing techniques for objective image alignment of digital autoradiograms for 3-D reconstruction. The techniques used were principal axis transformation and cross correlation, of which the latter proved the more effective. Where no form of fiducial markers is available these techniques probably have the best chance of producing good alignment. It is important to realise, however, that the optimum computational alignment scheme will be dependent on the characteristics of the images to be aligned. Completely general methods applicable to all types of data are unlikely to be identified.

The methods described above all assume that distortions are due to misalignment. In practice for soft tissue there may be additional distortion created by the staining or fixation techniques or by the sectioning process due to compression and shearing. Some attempts have been made to deal with these problems but they present formidable difficulties. The effects of artefacts due to histotechnic procedures can be compensated for by recording the section digitally before sectioning and staining and after all the histochemical procedures have been applied. The use of multiple reference points in a grid structure is one approach, calculating for each point on the grid a vector representing the correction to be applied at that point (Laan *et al.*, 1989). Using these vectors and treating the image mathematically as an elastic plate undergoing deformation it is possible to calculate corrections to be applied over the whole image (Durr *et al.*, 1988).

Estimating section separation

Estimating the distance between sections may also be a source of difficulty. Cutting techniques usually cause loss of material and so specific markers need to be incorporated to indicate depth. For soft materials, if the section thickness is known and no sections have been lost, the z parameter can be obtained by summation, i.e. adding the thicknesses of all the slices. This is, however, a dangerous procedure since if thicknesses derived using this method are summed they rarely accurately match the measured object thickness before sectioning. If the dimensions of the unprocessed tissue sample are known, allowances can be made for distortion, compression and tissue loss.

For hard tissues, where alignment is assured by parallel milled grooves as described earlier, a third reference can be provided running diagonally across the block between the two parallel grooves (Fig. 1). Simple trigonometry then allows the calculation of the position of the section in the block (Gillings & Buonacore, 1961).

In some circumstances, for example with sawn or ground sectioning, precise

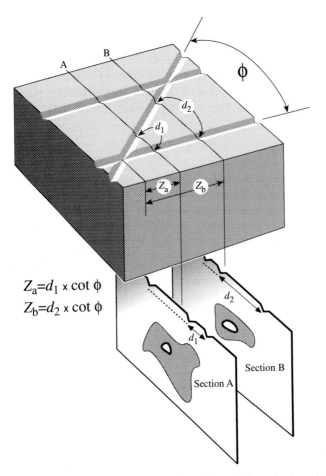

$$Z_a = d_1 \times \cot \phi$$
$$Z_b = d_2 \times \cot \phi$$

Fig. 1. Grooving system used to assess depth in serial sectioning of embedded material.

measurement of the z value is often more difficult. For hard materials which are ground to produce sections, the accuracy of the z variable depends on how accurately the grinding machine can be set. Typically, micrometer settings are used to ensure sufficient accuracy. As a last resort for section material which does not have fiducial markers, estimates or measurements of the thickness of the saw cut may be used to calculate the approximate thickness of the missing material.

Data acquisition for geometric models

In order to produce 3-D reconstructions by computer from the 2-D sections of the object under examination, a 3-D representation must be produced by recording the positions of parts of the object, volumes or surfaces of interest as numerical values or coordinates in 3-D space. Various devices are commonly used to collect digitized data for computer processing.

Digitization of boundaries of structures

For 2-D images of physical sections, especially cut section surfaces, for example those produced by sectioning by grinding away and polishing, the appropriate representation of the structures within the section is the visible edges. In cases where the section thickness is very small in relation to the separation between sections in the z-axis to be used for the reconstruction (i.e. the sampling frequency in the z direction), the 2-D images can be considered as 'true' 2-D representations. From the physical slices, the images of the 2-D slices may be visible through the microscope or in micrographs. With a drawing arm, microscope images can be traced and digitized using a digitizing tablet on which the image is projected. The cursor is used to 'draw' the structures of interest (i.e. to transmit the successive x, y coordinates of the cursor on the tablet to the computer). An effective way of using a digitizing tablet is to make a drawing by tracing around the images on a photomicrograph or projection arm drawing system and then to digitize these drawings. Separation of the identification of the contour from its digitization makes the digitization process less subject to error. It is essential to be able to identify to the system reference points on each slice so that the program can use them to align the slice with respect to reference points on the adjacent slices. A scale is needed if measurements are to be made.

The use of projection drawing systems is prone to error since the outlines are often faint and may be difficult to follow. Micrographs may be captured into the computer system using a video camera with a framegrabber card which records the image the camera acquires, typically with a 256×256 or 512×512 pixel resolution. Each image has to be accurately aligned prior or subsequent to capture. For quantitative work the characteristics of the camera and imaging system should be determined so that allowance can be made for instrumental errors. With micrographs, cameras and projection drawing systems there may be distortion at the edges of the field due to barrel or pincushion distortion in the optical system. These errors can be avoided by using a digitizing microscope (Dykes & Clement, 1980), which uses cross hairs in the centre of the field of view to define the points to be digitized thereby avoiding problems due to optical distortion.

In general there are two methods of data entry: 'horizontal' data entry, in which all the components on a slice are put in before moving on to the next slice, and 'vertical', in which each component must be followed through the slices individually. In the former either the model creation program makes assumptions about which components are connected or it does not use continuity between adjacent sections in the creation of the model. In what may be termed 'longitudinal' data entry, the operator has to decide which components are connected and how they are to be joined. Checking connectivity by hand is slow, but can exploit the reconstructor's knowledge of the anatomy. Approaches are being made to use mathematical methods to assess connectivity, artificial intelligence techniques, intelligent knowledge based systems, or expert systems for this task. Such research is still in its infancy and it will be some years before it results in practical applications. In more rudimentary modelling systems, structures are composed of separate individual discrete components. Since the continuity of the surface across a sequence of serial sections is not preserved, difficult decisions about the joining of surfaces on adjacent sections are not required. These model creation systems trade off ease of model creation against quality and accuracy of the 3-D model. The most important point concerning data entry is to realise that decisions taken at this stage can critically determine the model creation techniques which may subsequently be applied.

Boundaries derived from images from scanning systems

Contour data can be extracted from scanning systems such as confocal scanning laser microscopes (CSLM), although the extraction of contours presents problems. A major problem is determining the edges in the image. Edges may be extracted from these data as from scanner data by 2-D or 3-D edge detection algorithms, or by manual delineation. The automatic detection of edges in images with a low signal-to-noise ratio can be difficult. Using thresholding to produce bi-level images allows the effects of different threshold values on the accuracy of edge determination to be examined. Edge detection can be performed using Laplacian, Sobel or Roberts filters in two or three dimensions (Gonzalez & Wintz, 1987). Median smoothing allows subjective improvement in the image quality but with loss of edge clarity. Automatic methods for generating contours may be computationally tractable but are subject to failure, particularly when dealing with laminar or complex structures. For these reasons, manual methods such as digitizing tablets are often preferred for data entry. The tracing of the contours from the scanned image by using a graphics tablet allows the user to apply his or her judgement to the location of the boundaries of the objects. Since these boundaries are frequently inadequately represented by changes in adjacent voxel values, this allows the experimenter to use this higher level knowledge of the structures to make meaningful representations of the individual objects. This method is however time consuming.

Model construction for geometric models

Contour based models

The output from digitizing tablets and similar devices is a set of points in 3-D space that represent the boundary of an object. The simplest models representing surfaces use drawn sets of points or boundary lines in 3-D space. These models cannot represent 3-D surfaces adequately no matter how sophisticated the display algorithms used since they have lower dimensionality than the structure being modelled. A better method for modelling surfaces is to use a representation having the same dimensionality as the surface.

The most common method to produce a polygonal model of an object surface uses triangles. A triangulation algorithm is used to reconstruct the surface between adjacent contours in the form of a strip of triangles producing a 3-D surface model of each individual structure. For simple contours the generation of the strip of triangles joining the contours can be completely automated. Difficulties arise where branches and joins between multiple objects are to be created.

The problem of approximating the surface spanning a given set of 3-D points as a polyhedron of triangular faces (known as facetting or triangulation) is important in several computer graphical domains. It has been postulated that the problem of finding the optimum approximation of an object defined by an arbitrary set of 3-D points is intractable. By restricting the distribution of points onto parallel planar closed contours, the connectivity of whose points are defined by their ordering, a variety of solutions which are both optimal and heuristic can be found. Such methods normally terminate when some mathematically defined criterion of acceptability has been fulfilled. Normally such techniques require a heuristic step at the end to improve the triangulation produced.

Fuchs *et al.* (1977) developed the first algorithm applicable to surface construction from planar contours. Their contribution consisted of a method for connecting simple closed contours. It could not however deal with joining multiple contours on adjacent planes, partial contour mappings or open (i.e. non-closed) contours.

Other algorithms have been produced including some that allowed the connection of multiple contours usually with manual intervention. Shantz & McCann (1978) proposed an algorithm which was capable of handling highly branched objects with holes. The resolution of ambiguities occurring in multiple contour cases, however, requires human interaction. As one would expect, and as Shantz states, this is extremely labour intensive. In particular, Shantz cites the case of the set of contours from the Livingstone brain database which required some 80 hours of contour splitting with an interactive cursor.

Shantz's and similar algorithms have a number of serious limitations. They are still unable to handle cases of open contours and partial contour mappings. In addition, in Shantz's case multiple contours on adjacent planes can be joined only when a composite contour can be formed; if not, ambiguities must be resolved by human interactions.

Other attempts on the problem have been made by Ganapathy & Dennehy (1982) and Zyda *et al.* (1987). All these methods provide incomplete resolutions to the problems described earlier. The problem is that no general method of triangulation allows optimal connections to be found by local decision making. A general method of triangulation which is robust and provably correct is therefore needed. Reliable automated triangulation procedures are under development, the most promising of which uses the creation of a 3-D Delaunay triangulation (tetrahedronalization) (Boissonat, 1988). This method produces good triangulations of objects without the limitations of previous methods. However, the method is still dependent upon some coherence between structure in adjacent slices.

Any automated procedure must be based on sufficiently frequent sectioning to resolve ambiguities. If the frequency of sectioning is inadequate, decisions concerning the relationships between features visible in consecutive sections must be made using higher level knowledge of the nature of the structures being modelled. For this reason, although triangulation can be performed automatically, it is essential that provision is made for optional human intervention.

Creation of models based on volume elements

Although the output from scanning systems resembles superficially that of the 2-D images referred to above, it differs in significant ways. The scanned image does not represent a surface because each building block of the image represents the average or integrated intensity of some parameter over a small finite volume of space, a voxel or volume element. Thus the image seen is the 2-D projection of a 3-D volume.

In scanning systems, the sampling frequency in the $x-y$ plane is commonly higher than in the z-direction. To avoid the distortion caused by anisotropy in sampling, interpolation of extra slices may be used to provide models based on cubic elements. Linear interpolation is commonly used to compute these but this may be inaccurate and may not be scientifically justified. Interpolating extra slices in the dataset increases the storage requirements markedly and is, of course, creating fictitious data. However, not interpolating usually results in models that when displayed, give images of poor quality.

Serial section production by scanning systems

The production of serial sections from scanning systems avoids many of the problems with physical slicing. In particular, correct alignment of the image is usually performed automatically. There are, however, some problems with the acquisition of 3-D datasets in this form. The first problem is that the characteristics of signal generation and detection in the scanning system need to be fully understood. For medical imaging systems such as PET, MRI or CT there are well-developed theories describing the nature of the signals and their detection. For confocal laser scanning microscopy there is a less-developed body of theory. For medical imaging, failure to understand the nature of the imaging process can lead to serious errors. The same may be expected to be true for confocal microscopy.

Many factors influence data collection. These include instrumental factors, accurate alignment of optical components, optical distortions in beam scanning systems, bleaching of the specimen and uniformity of scanning. Particularly serious can be loss of signal from deeper regions within the viewed volume of the specimen. Although manipulations can produce perfectly readable 2-D images, this effect is serious for producing accurate 3-D datasets. In generating confocal microscope images the loss of information from regions increasingly deep within the tissue can arise from more than one source (Tanke *et al.*, 1982; Carlsson, 1991; Visser *et al.*, 1991). First, such depth dependent losses can result from the inner filter effect where a progressive reduction in the intensity of the excitatory illumination at lower levels of the section results from the absorption of the illumination by the upper layers. Second, re-absorption of the fluorescent emission from lower layers by the upper layers can result in depth-dependent losses of information. Third, a variety of aberrational effects that result from visualizing media of differing refractive index can cause depth-dependent reductions in both intensity and resolution. When examining fluorescence in thick structures both of the first two effects will play a role in the loss of information with increasing depth. Further, both of these effects will be most apparent in regions where the tissue is most densely packed. Severe and rapid loss of resolution with depth can occur, at depths greater than 50 μm, when samples are visualized with confocal microscopes (Visser *et al.*, 1991) and these losses are almost certainly due to aberration-induced effects (Carlsson, 1991; Visser *et al.*, 1991). However, the most severe losses of this type occur when there is a dramatic alteration in the refractive index of the media through which the light passes. The uncritical creation of 3-D models without consider-ing these problems would be expected to compromise the validity of models of structures deep within the sensed volume. The naive expectation for 3-D imaging of 3-D CSLM datasets was that simple error-free models would be produced. In fact, new problems arise whose significance is only now being understood. This emphasizes the need for a good experimentally verified theory for signal generation, propagation and detection.

Data acquisition for volumetric data

Data arrays derived from scanning systems

Slice data from scanning systems (CT, MRI or CSLM) is usually acquired in the form of arrays of numbers each of which represents the value of a volume element or voxel. The voxels of each slice form a 2-D array of numbers representing the values of some parameter such as absorbance throughout the thickness of a slice. For a single slice with a reasonable resolution of 512×512 voxels, for example, over 250 000 numbers have to be stored. For the number of slices needed to form a 3-D reconstruction, the computer storage require-ments may be considerable, especially for confocal laser scanning microscopy.

Datasets of 10 MBytes to 100 MBytes in size may easily be generated. Since the processing of large volumes of data is computationally intensive, systems to process these data must have large memories, large disk sizes and high-speed processing power. Manipulating these data requires expensive computer systems if results are to be obtained within reasonable time scales.

For systems that base their imaging on the display of collections of voxels, methods for the isolation of the collections of voxels of interest are needed. The process of identifying separate regions is termed segmentation. Numerous algorithms for image segmentation are available, but the problems are formidable and in general far from solved. Segmenting data simply on the values of voxels is not usually sufficient since differences in data values in the image may not accurately reflect the boundaries of structures as identified anatomically.

Quantitative measurements

Two types of quantitative data, surface areas and volumes, are commonly acquired from 3-D models. Calculation of areas and volumes requires a scale and knowledge of slice thickness. The construction of a model of the surface as triangular elements can give good area estimates, although there are pitfalls, notably that in some circumstances increasing the numbers of triangles may result in a less accurate estimate of area (Funnell, 1984; Fahle & Palm, 1983).

A number of methods have been applied for volume measurement of contour-based models. Early methods involved measuring the principal dimensions of the subject to be measured and calculating its volume considering it as an approximation to a standard geometric construct, such as a sphere, ellipsoid or similar object. These approaches have the merit of simplicity and ease of calculation. However the errors can become very large, as much as 40–50%. A more accurate approach is to calculate the area of the object to be measured on adjoining sections, calculate the mean of the two areas and multiply by the distance between the sections and continue this throughout the whole sectioned volume of the structure of interest. The existence of a model of the surface as a collection of triangles suggested a method of obtaining volumes directly by calculating the volumes of the prisms obtained by projecting the triangles onto one of the axes. Commonly the axes were translated in 2-D space so that minimum x and y values of the section were located on the x and y axes. This avoids numerical problems where the dimensions of the object to be measured are small in relation to its x, y coordinate values. A high degree of accuracy (better than 1% error) is obtainable using this method.

It should be noted that the collections of voxels that form one slice from a scanning system represents a digitized image. Taking the scan, and digitizing it, as is frequently done using a digitizing tablet, for example, is a re-digitizing process. As such it may be expected to introduce error. The size of the error depends on the sampling density and the accuracy of estimating the true contour of the object of interest. Re-digitizing scanner data is acceptable only if quantitative assessment of the errors induced is performed.

Conclusion

In the early days, computer based 3-D reconstruction techniques were difficult and time consuming to use. For this reason the production of a 3-D model was sufficient justification for its publication. With current technology, however, computer based 3-D reconstruction techniques are proving to be much quicker, simpler and more widely available. For this reason the biological justification for 3-D reconstruction projects must be sound. If the 3-D reconstruction is intended to improve understanding of 2-D material, then such material should be published with the 3-D model. If the object is to display 3-D datasets adequately, a wide variety of images using different viewing parameters need to be published to give an accurate view of the structure. If the intention is to measure 3-D models they should be published as images together with the quantitative results.

New developments in the automated production of 3-D models by triangulation mean that the speed of model building will be very rapid. Whereas in the past creation of models with voxel based systems had significant advantages of speed, these advantages are likely to disappear. The application of new technology, such as parallel processing systems on simple workstations, will mean that very fast reconstruction and display will be possible. This allows the use of the most significant 3-D cue derivable from 2-D images – the kinetic depth effect. The ability to animate rather than simply view, static images gives by far the most effective cue to 3-D understanding. The publication of such animations is however, at present, problematic.

In most reconstruction projects from physical sections the computer stages, especially the model building, are not the rate-limiting steps. The acquisition of good 2-D sections in appropriate alignment to form a 3-D dataset remains the most difficult and time consuming task.

References

Augustine, J. R. (1981). A lucite plate method for 3-dimensional reconstruction of neuronal populations. *Journal of Neuroscience Methods*, **4**, 63–71.

Boissonat, J.-D. (1988). Shape reconstruction from planar cross sections. *Computer Vision, Graphics and Image Processing*, **44**, 1–29.

Bron, C., Gremillet, P., Launay, D., Jourlin, M., Gautschi, H. P., Bachi, T. & Schupbach, J. (1990*a*). Scanning transmission and computer aided volumic electron microscopy: 3-D modelling of entire cells by electronic imaging. *SPIE Proceedings Biomedical Image Processing*, **1245**, 61–7.

Bron, C., Gremillet, P., Launay, D., Jourlin, M., Gautschi, H. P, Bachi, T. & Schupbach, J. (1990*b*). Three dimensional electron microscopy of entire cells. *Journal of Microscopy*, **157**, 21–35.

Burston, W. R. & Thurley, K. (1957). A technique for the orientation of serial histological sections. *Journal of Anatomy*, **91**, 409–12.

Carlsson, K. (1991). The influence of specimen refractive index, detector signal integration and non-uniform scanning speed on the imaging properties in confocal microscopy. *Journal of Microscopy*, **163**, 167–78.

Deverell, M. H. & Whimster, W. F. (1989). A method of image registration for three-dimensional reconstruction of microscopic structures using an IBAS 2000 image analysis system. *Pathology Research and Practice*, **185**, 602.

Durr, R., Peterhans, E. & Von der Heydt, R. (1988). Correction of distorted image pairs with elastic models. *European Journal of Cell Biology*, Supplement 25, **48**, 85–8.

Dykes, E. & Clement, J. (1980). The construction and applications of an X-Y co-ordinate plotting microscope. *Journal of Dental Research*, (Special Issue D, Part 1), **59**, 1800.

Fahle, M. & Palm, G. (1983). Calculation of surface areas from serial sections. *Journal of Neuroscience Methods*, **9**, 75–85.

Fuchs, H., Kedem, Z. M. & Uselton, S. P. (1977). Optimal surface reconstruction from planar contours. *Communications of the ACM*, **29**, 693–702.

Funnell, W. J. (1984). On the calculation of surface areas of objects reconstructed from serial sections. *Journal of Neuroscience Methods*, **11**, 205–10.

Ganapathy, S. & Dennehy, T. G. (1982). A new general triangulation method for planar contours. *Computer Graphics*, **16**, 69–75.

Gaunt, P. M. & Gaunt, W. A. (1978). *Three-dimensional Reconstruction in Biology*. Baltimore: University Park Press.

Gillings, B. & Buonacore, M. (1961). An investigation of enamel thickness in human lower incisor teeth. *Journal of Dental Research*, **40**, 105–18.

Gonzalez, R. C. & Wintz, P. (1987). *Digital Image Processing*. Reading, MA: Addison-Wesley.

Gough, N. G. (1967). A method for the accurate localisation and orientation of structures studied by the use of serial microscopic structures. *Journal of the Royal Microscopical Society*, **88**, 291–300.

Hibbard, L. S. & Hawkins, R. A. (1988). Objective image alignment for three-dimensional reconstruction of digital autoradiograms. *Journal of Neuroscience Methods*, **26**, 55–74.

Kimura, O., Dykes, E. & Fearnhead, R. W. (1977). The relationship between the surface area of the enamel crowns of human teeth and that of the dentine-enamel junction. *Archives of Oral Biology*, **22**, 677–83.

Laan, A. C., Lamers, W. H., Huijsmans, D. P., Te Kortschot, A., Smith, J., Strackee, J. & Los, J. A. (1989). Deformation-corrected computer-aided three-dimensional reconstruction of immunohistochemically stained organs: application to the rat heart during early organogenesis. *Anatomical Record*, **224**, 443–57.

Shantz, M. J. & McCann, G. D. (1978). Computational morphology: Three-dimensional computer graphics for electron microscopy. *IEEE Transactions in Biomedical Engineering*, **25**, 99–103.

Spacek, J. (1971). Three-dimensional reconstruction of astroglia and oligodendroglia cells. *Zeitschrift für Zellforschung und Mikroskopishe Anatomie*, **112**, 430–42.

Tanke, J., van Oostvelt, P. & van Duijn, P. (1982). A parameter for the distribution of fluorophores in cells derived from measurements of inner filter effect and reabsorption phenomena. *Cytometry*, **2**, 359–69.

Visser, D., Groen, F. A. & Brakenhoff G. J. (1991). Extinction correction in confocal microscopy. *Journal of Microscopy*, **163**, 189–200.

Werner, G. & Morgenstern, E. (1980). Three-dimensional reconstruction of human blood platelets using serial sections. *European Journal of Cell Biology*, **20**, 276–82.

Zyda, M. J., Jones, R. A. & Hogan, P. G. (1987). Surface reconstruction from planar contours. *Computers and Graphics*, **1**, 393–408.

18

Three-dimensional visualization

M. J. COOKSON, R. A. REYNOLDS and
D-C. ABRAMS

Introduction

As discussed in Chapter 17, the same biological structures can be represented in a number of fundamentally different ways, depending on the uses and applications to which the data will be put. In this chapter we analyse methods of visualizing biological structures, in the sense of making the information contained within biological datasets visually accessible to the human observer. The problems of interpreting such datasets are formidable. It is difficult to create in the mind a three-dimensional (3-D) image of an organ after it has been sliced, or a tubular structure that has been opened, or a solid structure that has been serially sectioned, and it is virtually impossible to understand the spatial relationships between components and subunits embedded within these structures. Such mental reconstructions are seriously limited, since their accuracy is not accessible to independent verification or measurement, and the results of these studies are difficult to communicate accurately to others.

Many different types of models (physical, conceptual, or computer) can be created from serial sets of two-dimensional (2-D) data making up one or more 3-D datasets. Physical models were popular in the 19th century and in the early part of this century, and are still created occasionally today (Werner & Morgenstern, 1980; Augustine, 1981). Physical models are time consuming to build and difficult to handle, since they are often large and fragile, and photography of such models does not always provide enough views for the 3-D structure to be fully understood. The need for quantitative measurement of 3-D structures means that conceptual models are inadequate, and mathematical or computer models are the method of choice today.

The central problem of 3-D visualization is to provide realistic 3-D cues in a 2-D image of a 3-D structure. The successful comprehension of the data depends largely on the effectiveness of these visual cues. Three parts to the problem can be identified: producing the computer model; creating the illusion of 3-D using the computer display system; and ensuring that it conveys an accurate understanding of the structure. It is easy to produce models that are

313

inaccurate, or images that are misleading about certain aspects of the model, such as concavity/convexity, surface texture, and detail.

Three-dimensional datasets can generally be visualized in one or more of the following ways:

1 2-D cross-sections through the data can be viewed slice by slice.
2 The entire dataset can be projected onto a single plane, as in conventional radiography.
3 Shaded 3-D images (or more accurately $2\frac{1}{2}$-D images, see below) can be generated using computer graphics techniques.
4 True 3-D images can be created in space.

These approaches are considered in detail in this chapter.

Data acquisition from biological specimens

In biological microscopy, the interpretation of 3-D datasets allows geometrical and spatial parameters of tissues, cells and organelles to be elucidated. Such information is useful in supporting cytochemical (Maure *et al.*, 1990), histological (Muller, 1984) and stereological data (Howard, 1990). The confocal scanning laser microscope (CSLM) has the ability to discriminate against light originating from out of focus specimen planes, coupled with the ability to produce perfectly registered digitized images (Stelzer & Wijnaendts-van-Resandt, 1990). These features result in excellent datasets for 3-D visualization (Sheppard & Cogswell, 1990). The principles of confocal microscopy have been described in Chapter 10; the purpose of this section is to introduce some practical techniques that are useful for 3-D dataset acquisition.

To obtain the maximum benefit from 3-D visualization, the datasets must consist of good quality images. In 2-D microscopy the acceptability of an image may simply be judged by its visual appearance; in 3-D microscopy such a subjective criterion is insufficient for effective visualization. The nature of the dataset is of paramount importance and this depends not only on the acquisition system, but also on the original sample (see Chapter 8). Staining protocols, for example, are appropriate only if they reveal structures of interest, so that many conventional staining protocols may be unsuitable. Thick tissue sections (150 μm) or whole mounts are usually examined with the confocal microscope, and therefore existing microtomy and staining techniques may have to be optimized to contend with these atypical samples.

Owing to selective discrimination in the CSLM, images tend to be significantly reduced in intensity when compared against similar images obtained from conventional fluorescence microscopy. This reduction in brightness must be taken into consideration during sample preparation. The microscopist must also be aware that high intensity staining often augments background fluorescence, which frequently causes problems during 3-D visualization. Under certain conditions the incorporation of anti-fade reagents may be necessary, to retard fluorescence bleaching of the fluorochromes. Such reagents have proved to be invaluable in the field of confocal epifluorescence microscopy. Prior to imaging, the microscope should be adjusted so that the minimum pixel value is just above 0 and the maximum pixel value is just below 255. Employing the full dynamic range of the greyscale (256 greylevels) in this manner improves the signal-to-noise ratio and prevents pixel saturation and resulting distortions. Remapping pixel values to pseudocolours, with the aid of a lookup table, enhances the visualization and is useful for setting the maximum and minimum intensities.

The effectiveness of the CSLM is predicated on its confocal property. For a reflection system, Xiao & Kino (1987) showed that the optical thickness of a slice ($Z_{1/2}$) is given by:

$$Z_{1/2} = \frac{0.45\lambda}{n(1 - \cos(\sin^{-1}(NA/n)))},$$

where λ is the wavelength of the light,
$\quad$ n is the refractive index of the immersion medium and
$\quad$ NA is the numerical aperture of the objective lens.

The imaging system should be as confocal as possible, and therefore all of these factors must be optimized.

Illumination and detector characteristics are highly dependent on the integrity of the optical system. This includes all objects that lie within the optical path, for example, the specimen, the coverslip and the immersion media. The optics of the microscope should be correctly aligned and the back aperture of the objective lens overfilled. In order to minimize aberrations, it is critical that lenses are used under the conditions for which they were manufactured. The immersion medium should be carefully chosen, to avoid mismatches in refractive indices as light propagates through the immersion medium, the mounting medium and the sample (Carlsson, 1991). Visser *et al.* (1992) used fluorescent beads mounted in media of various refractive indices to show how the mismatch can affect axial measurements. They concluded that this anomaly can alter the axial measurement by a factor of 2.5, clearly of great consequence in 3-D visualization and volumetry.

Multidimensional datasets and their manipulation

The field of visualization is concerned with the display, manipulation, and analysis of multidimensional datasets. In most cases, the datasets are 3-D, that is they represent some physical property (such as brightness, colour, or density) measured or computed at discrete points in 3-D space. In other cases the data may represent digitized contours derived from serial sections. A sequence of 3-D (also called volume) datasets acquired at successive time intervals would constitute a four-dimensional (4-D) dataset. Regardless of the dimensionality of the acquired data, in the vast majority of cases (with some exceptions given below) the display and manipulation is carried out via a 2-D computer screen.

As an initial stage in 3-D reconstruction, it is essential to be able to visualize the 3-D data as a sequence of 2-D planes or slices. This allows gross errors in data acquisition to be identified. In many cases, datasets are initially collected in this fashion. The most obvious orientation for the slices is perpendicular to the long axis of the structures of interest, in which case these are called transverse slices. Slices parallel to the long axis are termed longitudinal (or paraxial in the special case of slices that pass through the long axis). Any other slice is termed oblique.

It is possible to acquire data originally sectioned in one set of planes and transform it so that it is oriented as if sliced in another. Such an ability is called multiplanar reformatting. Programs for performing multiplanar reformatting are generally based on linear (or tri-linear) interpolation (Glenn *et al.*, 1975; Herman & Liu, 1977; Rhodes *et al.*, 1980) although methods based on Fourier transforms have been reported. Most multidimensional visualization packages such as Analyze™, SunVision™ and VoxelView™ incorporate multiplanar reformatting capabilities as a matter of course.

Creating the illusion of solidity

A growing number of computer techniques seek to create the illusion of the third dimension. The resulting images are still two-dimensional, in the sense that they are presented to the observer as brightness values at each pixel of a 2-D display. However, the brightness may be used to convey depth information, so they might be classified as 'two-and-a-half dimensional' ($2\frac{1}{2}$-D) images.

Generating depth cues

Several visual cues, both static and kinetic, can be used to create the illusion of three-dimensionality on a 2-D screen. Realistically simulated lighting and surface textures (known collectively as shading) are used to provide strong, static, visual depth cues, intended to give the impression of looking at a photograph of a 3-D scene. Shading can be used to indicate depth or shape of surfaces. Shadow generation can be used to create the impression of depth, surface relief or relative size. Perspective projection rather than orthographic projection gives the effect of recession with distance. It is thus a strong cue of position and size, but is more useful for geometric objects rather than fairly amorphous biological ones. The removal of hidden lines or surfaces when they should be obscured by others provides an indication of the ordering of objects within a scene. However, the creation of each of these cues has a computational cost, which can be high. Some are stronger in effect than others: shadow generation is a less effective cue and can prove confusing, although it has been applied to confocal microscope images (Van der Voort *et al.*, 1989). Some of these cues are mutually reinforcing and considerably enhance image understanding when used together. For biomedical applications, the cues appropriate for photorealistic rendering are rarely appropriate, since the improvement in understanding is not worth the computational expense.

A powerful static cue can be generated by exploiting the binocular nature of the human visual system. If a pair of $2\frac{1}{2}$-D images are generated with a small angular difference in viewpoint (3–12°) and presented one to each eye, the resulting stereoscopy provides an additional and very effective depth cue. Another powerful depth cue is a kinetic one, called motion parallax. This is based on the familiar observation that objects within a 3-D scene change their relative positions as the viewpoint is moved. This is often exploited by depicting rotating or tumbling objects on the computer screen. The combined depth cues from stereoscopic vision and motion parallax are so powerful that helmet-mounted displays (where the stereoscopic views are recomputed dynamically as the wearer moves his or her head) are widely used in the rapidly growing field of virtual reality.

There are other situations where dynamically changing images are appropriate. For example, from a 4-D dataset representing 3-D volumes captured at successive instances in time, movies of dynamically changing 2-D or $2\frac{1}{2}$-D images can be generated. Movies are also used to show the effect of changing one rendering parameter while others are kept constant.

True 3-D images

Although almost all visualization relies on cues incorporated into images presented on a 2-D screen, it is in fact possible to create truly 3-D, space-filling images. Like familiar 3-D objects, such images exhibit motion parallax and can be viewed from different vantage points by more than one person at a time. The interested reader is referred to the article by Budinger (1984) for a comprehensive overview of true 3-D display techniques.

Holograms are the most familiar type of 3-D image, but are usually difficult and time consuming to prepare and awkward to view. Computer generated holograms have been demonstrated (Benton, 1982) but affordable, real time, computer generated holographic output is still a long way in the future.

The varifocal or vibrating mirror (Fuchs *et al.*, 1982) might be described as a 'poor man's hologram'. It consists of a thin, reflecting membrane which is vibrated at a low frequency, often by means of a modified loudspeaker coil. Images presented on a computer screen are reflected off the membrane and synchronized in such a way that the back of the 3-D scene is displayed when the membrane is furthest from the observer, and the front is displayed when the membrane is closest to the observer. By rapidly changing the images the entire scene can be visualized, because of the persistence of vision. Varifocal mirror systems suffer from a number of drawbacks: bandwidth is limited, opaque objects cannot be depicted effectively, and the display can be observed from only a limited number of vantage points. Nevertheless these systems have been sold commercially, with reasonable success.

Stages in the visualization process

Although true 3-D or even 4-D display techniques may become more important in the future, the vast majority of 3-D datasets today are viewed by projection on a 2-D screen.

The first stage in the visualization process is data acquisition. Two basic types of data can be acquired, volume data or contour data. Contour data consist of ordered collections of x, y, z coordinates of points sampled from surfaces in 3-D space. These usually represent the edges of objects (where surfaces intersect the planes of the slices) and are input, for example, by hand-digitizing micrographs or tracing using a digitizing tablet.

Volume datasets can be captured in a number of ways and in several formats, and can even be computed from first principles. Most frequently however, volume datasets arise from properties of real objects that are measured at discrete points in 3-D space, often on a regular x, y, z grid. These measurements might be obtained by physically slicing an object and digitizing data from the slice, from a CSLM, or by using special non-destructive sensors or scanners. For volume data the value of the property measured at each sample point controls the brightness of the corresponding pixel when the slices are displayed. This value is often called the density although some other physical properties (e.g. colour or brightness) may in fact be represented.

Data acquisition is often followed by some slice-by-slice image processing or enhancement. This may be performed to filter the data, expand the contrast, or perhaps re-sample (interpolate) the data points to fit a finer or a coarser grid.

The next stage is to stack the 2-D slices in the correct sequence to form a 3-D dataset, a process referred to as reconstruction. It is essential to ensure that digitized information from each slice is correctly oriented and scaled relative to neighbouring slices. Very frequently, the spacing between the slices is not the same as the spacing of the sample points (pixels) within the slice. This is a potential problem which causes inaccurate volume representation. To overcome this it is imperative that the distance between sample points should be calculated and the $x : y : z$ aspect ratio determined. Armed with this information, it is possible to insert new slices (by interpolation) or to remove pixels in the plane of each slice (by filtering followed by subsampling). These techniques allow the investigator to produce uniformly spaced sample points called voxels (a voxel is the 3-D analogue of a 2-D pixel).

In confocal microscopy the $x : y$ aspect ratio is easily determined and is generally 1:1, however the $x : y : z$ ratio requires a knowledge of the thickness of the optical section ($Z_{1/2}$ in the equation above). This information is usually obtained by measuring the full width at half maximum (FWHM) of the point spread function (Shaw & Rawlings, 1991). The voxel aspect ratio determines whether the dataset should be resized by interpolation or by subsampling. Under ideal conditions the acquired voxel aspect ratio would be 1:1:1 and no resizing would be necessary.

If each slice in the volume is represented by a 2-D array of pixels, then new slices can be created by linear (or higher order) interpolation of the pixels along the z axis between the slices. In this case, interpolation to produce new slices from old is relatively simple. If, however, a different representation has been chosen (e.g. if contour data have been acquired or extracted from 2-D arrays of pixels) then interpolation between the slices can be very difficult. In theory, interpolation is always possible since from a 3-D Delaunay triangulation of the contours, a triangulation of the volume between the slices can always be produced (Boissonat, 1989). In practice, triangulation can produce counter-intuitive results that do not always correspond to the original biological structure. An alternative approach, termed shape based interpolation, has since been developed (Raya & Udupa, 1990). All interpolation schemes require making assumptions about the data between the acquired slices, and assumptions about linear relationships are not scientifically justifiable in general. The greater the amount of interpolation required, the less the reliability of the reconstruction.

Once a 3-D array of voxels has been achieved, further enhancement, together with manipulation, can be applied. These operations come under the heading of scene processing and include 3-D image processing (e.g. low pass, high pass, or median filtering), and sub-regioning (creation of a new, smaller, scene that excludes irrelevant regions of the original scene, typically to reduce storage). Sub-regioning can be very important as the storage space required for 3-D datasets can be very large (20 MBytes to 100 MBytes being not uncommon). For contour data this step is not usually necessary, since comparatively few points are stored.

The next stage in the process is classification, or more generally, segmentation. Segmentation in this context refers to the set of techniques used for classification, identification, and extraction of biological structures of interest. For contour data, segmentation is usually performed either manually or automatically at data entry time, so further action is not needed. For volume data, two types of segmentation can be employed: boundary based, which produces boundary information directly, and region based, which identifies the voxels inside the boundary. Techniques are available to convert between boundary and voxel representation.

One simple form of segmentation which sometimes works well classifies each voxel into one or more material types, based solely on the numerical value or density of the voxel. More sophisticated classifiers use additional information such as the location of the voxel, the values of neighbouring voxels, and *a priori* knowledge of the data. The classification can be binary, in which case it is accomplished by thresholding. Voxels with densities below the threshold map to zero and are treated as fully transparent (i.e. invisible); voxels with densities above the threshold map to a value 1 and are fully opaque. More generally, a non-binary classification can be performed and the voxel density is mapped to an opacity or alpha that is intermediate in value between 0 and 1.

Additional properties that affect the rendering and shading algorithms (such as brightness and colour) can be assigned to each voxel based on the percentage of each type of material that it contains. Non-binary classification is very important for certain volume rendering algorithms. Fully automatic implementation of the segmentation process has not yet been achieved, except for the most simple types of data. Very often manual intervention is required.

The next step is a mapping operation that allows the choice of display primitives to be selected or changed. This can be combined with previous steps, e.g. many segmentation schemes output a set of contours as a means of identifying structures of interest within the scene. Structures can also be identified using tag bits as part of the voxel values (Reynolds *et al.*, 1991). In general, any set of display primitives (points, lines, surfaces or volumes) can be converted to any other set; the choice depends largely on whether point, line, surface or volume rendering will be used, and the visualization effects that one wishes to create. Of course, the most efficient mapping is to leave the dataset in its original representation and not perform any conversion at all.

Once the display primitives have been chosen, the viewing step can be performed. Several sub-steps are needed to accomplish this. First, coordinate transformations are applied to translate, rotate and scale the object to produce the desired view. Then, an orthographic or perspective projection is applied, collapsing the 3-D object onto the 2-D screen. Prior to, or as part of, the projection process, hidden parts (i.e. those that should be obscured by others) are eliminated and visible parts retained. This visible-object determination forms the central core of the viewing process, and rendering algorithms are often divided into categories according to the way in which visible-object determination is performed.

Conceptually, shading is the last step in the visualization process, although in practical implementations it may be combined with one of the previous steps. The type of shading that can be applied again depends in large measure on the object representation that is used. For some representations (e.g. polygons), parts of the shading (e.g. surface normals) can be pre-computed and stored with the object representation. For others (e.g. binary voxels), no pre-processing is possible and shading is deduced from the 2-D image (Gordon & Reynolds, 1985). As an addendum to the shading step, anti-aliasing can be applied by judicious blending of the object with the background to ensure that the object has no jagged silhouette edges. Antialiasing is more important for surface rendering than for volume rendering, as aliasing errors are minimized earlier during volume rendering.

Basic principles of computer graphics display

The last three stages in the visualization pipeline (Kaufman, 1991) – viewing, shading, anti-aliasing – are considered in detail in this section. Although presented separately here, these stages are often combined in practice. Any software or hardware system that displays 3-D objects by projection onto a 2-D screen must perform the following steps, not necessarily in the order given:

1 A coordinate transformation to rotate, translate and scale the object to the desired orientation, position and size.
2 A perspective or parallel projection onto the 2-D screen, often combined with clipping.
3 Visible object determination: eliminating from the image parts of the object that should be obscured by others.
4 Scan conversion: pixels within the area of the screen defined by each clipped, projected, transformed object primitive must be identified and filled in. The intensity assigned to each pixel is determined by the shading.
5 Realistic shading: the shading algorithm may be made more or less complex depending on the degree of realism required, and the colours, opacities and textures of the materials to be simulated.
6 Anti-aliasing: suppression of artefacts arising from discrete sampling of the scene. To achieve anti-aliasing correctly, the contributions of all visible objects (even small ones) that can project onto a given pixel should be taken into account.

Details of projection and clipping may be found in standard texts (e.g. Foley *et al.*, 1990). The other operations are addressed in detail here.

Coordinate transformation

One way of describing the steps in the visualization process is in terms of the transformations the dataset undergoes from its initial to its final form. Scene space represents the coordinate system in which the original data are acquired. Object space is the coordinate system in which objects of interest are defined, typically at the segmentation stage. Image space is the 3-D coordinate system in which the image is assembled, prior to projection. View space includes the actual computer screen.

Coordinate transformations are used to perform the transformations from object space to image space. A general coordinate transformation (M) can be expressed as the product of translations, rotations, dilations (scaling) and projections:

$$M = T_i S_i P R_3 R_2 R_1 S_o T_o,$$

where T_i and S_i are translations and dilations in image space,

P is a projection matrix which can be either orthographic or perspective as the viewing needs dictate,

R_1, R_2 and R_3 are rotations and

S_o and T_o are dilations and translations in object space.

Although we are dealing with rotations in 3-D space, it is convenient to use 4×4 matrices for all operations. This is because 3-D translations can be expressed with a 4×4 matrix (but not with a 3×3 matrix) and perspective transformations can be conveniently expressed through the use of 4-D homogeneous coordinates (Foley *et al.*, 1990). The homogeneous coordinate system represents the point x,y,z by the 4-vector (hx,hy,hz,h). Viewing angles can be specified in any of a number of ways and are frequently expressed differently in different computer programs. Usually, angles are specified in terms of rotations of the object relative to the observer, although alternatively (and equivalently) the observer's position can be specified relative to the object.

To specify a general rotation (that is, any desired orientation of an object for display) requires three angles, corresponding to three degrees of freedom. One way of specifying these is to use two angles to establish the direction of an axis through the centre of the object, and the third to specify a rotation about this axis. An alternative is to decompose the rotation into the product of three rotations about three pre-determined axes in space. It can be shown that any rigid body can be rotated from one orientation to another by performing at least three rotations about at least two of the coordinate axes (Higman, 1955). The exact choice of which axes to use can be completely arbitrary, so long as the axes are distinct.

Object space angles describe rotations about axes which can be thought of as rigidly fixed to the object (i.e. they move with the object when it is rotated). The X, Y and Z principal axes of the object are usually chosen for convenience. In general, 3-D rotations do not commute, so the order in which the rotations are applied must be clearly specified. Let us suppose that R_X is to be applied first, followed by R_Y, followed by R_Z. From the point of view of a stationary observer, R_X will have the effect of moving the object's Y and Z axes to new locations, and it is these new axes that are to be used for R_Y and R_Z.

Image space angles describe rotations about axes which can be thought of as fixed to the observer (or, equivalently, the computer screen). Thus, these axes *do not move* when the object is rotated. After the first rotation they are no longer parallel to the natural X, Y and Z axes of the object; instead, they remain parallel to the edges of the computer screen. Matrix expressions for the various rotations have been given in detail by Reynolds (1985).

Visible object determination

A considerable number of algorithms for visible object determination have been developed over the years, mostly for use with surface rendering, where they are referred to as hidden-surface removal algorithms. Some, but not all, can be used with point, line and volume primitives as well. Visible object determination can conveniently be considered under the following four headings: scanline algorithms, z-buffer algorithms, priority algorithms and ray tracing.

Scanline algorithms

Scanline algorithms generate visible pixels in sequence from left to right, top to bottom, in the same sequence that the computer display scans from its image buffer. Scanline algorithms apply only to surface representations (polygons or surface patches). This is because these algorithms combine scan conversion with hidden-surface removal by making visibility determinations one pixel at a time. Scanline algorithms are the method of choice for scenes composed of a moderate number of polygons. They employ sophisticated linked list data structures to exploit the maximum coherence of the scene. Sorting operations are central to scanline algorithms (Sutherland *et al.*, 1974). For complex scenes the sorting will dominate the other computations, so the execution time of a scanline algorithm is typically proportional to $(N \log N)$, where N is the number of display primitives. For a small number of primitives, scanline algorithms can be very efficient.

Z-buffer algorithms

The z-buffer algorithm, first set down by Catmull (1974) performs no explicit sorting and therefore the work required to render a scene is a linear function of the number of primitives. This reduction in time complexity, from $(N \log N)$ to (N), is achieved at the expense of increased storage space. Two buffers, each the size of the final image, are set aside: one (the framebuffer) accumulates the final image, while the other (the depth buffer or z-buffer) records the distances to the closest primitives rendered so far. The z-buffer algorithm is not restricted to surface primitives. When each primitive is rendered, a test is made at each pixel it projects onto, by looking into the z-buffer to see if the new primitive is closer than what was previously rendered there. If it is, then the new primitive obscures the old one, and the image buffer and the z-buffer are both updated with values pertaining to the newly rendered primitive. One advantage of the z-buffer algorithm (apart from improved performance for complex scenes) is that primitives can be processed in any order. One disadvantage (apart from the large amount of storage that is required) is that transparency and anti-aliasing are hard to implement correctly.

Priority algorithms

Priority algorithms work by sorting the primitives into priority order, for example, by distance from the observer. If 'painted' into a framebuffer in the opposite order, then objects with high priority will automatically paint over objects with a lower priority, obscuring hidden parts of the object appropriately. For obvious reasons this approach is referred to as the painter's algorithm. If the high priority objects are not wholly opaque, or if they are small and do not completely obscure the low priority objects, then relative contributions are accumulated so that transparency and anti-aliasing are correctly achieved.

In the simplest depth sort algorithm, the priority list must be re-sorted each time the observer's viewpoint changes. However Fuchs *et al.* (1980) showed that, for polygons, a special data structure called the Binary Space Partitioning (BSP) tree has the property that it can be used for all viewpoints without resorting. A related data structure, called an octree, was devised (independently) for volume datasets by Meagher (1982) and others. At display time, the tree is not changed but is simply traversed in a sequence that depends on the current viewpoint. The time complexity of the BSP tree and octree algorithms is also linearly proportional to the number of primitives to be processed. Tree structures and priority algorithms provide one of the most efficient ways of performing visible object determination.

Ray tracing

Ray casting is perhaps the most intuitive method of visible object determination, especially for volume datasets. This algorithm starts at the front of the object and works towards the back, stopping when the pixels on the screen have been painted in. This may be accomplished by looping over the pixels of the screen and for each pixel, casting a ray into the object to see which primitives it intersects. Ray casting stops here, but ray tracing goes one step further, taking account of reflections and refractions at each object surface by tracing further rays from the point of intersection back to each light source. In this manner, very complex lighting conditions can be simulated.

Ray tracing has been used to produce some of the most realistic images in computer graphics. While primarily a method of visible object determination, it lends itself well to modelling special effects such as reflections, refractions, transparency and shadows. Most modern ray tracing approaches are based on the work of Whitted (1980) and Glassner (1984). Ray tracing is capable of generating very realistic renderings but its main disadvantage is that its performance is relatively slow.

Scan conversion

The projection of an object primitive onto the screen generally covers an area consisting of several pixels. The task of the scan conversion algorithm is to determine which pixels lie within this area; the intensity to be assigned to these pixels is then computed by the shading procedure. Although not all primitives are bounded by straight lines, their projections can usually be represented sufficiently accurately by polygons with straight edges. Therefore, most scan conversion algorithms address the issue of finding the pixels that lie inside such polygons.

A simple polygon scan conversion algorithm consists of two nested loops, with the outer (y) loop over scanlines of the image and the inner (x) loop over pixels. The limits of the inner loop are determined from the intersections of the current scanline with the appropriate polygon edges. Such an algorithm will work for any simple, closed polygon, concave or convex, provided special cases (such as vertices falling on scanlines) are handled correctly. Detailed discussions of polygon scan conversion algorithms are given in standard texts (e.g. Newman & Sproull, 1979).

Shading

Once the pixels lying within the projection of the primitive have been determined, their intensities can be computed by an appropriate shading algorithm. The ultimate goal of shading is to provide a $2\frac{1}{2}$-D image that is practically indistinguishable from a photograph of the real object, but retains all its minute details, which may be of great scientific importance. Many shading schemes are described in the computer graphics literature. We distinguish between the shading model, which describes the types of object materials (smooth, faceted, textured, diffuse, shiny, coloured) and light sources to be simulated, and the shading method, which provides an algorithm by which the desired effects can be realized.

The simplest form of shading is called distance-only or depth shading. In this case the surface properties are ignored and objects far from the light source simply appear darker. More sophisticated shading models distinguish between diffuse reflection (where the surface scatters light equally in all directions) and specular reflection (where a glossy surface exhibits highlights which vary with the viewing angle). Diffuse surfaces appear to have the same brightness from all directions; this brightness depends on the illumination (I) given by:

$$I = I_{max} \cos \theta$$

where I_{max} is the maximum illumination, which results when $\theta = 0$ and
$\quad \theta$ is the angle between the incident light and the normal to the surface.
This equation can be rewritten as:

$$I = I_{max} \hat{N} \cdot \hat{L},$$

where $\hat{N}$ is the unit vector normal to the surface and $\hat{L}$ is the unit vector along the line from the surface to the light source. In theory, illumination falls off with the square of the distance to the surface from a point light source, but in practice, a factor of $1/d^2$ does not produce natural looking images, and $1/d$ is often used instead. Also, the $\cos \theta$ term creates a harsh angular dependence and may be replaced by $(\cos \theta)^p$ where p is an empirically determined parameter. The following expression is often used (Chen *et al.*, 1985):

$$I = \frac{(I_{max} - I_a)(D - d)(\cos \theta)^p}{D} + I_a,$$

where I_a is the ambient light,

D is the distance at which the illumination falls to zero (D can be considered to be the diameter of a sphere enclosing the object) and

d is the distance from the light source.

For a discussion of more advanced shading models, the reader is referred to the work of Foley *et al.* (1990).

Having established an expression to be used for computing the intensity, it remains to discuss methods of estimating the surface normal $\hat{N}$. If the surface is represented by a polygonal mesh and a faceted appearance is desired, each polygon can use its own local normal, computed geometrically. This is called constant shading. Pixel intensities are computed independently for each polygon based on its local normal, without taking neighbouring polygons into account.

If the polygons are intended to approximate a smoothly curving surface, then constant shading results in undesirable intensity discontinuities at the edges where polygons meet. Gouraud shading was designed to eliminate these discontinuities by finding the resultant normal at each vertex. From these vertex normals, intensities are computed and interpolated smoothly across all polygons which are adjacent at that vertex. Phong shading is similar to Gouraud shading, but interpolates the vertex normals rather than the vertex intensities, thus obtaining an effective normal at each pixel from which the intensity can be calculated. Phong shading produces a smoother, higher quality image than Gouraud shading, and is often used as the reference technique in comparisons of shading algorithms. It is however significantly more expensive in computational terms than Gouraud shading.

The above methods are applicable when the object is represented by surface primitives. With volume primitives these normals cannot be calculated from the geometry, but must be estimated from some numerical property of the volume data. There are two ways of accomplishing this; both involve taking the gradient of some function. In image based volume shading methods, the gradient of the distance to the visible voxels is computed; in object based methods, the gradient of the density values is computed.

Distance gradient shading (Horn, 1982; Gordon & Reynolds, 1985) is an image space method that takes the gradient of the distances from the observer to the front surfaces of visible objects. This is accomplished by running a gradient operator over a depth shaded pre-image, often computed from the contents of the z-buffer. The gradient provides an estimate of the surface normal, which (with a suitable weighting function) can then be used to shade each pixel. Distance gradient shading provides a dramatic improvement over distance only shading, and is capable of very satisfactory results when implemented carefully. It is the method of choice with binary datasets and when no additional shading information is available.

Density gradient shading (Hohne & Bernstein, 1986; Schlusselberg, Smith & Woodward, 1986) is an object space method that uses voxel values rather than their distances or location. This method takes the gradient of the voxel values (densities) in a 3-D neighbourhood surrounding the voxel of interest as an estimate of the normal vector at that voxel. The resulting normal is then used to shade the pixel onto which this voxel is projected. Strictly speaking, the density gradient is a good approximation to the surface normal only when the voxel forms part of an isodensity surface. The method does not work correctly for thin objects, or at manually created surfaces such as at clipping planes. When applied correctly however, the method results in smooth shading and very good image quality.

Anti-aliasing

The term aliasing is used to denote a multitude of anomalies that result from the discrete sampling of 3-D scenes at various stages of the visualization process. When dynamically changing images are created, there is sampling in both space and time domains, resulting in additional errors and anomalies. Problems result if there are high spatial or temporal frequencies in the representation, in the form of sharp edges or rapid motion. According to the Nyquist criterion, unless the sampling frequency (pixel spacing or image update rate) is more than twice the object frequency, the scene cannot be rendered correctly and aliasing will result.

Symptoms of aliasing in computer generated images include the following (Catmull, 1978):

1 Jagged edges along object boundaries (also known as 'rastering' or 'staircasing').
2 Small objects disappearing and reappearing as the viewpoint is changed slightly.
3 Field interlace problems. A standard television frame is composed of two fields which contain the odd and even scanlines respectively (see Chapter 3). The fields should be computed independently, with moving objects occurring in slightly different positions in each.
4 Beat frequencies occurring when periodic motion is close in frequency to the field or frame update rate. This results in the familiar phenomenon of wagon wheels in movies turning slowly or even backwards.

Methods of preventing or at least mitigating aliasing errors, which are known collectively as anti-aliasing algorithms, have been developed by Catmull (1978), Crow (1981) and others. These methods fall into one or other of the following categories: pre-filtering the scene to remove high frequencies, or supersampling at sub-pixel intervals, followed by averaging or post-filtering.

The supersampling approach involves dividing each pixel into a number of smaller sub-pixels and averaging the intensity calculated for each one separately. This approach cannot hope to remove aliasing errors completely, since it is still possible for very small objects to miss all sub-pixels and 'fall between the cracks' at certain orientations, while being fully visible at others. The prefiltering approach regards each pixel as a window against which all primitives visible or partly visible at that pixel should be clipped. The contribution of each visible fragment is then weighted by its area within the window.

Rendering algorithms

Object representations can be categorized according to the dimensionality of the geometric primitives on which they are based. One such classification would be: points, lines, surfaces and volumes. Rendering algorithms can be similarly categorized, based on the object representations to which they are best applied: surface representations, for example, are most easily visualized via surface renderings. The correspondence is not absolute, however, since it is possible to convert from one representation to another: objects represented by voxels can be visualized via surface rendering, provided that surfaces are extracted and converted to a polygon representation first (Artzy *et al.*, 1981; Lorensen & Cline, 1987).

A second criterion is the type of information that one wishes to convey. With suitable segmentation, objects represented by points, lines and surfaces can be extracted from volume datasets. The appearance of these structures, however, will be very different depending on the type of rendering that is employed. In this respect the choice of point, line, surface, volume, or even hybrid rendering depends primarily on the specific visualization task, and the different approaches are largely complementary.

Point rendering applies to zero-dimensional primitives or particles (Csuri *et al.*, 1979; Reeves, 1983; Cline *et al.*, 1988). The object representation is an unordered collection of independent points, with x,y,z coordinates stored explicitly, unlike the voxel representation where the coordinates are implicit because the points are spaced uniformly on a 3-D grid. Usually, there is no density value associated with point primitives. Point primitives are used to represent fuzzy objects such as fire, clouds and water, and other objects whose form or shape changes over time, often in a stochastic or non-deterministic manner. Point representations and voxel representations are conceptually quite similar, but point rendering and volume rendering produce quite different results. Point rendering is designed to convey the independent nature of each particle, whereas volume rendering conveys the volume nature of the object as a whole.

Points with associated normal vectors can be thought of as the limiting case of small surface patches. As the complexity of an object increases, the size of the polygons needed to represent its surface decreases until each covers little more than one pixel of the display. It then becomes more efficient to render point primitives instead of surface primitives. The dividing-cubes algorithm generates a large cloud of points which can approximate a surface very accurately (Cline *et al.*, 1988). Point rendering involves the coordinate transformation, projection, and visible object determination steps outlined above, but avoids the need for scan conversion. Normal vectors associated with each point (if available) are used for the shading computation.

Line rendering consists of generating so called wire frame images, which may or may not have hidden lines removed. Either vector graphics or raster graphics methods may be used, depending on the type of hardware to be employed. Vector graphics devices can illuminate any of a continuum of points on the screen, so that lines can be drawn by simply specifying the coordinates of their endpoints. Raster graphics devices can only address discrete points (pixels), so that lines have to be scan converted in software before they can be drawn.

The more primitive line rendering programs show boundaries of objects as piecewise-connected lines after rotation and scaling in three dimensions. These can be drawn as they would appear from different viewpoints. The more sophisticated programs perform hidden line removal; that is, lines that would be obscured by opaque slices from the current viewing position are not drawn. This improves the 3-D illusion by providing better depth cues. Many such programs have been developed for large computers (Cahan & Trombka, 1975; Johnson & Capowski, 1983; Dykes & Afshar, 1982), and more recently for microcomputers (Vanden Berghe *et al.*, 1986; Gras, 1984).

When an object is represented by a line drawing of its boundaries, reconstruction of the surface connecting the boundaries is dependent on the imagination and experience of the viewer. If the boundaries overlap from the chosen viewpoint and the object is fairly simple, the illusion of 3-D can be sustained by hidden line removal and the image is usually relatively easy to interpret. Difficulties arise when the scene is more complex or the boundaries do not significantly overlap. When several objects are present, confusion can arise over which boundaries belong to which object. These difficulties are due to the lack of adequate depth and shape cues. One solution is to draw the sections as flat-shaded filled contours (Runham *et al.*, 1990). This requires a change in object representation (from line to volume). Filled contours provide significantly better cues than line drawings since colour can be more effectively used to shade different structures. A related approach is to extrude each serial section as a solid slice. This capability is provided, for example, by the AT-Videoplan^{TM}. This approach, although technically simple to achieve, gives only limited object visualization and, like line rendering, can reveal no surface detail.

Line rendering involves the coordinate transformation and projection steps, and may or may not involve visible object determination (hidden line removal). As with point primitives there is no need for scan conversion. Depth or distance only shading (lines further from the light source appear darker) is the only type of shading generally applied.

Surface rendering requires the existence of an underlying surface represent-ation. Surfaces are most frequently represented by plane polygons, although curved surface patches are also used. Surfaces are often constructed from object boundaries, which are obtained as contours by manual tracing of 2-D slices or by semi-automatic segmentation of volume data. The boundaries are then interconnected to form surfaces. The most common approach is to triangulate the surface between the boundaries. For simple boundaries the generation of the connecting strip of triangles can be completely automatic. However, difficulties arise where branches and joins between multiple objects are to be created and manual intervention in the triangulation process is usually necessary in these cases. Automated triangulation procedures have been under development for many years, but so far have not been applied widely enough for potential users to be assured that they will work satisfactorily in practice. An important part of the surface construction process is to associate normal vectors with each primitive triangle, based on the geometrical organization of this surface.

Steps in the surface rendering process are as follows: coordinate transforma-tion, projection, scan conversion, visible object determination, shading and anti-aliasing. These have been described in previous sections.

Volume rendering, as the name implies, is based on volume representations and seeks to convey the volume nature of the object to be displayed. Origin-ally, the term volume rendering was applied to any method that traversed the volume representation at display time, making visible object determinations in the process (Reynolds, 1985). More recently, however, it has been associated with generalized transparency models, where all voxels in the object contribute something to the final image (Drebin *et al.*, 1988; Levoy, 1988). Unlike surface rendering, volume rendering permits boundaries to be defined at display time, if they are explicitly defined at all. Many volume rendering methods rely on a technique known as volumetric compositing: thin slices of the object, refor-matted if necessary, are combined to produce a view of the object in its entirety, including visualization of surfaces and internal structures to which traditional shading algorithms are applied.

In the compositing approach, the scene is (conceptually) represented by a block of translucent, coloured 'jelly' whose colour and opacity may be adjusted for different tissue types. One advantage of volume rendering is that no *a priori* decisions need be made about the geometry or structural relationships in the volume. At the classification stage, each voxel is assigned an opacity and a colour based on a number of factors including densities and gradients (Levoy, 1988), estimated tissue mixtures (Drebin *et al.*, 1988), or fuzzy classification schemes (Barillot *et al.*, 1991). The effect is to make thin structures (which have an anomalously low density, due to the partial volume effect) almost translucent, so that only the trained observer can distinguish, for example, thin bone from thick tissue in the 3-D presentation. For visualization purposes this may be an advantage, since the fuzziness of the rendering conveys the uncertainty of the classification.

For volume rendering, non-binary material classification is generally used. Classification for volume rendering may assign optical properties such as light attenuation (i.e. opacity) and brightness (colour, light emission) to each voxel in the dataset. These optical properties are assigned to each voxel on the basis of its value, the percentage of material present in the voxel, the position of the voxel, and *a priori* knowledge of the material. Different classifiers require different kinds of rendering algorithms and result in different kinds of images. The resulting coloured translucent gel is then projected by carefully resampling and compositing all the voxels along each projection ray to form the corresponding pixel. Two different approaches to volume rendering have been devised:

1 Image order (the ray casting method).
2 Object order (the compositing or splatting method).

In the ray casting approach, which operates entirely in image order, rays are driven through the volume from front to back, accumulating visual attributes of the volume as voxels are encountered (Levoy, 1988). This method requires more calculations than the compositing approach, and may also introduce errors, since new voxel densities must be re-sampled at arbitrary locations from the surrounding voxel values.

In the compositing approach (pioneered by Pixar Inc, San Rafael, California and similar to the method currently used in Vital Images' VoxelView^{TM}), voxels are stacked in order, back to front, and then projected or composited into a 2-D picture. Thus the image is built up layer by layer on the screen. The work at Pixar, described in general terms by Smith (1987) and presented in detail by Drebin *et al.* (1988), transforms slices in sequence but uses a scanline method (Catmull & Smith, 1980) for resampling the voxels in each slice. Thus it may be considered a hybrid of image order and object order approaches.

The splatting approach operates entirely in object order. Westover (1990) transformed each voxel from object space to image space, performed shading to obtain a colour and opacity, applied blurring and blending using lookup tables to obtain a 2-D footprint spanning multiple image pixels, and blended or 'splatted' the footprint into the image array. All of these methods make use of the image compositing algebra developed by Porter & Duff (1984) and the object modelling concepts established by Blinn (1982).

One way of creating 2-D images from a 3-D scene, usually classified as volume rendering although it does not quite fit into any of the rendering algorithm classifications discussed above, is by re-projection. In the summed voxel projection method, pioneered by Harris *et al.* (1979), the greylevel assigned to each pixel is obtained by taking a line integral through the 3-D scene; in effect, each pixel receives the sum of the densities of the voxels which project onto it. The advantage is that familiar, projected views are obtained that are similar to conventional radiographs, but obscuring structures can be removed. In the maximum intensity projection, only the brightest voxel encountered along each line is retained. This is useful for extracting weak signals from a noisy background, for example in magnetic resonance angiography, but suffers from a lack of adequate depth cues especially in static images.

Image interpretation

Different rendering schemes exploit different visual cues concerning 3-D structure, and recognizing these cues is important in interpreting the image correctly. As an example, consider the re-projection methods maximum intensity projection and summed voxel projection provided in the Analyze™ package. In both cases the projection onto the 2-D screen contains no explicit depth information such as distance shading, so other depth cues must be used. In a recent application involving confocal microscopy images of the alveolar duct system of the human lung rendered using maximum intensity projection, animation was used to convey some depth information. Based on static views, the structure was originally thought to be a spiral; however, this was shown in the animation to be a set of rings (Cookson *et al.*, 1994). As another example, static depth cues, such as shading, based on local proportions of the object or image may lead to confusion in interpreting order relations between non-overlapping structures. Animation and kinetic depth cues are powerful ways of resolving such conflicts.

Conclusion

An important factor in selecting an appropriate visualization technique is the overall characteristic of the structure that one wishes to convey. Volume datasets can be displayed as complete entities using volume rendering, or selected structures can be identified and their surfaces extracted and displayed in isolation using surface rendering. Although the starting point may be the same, the resulting images will be very different.

References

Artzy, E., Freider, G. & Herman, G. T. (1981). The theory, design, implementation and evaluation of a three-dimensional surface detection algorithm. *Computer Graphics and Image Processing*, **15**, 1–24.

Augustine, J. R. (1981). A lucite plate method for 3-dimensional reconstruction of neuronal populations. *Journal of Neuroscience Methods*, **4**, 63–71.

Barillot, C., Lachman, F., Gibaud, B. & Scarabin, J. M. (1991). Three-dimensional display of MRI data in neurosurgery: volume sampling, segmentation, and rendering aspects. *Proceedings of the Society of Photo-Optic Instrumentation Engineers*, **1445**, 54–65.

Benton, S. A. (1982). Survey of holographic stereograms. *Proceedings of the Society of Photo-Optic Instrumentation Engineers*, **367**, 15–19.

Blinn, J. F. (1982). Light reflection functions for simulation of clouds and dusty surfaces. *Computer Graphics*, **16**, 21–9.

Boissonat, J. D. (1989). Shape reconstruction from planar cross sections. *Computer Vision, Graphics and Image Processing*, **44**, 1–29.

Budinger, T. F. (1984). An analysis of 3D display strategies, *Proceedings of the Society of Photo-Optic Instrumentation Engineers*, **507**, 2–8.

Cahan, L. D. & Trombka B. T. (1975). Computer graphics – three-dimensional reconstruction of thalamic anatomy from serial sections. *Computer Programs in Biomedicine*, **5**, 91–8.

Carlsson, K. (1991). The influence of specimen refractive index, detector signal integration, and non-uniform scan speed on the imaging properties in confocal microscopy. *Journal of Microscopy*, **163**, 167–78.

Catmull, E. A. (1974). *A Subdivision Algorithm for Computer Display of Curved Surfaces*. PhD Thesis, Department of Computer Science, University of Utah, UT.

Catmull, E. A. (1978). A hidden-surface algorithm with anti-aliasing. *Computer Graphics*, **12**, 6–9.

Catmull, E. A. & Smith, A. R. (1980). 3D transformations of images in scanline order. *Computer Graphics*, **14**, 279–85.

Chen, L. S., Herman, G. T., Reynolds, R. A. & Udupa, J. K. (1985). Surface shading in the cuberille environment. *IEEE Computer Graphics and Applications*, **5**, 33–43.

Cline, H. E., Lorensen, W. E., Ludke, S., Crawford, C. R. & Teeter, B. C. (1988). Two algorithms for the three-dimensional construction of tomograms. *Medical Physics*, **15**, 320–7.

Cookson, M. J., Davies, C. J., Entwistle, A. & Whimster, W. F. (1994). The microanatomy of the alveolar duct of the human lung imaged by confocal microscopy and visualised with computer-based 3D reconstruction. *Computerised Medical Imaging and Graphics* (in the press).

Crow, F. (1981). A comparison of anti-aliasing techniques. *IEEE Computer Graphics and Applications*, **1**, 40–9.

Csuri, C., Hackathron, R., Parent, R., Carlson, W. & Howard, M. (1979). Towards an interactive high visual complexity animation system. *Computer Graphics*, **13**, 289–99.

Drebin, R. A., Carpenter, L. & Hanrahan, P. (1988). Volume rendering. *Computer Graphics*, **22**, 65–74.

Dykes, E. & Afshar, F. (1982). Computer generated three-dimensional reconstruction from serial sections. *Acta Stereologica*, STEREOL **82**, 289–96.

Foley, J. D., van Dam, A., Feiner, S. K. & Hughes, J. F. (1990). *Computer Graphics Principles and Practice* (2nd edition). Reading, MA: Addison-Wesley.

Fuchs, H., Kedem, Z. M. & Naylor, B. F. (1980). On visible surface generation by a priori tree structures. *Computer Graphics*, **14**, 124–33.

Fuchs, H., Pizer, S. M., Tsai, L. C., Bloomberg, S. H. & Heinz, E. R. (1982). Adding a true 3D display to a raster graphics system. *IEEE Computer Graphics and Applications*, **2**, 72–8.

Glassner, A. S. (1984). Space subdivision for fast ray tracing. *IEEE Computer Graphics and Applications*, **4**, 15–22.

Glenn, W. V., Johnston, R. J., Morton, P. E. & Dwyer, S. J. (1975). Image generation and image display techniques for CT scan data. *Investigative Radiology*, **10**, 403–16.

Gordon, D. & Reynolds, R.A. (1985). Image space shading of 3-dimensional objects.

Computer Vision, Graphics, and Image Processing, **29**, 361–76.

Gras, H. (1984). A hidden-line algorithm for 3D reconstruction from serial sections: an extension of the neurec program package for a microcomputer. *Computer Programs in Biomedicine*, **18**, 217–26.

Harris, L. D., Robb, R. A., Yuen, T. S. & Ritman, E. L. (1979). Display and visualization of three-dimensional reconstructed anatomical morphology: experience with the thorax, heart and coronary vasculature of dogs. *Journal of Computer Assisted Tomography*, **3**, 439–46.

Herman, G. T. & Liu, H. K. (1977). Display of three-dimensional information in computed tomography. *Journal of Computer Assisted Tomography*, **1**, 155–60.

Higman, B. (1955). *Applied Group-Theoretic and Matrix Methods*, London: Oxford University Press.

Hohne, K. H. & Bernstein, R. (1986). Shading 3D-images from CT using gray-level gradients. *IEEE Transactions on Medical Imaging*, **5**, 45–7.

Horn, B. K. P. (1982). Hill shading and the reflectance map. *Geo-Processing*, **2**, 65–146.

Howard, V. (1990). The confocal microscope as an instrument for measuring microstructural geometry. *Confocal Microscopy*, **10**, 285–303.

Johnson, E. M. & Capowski, J. J. (1983). A system for the three-dimensional reconstruction of biological structures. *Computers and Biomedical Research*, **16**, 79–87.

Kaufman, A. (1991). Introduction to volume visualization. In *Volume Visualization*, ed. A. Kaufman, pp. 1–18. Los Alamitos, CA: IEEE Computer Society Press.

Levoy, M. (1988). Display of surfaces from volume data. *IEEE Computer Graphics and Applications*, **8**, 29–37.

Lorensen, W. E. & Cline, H. E. (1987). Marching cubes: a high resolution 3D surface construction algorithm. *Computer Graphics*, **21**, 163–9.

Maure, A. G., Halton, D. W., Johnston, C. F., Shaw, C. & Fairweather, I. (1990). The serotoninergic, cholinergic and peptidergic components of the nervous system in the monogenean parasite, *Diclidophora merlangi*: a cytochemical study. *Parasitology*, **100**, 255–73.

Meagher, D. (1982). Geometric modelling using octree encoding. *Computer Graphics and Image Processing*, **19**, 129–47.

Muller, J. (1984). Morphometry and histology of gonads from twelve children and adolescents with the androgen insensitivity (testicular feminization) syndrome. *Journal of Clinical Endocrinology and Metabolism*, **59**, 785–9.

Newman, W. F. & Sproull, R. F. (1979). *Principles of Interactive Computer Graphics* (2nd edition). New York: McGraw-Hill.

Porter, T. & Duff, T. (1984). Compositing digital images. *Computer Graphics*, **18**, 253–9.

Raya, S. P. & Udupa, J. K. (1990). Shape-based interpolation of multidimensional objects. *IEEE Transactions on Medical Imaging*, **9**, 32–42.

Reeves, W. T. (1983). Particle systems: a technique for modelling a class of fuzzy objects. *Computer Graphics*, **17**, 359–76.

Reynolds, R. A. (1985). *Fast Methods for 3D Display of Medical Objects*. PhD thesis, Department of Computer and Information Science, University of Pennsylvania, Philadelphia PA.

Reynolds, R. A., Wyatt, E. D. & Peterson, M. A. (1991). Segmentation for 3D display. *Colloquium on Image Processing in Medicine*, IEE Digest 1991/081, 8/1–8/7. London: IEE.

Rhodes, M. L., Glenn, W. V. & Azzawi, Y. M. (1980). Extracting oblique planes from serial CT sections. *Journal of Computer Assisted Tomography*, **4**, 649–57.

Runham, N. W., Davies, D. A. & Roberts, D. (1990). Computer-aided three dimensional reconstructions from serial sections. *Microscopy and Analysis*, **16**, 15–18.

Schlusselberg, D. S., Smith, W. K. & Woodward, D. J. (1986). Three-dimensional display of medical image volumes. *NCGA'86 Technical Session Proceedings*, **III**, 114–23.

Shaw, P. J. & Rawlings, D. J. (1991). The point-spread function of a confocal microscope: its measurement and use in deconvolution of 3-D data. *Journal of Microscopy*, **163**, 151–65.

Sheppard, C. J. R. & Cogswell, C. J. (1990). Three-dimensional imaging in confocal microscopy. *Confocal Microscopy*, **4**, 143–69.

Smith, A. R. (1987). Volume graphics and volume visualization: a tutorial. *Technical Report 176*, San Rafael CA: Pixar Inc.

Stelzer, E. H. K. & Wijnaendts-van-Resandt, R. W. (1990). Optical cell splicing with the confocal fluorescence microscope: microtomoscopy. *Confocal Microscopy*, **7**, 199–212.

Sutherland, I., Sproull, R. & Schumacker, R. (1974). A characterization of ten hidden surface algorithms. *ACM Computing Surveys*, **6**, 1–55.

Van der Voort, H. T. M., Brakenhoff, G. J. & Baarslag, M. W. (1989). Three-dimensional visualisation methods for confocal microscopy. *Journal of Microscopy*, **153**, 123–32.

Vanden Berghe, W., Aerts, P., Claeys, H. & Verraes, W. (1986). A microcomputer-based graphical reconstruction technique for serially sectioned objects, with hidden line removal. *Anatomical Record*, **215**, 84–91.

Visser, T. D., Oud, J. L. & Brakenhoff, G. J. (1992). Refractive index and axial distance measurements in 3-D microscopy. *Optik*, **90**, 17–19.

Werner, G. & Morgenstern, E. (1980). Three-dimensional reconstruction of human blood platelets using serial sections. *European Journal of Cell Biology*, **20**, 276–82.

Westover, L. (1990). Footprint evaluation for volume rendering. *Computer Graphics*, **24**, 367–76.

Whitted, T. (1980). An improved illumination model for shaded display. *Communications of the ACM*, **23**, 343–49.

Xiao, G. Q. & Kino, G. S. (1987). A real-time confocal scanning optical microscope. *Proccedings of the Society of Photo-Optic Instrumentation Engineers*, **809**, 107.

PART 4

Applications

19

Quantitative immunocytochemistry

J. T. McBRIDE

Introduction

Immunocytochemistry is classically used to identify microscopic structures such as cells or granules by their immunoreactivity or to demonstrate that specific immunoreactivity is associated with a particular microscopic structure. Quantification has not been a major concern in most immunocytochemical studies: localization of immunoreactivity is often demonstrated definitively with one or more photomicrographs. However, it is often important to know not only that a particular compound is present in a specific cell type or granule, but to detect and quantify changes in local concentrations of such compounds. Intracellular levels of proteins or other molecules can be measured easily in cell culture studies, and tissue concentrations can be estimated precisely by radioimmunoassay (RIA), but the local concentration of antigen in a complex tissue cannot be measured by RIA if the antigen is not evenly distributed. Quantitative immunocytochemistry is often the only practical way to estimate local concentrations of immunoreactive molecules at the microscopic level.

Quantitative immunocytochemistry has been used comparatively infrequently. Many immunocytochemists are less comfortable with quantitative than with qualitative techniques. Investigators accustomed to the precision of radioimmunoassay have been discouraged by the limitations of quantitative immunocytochemistry. Tissue fixation and processing usually preclude absolute measurements of antigen concentrations. Because immunocytochemistry involves many steps and reagents, it is often assumed that variability compounded with each step would overwhelm the ability to detect even important differences in immunoreactivity. Finally, quantitative immunocytochemical studies are often labour intensive, time consuming and expensive because they typically involve analysis of numbers of slides from numbers of animals in each of a number of experimental groups.

On the other hand, as journal editors increasingly require conclusions supported by statistical analyses, quantitative immunocytochemistry is being used with increasing regularity. The widespread availability of economical and flexible image analysis systems has also been an important development in this

regard. In this chapter, I review general aspects of quantitative immunocytochemistry at the cellular level. Quantitative immunofluorescence, although not
specifically discussed, shares many of the principles which will be presented.
Stereology, the quantification of immunoreactivity in nervous tissue, and
technical aspects of image analysis are covered in depth elsewhere in this
volume.

The design of quantitative studies

In a typical quantitative immunocytochemical study, histologic slides from a
group of individuals (patients, animals, etc.) are compared with those of one or
more other groups. At the outset two questions must be answered:

1 How many observations (blocks/slides/fields, etc.) from each individual
will be needed to estimate the parameter of interest with adequate
precision?
2 How many individuals are needed in each experimental group to estimate
the group mean value with sufficient accuracy to detect the expected
difference between experimental groups?

These questions are important: underestimating these numbers results in an
inconclusive study; overestimation results in wasted supplies, animals and time.
The number of observations per individual is appropriate when the standard
error of the estimate for each individual is small relative to interindividual
variability. It is a waste of effort to estimate the value of a parameter to the
nearest 1% for each individual if interindividual variation within each group is
10%. The appropriate size of experimental groups depends on both the
magnitude of the experimental effect which is expected and the variability
among individuals. If immunoreactivity is expected to increase by 100-fold in
one experimental group, fewer animals will be necessary than if a 10% increase
is expected. Interindividual variability can be estimated easily from earlier
studies if a technique has been used previously. If the technique is new,
variability must be estimated from preliminary measurements on a number of
subjects. A reasonable number of individuals to include can be calculated with
a sample size equation (Snedecor & Cochran, 1967) once the magnitude of the
expected effect and interindividual variability are estimated. Because biological
variability between individuals within each group is often greater than the
variability between fields/slides/sections in any one individual, a common
mistake is to make too many measurements on too few animals.

Quantitative immunocytochemical techniques

Quantitative approaches to immunocytochemistry fall into two categories:

1 Those that involve counting or measuring immunoreactive structures
without regard to the intensity of the immunoreactivity.

2 Those that estimate or discriminate differences in the intensity of immunoreactivity.

The first approach is a natural extension of classical immunocytochemistry and will be dealt with only briefly here; in the bulk of this chapter I will deal with the second approach.

Counting of measuring immunoreactive structures

The simplest quantitative approach to immunocytochemistry is to count the number, or measure the area, of immunoreactive structures such as cells or nerve fibres within a tissue. The underlying assumptions are that all immunoreactive structures are stained and that the major experimental effect is a change in the size and/or number of such structures. The strategy for immunostaining, as in classical immunocytochemistry, is to maximize the intensity of specific staining and minimize background staining.

The challenge of this type of quantification is to use appropriate manual or automated morphometric techniques to estimate accurately the number, area, or volume density of immunostained structures. Comparable areas of tissue in individuals of various experimental groups must be sampled and stereologic and image analysis principles covered elsewhere in this volume followed. There are a number of considerations specifically relating to immunocytochemistry. An example is the Bigbee effect (Bigbee *et al.*, 1977): if the density of epitopes is excessive, the peroxidase–antiperoxidase technique may fail to demonstrate immunoreactivity because both immunoreactive sites of secondary antibodies bind to primary antibodies and neither is available for binding to third layer immunoglobulins. Accurately discriminating immunoreactive structures from background when staining is not intense can be technically difficult with image analysis systems.

Variation in staining intensity between individuals or between sections poses a particular problem for identifying immunoreactive structures objectively. Whether manual or automated image analysis techniques are used, intensely stained structures tend to appear artefactually larger than those stained less intensely and faintly stained structures may be overlooked altogether. This is especially true with structures such as nerve processes or fibres that are not easily delineated by characteristics other than immunoreactivity. If staining intensity varies between individuals, the importance of this effect can be estimated by immunostaining serial or identical sections with progressive dilutions of primary antiserum. A difference in the measured area of immunostaining between staining intensities that bracket those observed in experimental tissue suggests that this phenomenon needs to be taken into consideration. Sternberger & Sternberger (1986) have described an innovative approach which avoids this problem. This technique is discussed in the final section of this chapter.

Measuring the intensity of immunoreactivity

Quantitative immunocytochemistry usually refers to measurements of the intensity of immunoreactivity rather than the size or number of immunoreactive structures. Although most morphometric techniques are primarily useful for quantitating differences that are obvious on casual examination, measurements of the intensity of immunoreactivity are an exception to this rule because the human eye is a relatively poor densitometer. Although the eye can recognize differences in the intensity of staining between two structures in the same field of view, differences between structures examined sequentially in different fields or different slides are poorly judged. Therefore, quantitative measurements may document experimental differences that are not initially apparent.

The usual assumptions of this type of quantitative immunocytochemical technique are that the intensity of immunostaining reflects the density of immunoreactive epitopes and that the major experimental effect is a difference in the density of immunoreactive epitopes within structures rather than a difference in the number or size of the structures themselves. This section will discuss two such methods:

1 Microdensitometry or the direct measurement of the intensity of immunostaining.
2 The 'supraoptimal dilution' technique, a simple but sensitive adaptation of counting techniques which can be a useful screening procedure.

Microdensitometry

Microdensitometry is the direct measurement of the optical density of immunostaining of microscopic structures. Because it is often the only truly quantitative method for estimating the distribution of immunoreactivity among microscopic tissue compartments, microdensitometry has been used with increasing frequency. Although this approach has been validated in a variety of systems (Benno et al., 1982; Gross & Rothfeld, 1985; Rahier et al., 1989; McBride et al., 1990; van Schooten et al., 1991; Peretti-Renucci et al., 1991), neither the potential usefulness nor the limitations of this technique are widely appreciated.

The tacit assumption of immunocytochemical microdensitometry is that the intensity with which a structure is stained is directly related to the concentration of immunoreactive epitopes in that structure. Although not a necessity, a linear relationship between the intensity of staining and immunoreactivity is desirable. It is obvious that a greater density of epitopes usually results in more intense immunostaining (notwithstanding artefacts such as the Bigbee effect). However, a direct and linear relationship between epitope density in a microscopic structure in fresh tissue and staining intensity is potentially compromised in two ways:

1 Tissue fixation and immunocytochemical processing tend to decrease

immunoreactivity by altering or shielding epitopes and by eluting epitopes from tissue sections. Therefore, it is difficult, if not impossible, to estimate the precise concentration of immmunoreactive epitopes in microscopic structures in fresh tissue using immunocytochemical techniques.

2 All immunocytochemical techniques involve one or more immunologic and/or non-immunologic steps beyond the primary antigen–antibody reaction. For example, many methods include secondary and tertiary immunologic reactions and deposition of pigment by an enzymatic reaction. The amount of pigment deposited must then be estimated by microdensitometry. At each of these steps a linear relationship between immunoreactivity and the intensity of immunostaining can be violated.

A general approach to immunocytochemical microdensitometry

Immunocytochemical microdensitometry involves four steps:

1 Selecting an appropriate immunocytochemical method.
2 Making preliminary choices of appropriate reagent dilutions, development times, etc.
3 Documenting the relationship between immunoreactivity and the density of immunostaining.
4 Applying the technique to experimental tissue.

Of these steps, the third is the most critical and least familiar to most investigators. The simplest method of documenting a direct relationship between immunoreactivity and staining intensity is to process serial or similar sections of the pertinent tissue with progressive dilutions of primary antiserum. If the optical density of immunostaining is a quantitative function of antiserum dilution over a range of dilutions (Fig. 1), the minimal conditions necessary for quantitative immunocytochemistry are satisfied. If this is not the case, the technique must be modified or a different technique used. When these minimal conditions are satisfied, the next step is to use an antiserum dilution well within the linear range to immunostain a series of synthetic or biological standards with known concentrations of the epitope of interest. These data will formally define the relationship between immunoreactivity and staining intensity. Experimental sections are then processed in parallel with additional standard sections. Because immunocytochemistry involves many different reactions, reagents, and manipulations, it is preferable that all sections and standards are processed simultaneously with single batches of reagents.

The following sections consider the various steps of quantitative immunocytochemistry and sources for error in each. Although the peroxidase–antiperoxidase technique has been used most frequently, almost any immunocytochemical technique can be used for quantitative studies. The general principles outlined, if not the details, apply to each.

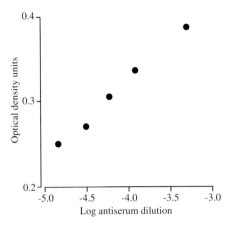

Fig. 1. Mean optical density of CGRP-like immunoreactivity in pulmonary neuroendocrine cells in serial rat lung sections stained with doubling dilutions of anti-rat-CGRP antiserum by the peroxidase–antiperoxidase technique. Optical density is an approximately linear function of the logarithm of antiserum dilution, demonstrating that minimal criteria for quantitative immunocytochemistry are satisfied. (Redrawn from McBride *et al.*, 1990).

Immunologic (antigen–antibody) reactions

Antigen–antibody reactions generally satisfy the assumptions of quantitative immunocytochemistry: for a given concentration of antibody, the number of bound antibody molecules will increase quantitatively over a broad range of increasing antigen concentrations. As in classical immunocytochemistry it is important to acknowledge the possibility of cross-reactivity: the presence of specific immunoreactivity does not guarantee the presence of a particular molecular species but only that an epitope similar to or identical with one characteristic of that molecule is present.

Steric hindrance is an important consideration in quantitative immunocytochemistry. The average diameter of the Fab fragment of an IgG molecule is approximately 5–10 nm. If immunoreactive epitopes are more closely spaced than this, antibody binding will be limited by the size of the immunoglobulin molecule rather than by the number of epitopes and a direct relationship between epitope density and staining intensity will be lost. The same consideration applies even more stringently to the second and third layers of many techniques (Sternberger & Sternberger, 1986). Enzyme complexes of the peroxidase–antiperoxidase technique are larger than individual immunoglobulin molecules and those of the avidin–biotin complex method are larger still. Therefore, the number of enzyme molecules or other markers bound to an epitope may be limited by the size of the complex rather than the number of bound primary antibodies. Steric hindrance should be considered if the relationship between staining intensity and primary antiserum dilution is lost. This problem can be remedied by using a relatively high dilution of primary antiserum or by substituting a technique that involves smaller complexes or single immunoglobulin molecules.

Enzymatic reactions

Many immunocytochemical techniques involve the deposition of an insoluble pigment by an enzymatic reaction. In order for staining intensity to be linearly related to the density of immunoreactive epitopes, the number of pigment molecules deposited must be linearly related to the number of enzyme molecules bound to the section. Proportionality between enzyme concentration and pigment density is the basis of many standard biochemical assays. The relationship holds, however, only within limits. For a given concentration of enzyme molecules, the pigment deposition increases approximately linearly with time until the reaction is inhibited by the build up of end product (Fig. 2(a)). The time at which pigment deposition departs from this pseudo-linear relationship is inversely related to enzyme concentration: the higher the concentration of enzyme, the faster pigment is deposited and the sooner the pseudolinear relationship between pigment production and time is violated (Fig. 2(b)). The proportionality between pigment deposited and enzyme concentration is satisfied only as long as the pseudolinear relationship with time is maintained for areas of the section with the highest concentration of enzyme (the most intense immunostaining). To ascertain that this condition is true, serial sections of experimental tissue expected to have the greatest immunoreactivity are immunostained with the concentration of primary antiserum and other reagents to be used for the quantitative study. Slides are developed for various periods of time and the intensity of immunostaining quantified (Fig. 2(c)). A development time well within the pseudolinear portion of this relationship is appropriate for subsequent studies.

Morphometry and microdensitometry

Economical image analysis systems suitable for quantitative microdensitometry are now widely available, but the proper use of such systems requires an appreciation of the basic technical aspects of these measurements. An image analysis system divides an image into a grid of individual pixels or points, each of which is assigned a position within the grid and a value proportional to the brightness or greylevel of the point. The first step of microdensitometry is to determine which pixels represent background tissue and which represent the immunoreactive tissue compartment of interest; the second is to calculate the average optical density of immunostaining of pixels constituting that compartment by comparing the brightness of pixels within the compartment, the brightness of pixels representing unstained tissue, and the intensity of the light illuminating the field.

Tissue compartments can be identified manually by an interactive process

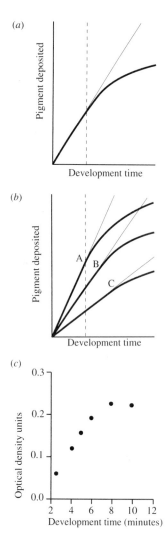

Fig. 2. (*a*) The theoretical relationship between the amount of pigment deposited and development time for the type of enzymatic reaction commonly used in immunocyto-chemistry. Pigment accumulation is approximately linear until the point indicated by the vertical broken line, at which time the reaction rate falls off. (*b*) Schematic illustration of the relationship between pigment deposition and time for three different concentrations of enzyme. So long as pigment deposition is a linear function of time, the quantity of pigment deposited at any one time is proportional to enzyme concentration (A > B > C). Pigment deposition deviates from an approximately linear function of time first for the highest enzyme concentration (A). Staining intensity is a valid measure of enzyme concentration only if development time is shorter than that indicated by the vertical broken line. (*c*) Mean optical density of CGRP-like immunostaining of pulmonary neuroendocrine cells in serial rat lung sections immunostained with the peroxidase–antiperoxidase technique and developed in 0.005% hydrogen peroxide and 0.02% diaminobenzidine for various periods of time. Staining intensity increases nearly linearly with times shorter than 6–8 minutes. A development time of 4.5 minutes was used for subsequent studies. (Redrawn from McBride *et al.*, 1990).

using a joystick or mouse, or automatically by image analysis techniques detailed elsewhere in this volume. For example, to quantify the calcitonin gene-related peptide (CGRP)-like immunoreactivity of pulmonary neuroendocrine cells (McBride *et al.*, 1990), images of immunostained sections were collected and groups of CGRP-immunoreactive neuroendocrine cells outlined manually using a mouse. It would have been possible to identify immunostained cells and determine their borders automatically. As mentioned earlier, it is important with either technique to be sure that the intensity of staining does not influence object identification. A tendency to underestimate the boundaries of cells with relatively low levels of immunostaining and to fail to identify faintly stained cells can be formally assessed by processing serial sections with progressive dilutions of primary antiserum. Both errors compromise quantitative measurements: the mean optical density of immunostaining is overestimated if areas with low levels of immunoreactivity are systematically neglected. When the experimental intervention being studied is not expected to alter the number or size of immunoreactive structures, it is reassuring to document that the number or area of structures per area of tissue is independent of immunoreactivity.

Measurements of the optical density of staining must be carefully standardized. The light transmitted through a structure is dependent on the intensity of light illuminating the field. Therefore, field illumination should not vary over time as multiple sections are analysed. Although many systems provide relatively stable levels of illumination, this level should be checked at regular intervals. Because light intensity is never evenly distributed across a microscopic field, the image analysis system should be able to measure the variation in light intensity across the field and compensate appropriately. While it is prudent to prepare sections as uniformly as possible, variation in section thickness has surprisingly little influence on microdensitometric measurements as long as the depth of field is shallow compared to section thickness; staining outside the depth of field has relatively little influence on the amount of light transmitted through the section. To measure the optical density of immunostaining, the amount of light absorbed by the tissue itself must be subtracted from the total light absorption. Thus it is preferable that sections are not counterstained. Counterstaining, if necessary to identify tissue compartments, should be as light as possible. An advantage of quantitative light microdensitometry is the relative stability of most pigments. Signal stability is an important consideration with immunofluorescence, but should be critical for light microscopy only in exceptional circumstances.

Standards for immunocytochemical microdensitometry

The validity of immunocytochemical microdensitometry depends critically on the preparation and analysis of standard sections. To measure the protein content of tissue samples biochemically, standard samples with known protein concentrations are run simultaneously and a calibration curve for the assay defined. Standards for quantitative immunocytochemistry serve the same purpose. Without standards it may be reasonable to conclude that a greater intensity of immunostaining suggests a greater density of epitopes. Conclusions about relative intensities of immunoreactivity or estimates of actual concentrations of an epitope depend, however, on standard measurements. The validity of quantitative conclusions depends on the degree to which the standards used resemble the experimental tissue.

Immunocytochemical standards can be either synthetic or biological. If purified antigen is available, synthetic standards can be prepared by binding known concentrations to a matrix suitable for histologic processing. Both agarose (Streefkerk *et al.*, 1975; McBride *et al.*, 1990) and nitrocellulose (Nibbering & van Furth, 1987; Peretti-Renucci *et al.*, 1991) have been used for this purpose. If purified antigen is not available, biological tissues that contain a range of measurable concentrations of antigen may be used. For example, Gross & Rothfeld (1985) correlated densitometric immunocytochemical estimates of hypothalamic and pituitary hormone concentrations before and after manipulation of gonadal steroid levels with values obtained by radioimmunoassay. Benno *et al.* (1982) compared immunocytochemical and biochemical measurements of tyrosine hydroxylase concentrations in the locus coeruleus of control animals and animals treated with reserpine to increase brain levels of this enzyme.

Fractional differences in optical density of immunostaining have corresponded closely to fractional differences in antigen concentration in standards in a number of settings. The optical density immunostaining for tyrosine hydroxylase bound to nitrocellulose strips (Fig. 3(*a*)) closely paralleled the concentration bound to the strips (Peretti-Renucci *et al.*, 1991). The relative optical densities of CGRP-immunostained agarose beads (Fig. 3(*b*)) slightly underestimated differences in the actual concentrations of CGRP (McBride *et al.*, 1990). Similar results have been demonstrated by a number of investigators using biological standards (Benno *et al.*, 1982; Gross & Rothfeld, 1985). The optical density of lung cell nuclei immunostained for specific DNA binding of an aromatic hydrocarbon (Fig. 1(*c*)), generally paralleled the concentration of DNA–hydrocarbon complexes measured by a radioactive assay (van Schooten *et al.*, 1991).

It may be difficult to prepare optimum standards for every study, particularly if purified antigen is not available. The validity of immunocytochemical standards is greatest if:

1 The actual level of the pertinent antigen in the standard is measured biochemically.
2 The intensity of immunostaining of standards brackets the intensity of staining in the experimental material.
3 The standard sections are treated identically and simultaneously with the experimental sections from fixation to microdensitometry.

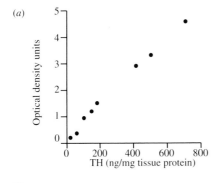

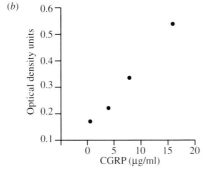

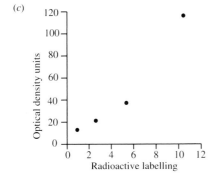

Fig. 3. (*a*) The optical density of immunostaining of nitrocellulose strips stained for tyrosine hydroxylase (TH) by the peroxidase–antiperoxidase method as a function of the amount of TH adsorbed to the strips. (Redrawn from Peretti-Renucci *et al.*, 1991). (*b*) The optical density of immunostaining of agarose beads immunostained for calcitonin gene-related peptide (CGRP) by the peroxidase–antiperoxidase technique as a function of the concentration of CGRP bound to the beads. The fractional change in optical density somewhat underestimates the fractional change in CGRP concentration over the range of optical density units from 0.25 to 0.5. (Redrawn from McBride *et al.*, 1990). (*c*) Staining intensity of mouse lung cell nuclei immunostained for the presence of benzo[a]pyrene-derived adducts in DNA as a function of adduct density measured by a radioactive technique. The relationship is roughly linear. Additional points between 40 and 120 optical density units would be desirable. (Redrawn from van Schooten *et al.*, 1991).

The supraoptimal dilution technique

The supraoptimal dilution technique is an alternative to microdensitometry that can be used to document differences in immunoreactivity between experimental groups but does not permit estimation of the extent of such differences (Taugner *et al.*, 1982; Vacca-Galloway, 1985). The 'optimal' dilution of primary antiserum in classical immunocytochemistry is that with which all structures with appreciable levels of immunoreactivity are stained. This presumably corresponds to that highest dilution with which all available epitopes are bound by specific antibodies. The supraoptimal dilution technique is based on the assumption that as the primary antiserum is progressively diluted, immunostaining of structures with relatively low densities of immunoreactive epitopes will disappear while structures with greater immunoreactivity will continue to stain.

The usual strategy of the supraoptimal dilution technique is to stain one set of sections with the optimal dilution of primary antiserum and a second set with a weaker or supraoptimal dilution. The fractional decrease in the area or number of immunostained structures (the number or area identified after staining with the supraoptimal dilution divided by that identified with the optimal dilution) should be inversely related to the level of immunoreactivity. Therefore, the hypothesis that one experimental group has less specific immunoreactivity than another is supported by a greater fractional decrease in the number or area of immunostained structures after staining with the supraoptimal dilution.

Several practical aspects of this technique deserve consideration. To choose an appropriate supraoptimal dilution, serial sections expected to have lower levels of immunoreactivity are immunostained with progressive dilutions of primary antiserum beginning with the optimal dilution. A suitable supraoptimal dilution is one with which the number or area of detectable immunostained structures is decreased by 50–75% from the value obtained with the optimal dilution. Because immunostaining is relatively weak with the supraoptimal dilution, discriminating immunostained structures from background may become difficult. This inevitably involves judgement, but does not compromise the technique so long as sections are randomized and the microscopist is strictly unaware of which sections are being analysed. Rather than processing separate sets of sections with optimal and supraoptimal dilutions, it is preferable to sequentially stain and analyse a single set of sections. Sections are first stained with the supraoptimal dilution of primary antiserum, coverslipped, and counted. The coverslips are then removed and the sections restained with the optimal dilution. This method eliminates the unavoidable difference in the number or area of immunostained structures between sections from the same tissue.

Springall *et al.* (1988) used this technique to investigate the influence of hypoxia on the CGRP-like immunoreactivity of pulmonary neuroendocrine cells in the rat. They found that the number of cells per area of lung section immunostained with the optimal dilution of anti-rat CGRP antiserum was similar between control rats and rats maintained in an hypoxic environment for three weeks (Fig. 4). The number of immunoreactive cells per unit area on sections stained with a supraoptimal dilution of primary antiserum fell by only 11% in hypoxic animals but decreased by 67% in controls, supporting the hypothesis that CGRP-like immunoreactivity in these cells was greater in hypoxic rats. In a subsequent study, McBride *et al.* (1990) demonstrated that the supraoptimal dilution technique was more sensitive than microdensitometry in detecting increased CGRP-like immunoreactivity in pulmonary neuroendo-crine cells in rats exposed to hypoxia for one week.

The supraoptimal dilution technique is a simple and surprisingly sensitive method to detect differences in immunoreactivity. It would be reasonable to use this technique to screen for differences in immunoreactivity between groups. When such differences are identified, microdensitometry can be used to estimate the extent of such differences.

An innovative method of quantitative immunocytochemistry: the Sternberger technique

An innovative method to measure the area and intensity of immunostaining, described by Sternberger & Sternberger (Sternberger, 1985; Sternberger &

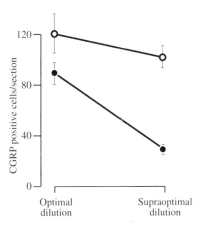

Fig. 4. The number of pulmonary neuroendocrine cells with calcitonin gene-related peptide (CGRP)-like immunoreactivity per section of whole lung in control rats (filled circles) and rats exposed to hypoxia for three weeks prior to sacrifice (open circles). Hypoxic rats have a slightly lower number of CGRP-reactive cells per unit area than controls when sections were immunostained with the optimal dilution (1:2000) of primary anti-rat CGRP antiserum. The fractional decrease in the number of CGRP-reactive cells after staining with a supraoptimal dilution of primary antiserum (1:50000) is greater in the control group than in the hypoxic group (Springall *et al.*, 1988).

(a)

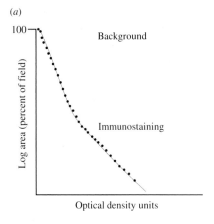

(b)

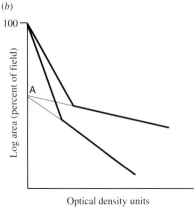

Fig. 5. (a) Logarithm of the area of immunostaining (y axis) with intensity greater than each given value of optical density (x axis) for one microscopic field of rat cerebellum stained with an anti-phosphorylated-neurofilament monoclonal antibody using the peroxidase–antiperoxidase technique. The plot can be resolved into two straight lines. The upper line represents background and the lower line specific immunostaining. The slope of each line is inversely related to staining intensity. Because the vertical axis is positioned at the optical density of the brightest pixel in the image, the upper line transects the vertical axis at the area of the entire section. The extrapolation of the lower line (not shown) crosses the vertical axis at a value characteristic of the total area of immunostaining. (b) Theoretical plot for area of immunostaining and optical density for a single section stained with two dilutions of primary antiserum. The slope of the line representing immunoreactive tissue is flatter for the section stained more intensely. Back extrapolation of the lines for immunostaining crosses the vertical axis at the same value (A), demonstrating that the measurement of area is independent of the intensity of immunostaining.

Sternberger, 1986), eliminates the need to discriminate immunostained structures from background. It is, therefore, particularly suited for studies of complex structures such as nerve or connective tissue fibres that are difficult to discriminate from background. The tacit assumptions of this technique are that there is only one type of immunoreactive element in the tissue, that the optical density of all pixels constituting immunoreactive structures is normally distributed around some mean value, and that the optical density of pixels constituting background are normally distributed around some lower mean value. When the optical density of each pixel is measured, a log-linear plot (Fig. 5(*a*)) is constructed such that each point represents (on the *y* axis) the logarithm of the number of pixels with an optical density greater than or equal to each value of optical density (on the *x* axis). The value corresponding to the optical density of the brightest pixel in the image will therefore be the total number of pixels and that for the optical density of the darkest pixels will be very small. Because the area of a structure is proportional to the number of pixels it comprises, the *y* axis corresponds to area.

If the assumptions are satisfied the plot comprises two straight lines. The lower line represents specific immunostaining and the upper, background. The slope of each line reflects the intensity of staining with a more horizontal slope corresponding to a greater intensity of staining. The point at which the plot reaches the optical density value of the brightest pixel is, by definition, the area of the entire image. When the line representing immunostaining is extrapolated back to the same point, its value will correspond to the area of specific immunoreactivity.

The appeal of this analysis is that the area of immunoreactivity is defined independently of the intensity of immunostaining. If identical sections are stained with different dilutions of primary antiserum, the apparent area of immunostaining might vary considerably and the slopes of the portions of the plots representing immunostaining differ, but the lines on the two plots should extrapolate to the same point (Fig. 5(*b*)). Although this is potentially most valuable for small complex structures, it might be useful whenever the apparent area of immunoreactivity varies with staining intensity or immunostaining is weak compared to background. The technique as originally described involved relatively laborious manipulations, but with modern equipment the plot can be generated nearly instantaneously. Although this method has great theoretical appeal, it has been used infrequently. A quantitative relationship between staining intensity as measured by this technique and epitope concentration in standard sections has not been documented.

References

Benno, R. H., Tucker, L. W., Joh, T. H. & Reis, D. J. (1982). Quantitative immunocytochemistry of tyrosine hydroxylase in rat brain. I. Development of a computer assisted method using the peroxidase-antiperoxidase technique. *Brain Research*, **246**, 225–36.

Bigbee, J. W., Kosek, J. C. & Eng, L. E. (1977). The effects of primary antisera dilution on staining of 'antigen' rich tissue with the peroxidase antiperoxidase technique. *Journal of Histochemistry and Cytochemistry*, **25**, 443–47.

Gross, D. S. & Rothfeld, J. M. (1985). Quantitative immunocytochemistry of hypothalamic and pituitary hormones. *Journal of Histochemistry and Cytochemistry*, 33, 11–20.

McBride, J. T., Springall, D. R., Winter, R. J. D. & Polak, J. M. (1990). Quantitative immunocytochemistry shows calcitonin gene-related peptide-like immunoreactivity in lung neuroendocrine cells is increased by chronic hypoxia in the rat. *American Journal of Respiratory Cell and Molecular Biology*, 3, 587–93.

Nibbering, P. H. & van Furth, R. (1987). Microphotometric quantitation of the reaction product of several indirect immunoperoxidase methods demonstrating monoclonal antibody binding to antigens immobilized on nitrocellulose. *Journal of Histochemistry and Cytochemistry*, 35, 1425–31.

Peretti-Renucci, R., Feuerstein, C., Manier, M., Orimeier, P., Savasta, M. Thibault, J., Mons, M. & Geffard, M. J. (1991). Quantitative image analysis with densitometry for immunohistochemisty and autoradiography of receptor binding sites-methodological considerations. *Journal of Neuroscience Research*, 28, 583–600.

Rahier, J., Stevens, M., de Menten, Y & Henquin, J-C. (1989). Determination of antigen concentration in tissue sections by immunodensitometry. *Laboratory Investigation*, 61, 357–63.

Snedecor, G. W. & Cochran, W. G. (1967). Statistical Methods (6th edition), pp. 58–9. Ames, IA: Iowa State University Press.

Springall, D. R., Collina, G., Barer, G. Suggett, A. J., Bee, D. & Polak, J. M. (1988). Increased intracellular levels of calcitonin gene-related peptide-like immunoreactivity in pulmonary endocrine cells of hypoxic rats. *Journal of Pathology*, 155, 259–67.

Sternberger, L. A. (1985). *Immunocytochemistry* (3rd edition), pp. 146–63, New York, John Wiley.

Sternberger, L. A. & Sternberger, N. H. (1986). The unlabeled antibody method: comparison of peroxidase-antiperoxidase with avidin-biotin complex by a new method of quantification. *Journal of Histochemistry and Cytochemistry*, 34, 599–605.

Streefkerk, J. G., van der Ploeg, M. & van Duijn, P. (1975). Agarose beads as matrices for proteins in cytophotometric investigations of immunohistoperoxidase procedures. *Journal of Histochemistry and Cytochemistry*, 23, 243–50.

Taugner, R., Hackenthal, E., Inagami, T., Nobiling, R. & Poulsen, K. (1982). Vascular and tubular renin in the kidneys of mice. *Histochemistry*, 75, 473–84.

Vacca-Galloway, L. L. (1985). Differential immunostaining for substance P in Huntington's Diseased and normal spinal cord: significance of serial (optimal, supra-optimal and end-point) dilutions of primary anti-serum in comparing biological specimens. *Histochemistry*, 83, 561–9.

van Schooten, F. J., Hillebrand, M. J. X., Scherer, E., den Engelse, L. & Kriek, E. (1991). Immunocytochemical visualization of DNA adducts in mouse tissues and human white blood cells following treatment with benzo[a]pyrene or its diol epoxide. A quantitative approach. *Carcinogenesis*, 12, 427–33.

20

Quantification of nerves and neurotransmitters using image analysis

T. COWEN

Introduction

A decade has passed since image analysis began to be used widely to quantify cellular features of the nervous system. The seminal studies of Agnati, Fuxe and their co-workers (Agnati & Fuxe, 1984) and others (Gardette, Mallet & Bisconte, 1981) demonstrated the possibilities of what could be achieved using these new methods in the central nervous system.

Catecholamine histochemistry generated high contrast fluorescence images of specific populations of central and peripheral nerves suitable for quantification (Falck *et al.*, 1962; Lindvall & Bjorklund, 1974). Early applications demonstrated that image analysis, with its ability to make many measurements rapidly on complex images, was ideally suited to work on the nervous system where the human eye is frequently defeated by the sheer numbers of fibres and cells.

Immunohistochemistry provided a new kind of information about neurotransmitter, structural and other markers specific to particular populations of nerve cells. Image analysis methods were modified in developmental and other studies using immunohistochemical labelling and were helped by a new generation of image analysers providing increased flexibility of operation and improved resolution (see Agnati & Fuxe, 1985; Zoli *et al.*, 1986).

One of the most challenging areas of image analysis has been in the development of densitometric techniques. Autoradiographic labelling of neuroreceptors, measurements of glucose utilization in nerves, and attempts to quantify neurotransmitter dynamics all require densitometric assessment. Image analysis, because it can combine cellular localization of labelling with densitometry, is well suited to such applications and several approaches have been developed.

Microscopists have striven to develop images ever more closely related to living biological stuctures. Confocal laser scanning microscopy can now provide 3-D images of, for example, the dendritic arbors of neurones (Wallen *et al.*, 1988). Low light video imaging has been used to demonstrate growth and retraction of living nerves. Image analysis will be important in quantifying information from these exciting new images of nerves. Molecular biological techniques such as *in situ* hybridization can also be quantified using image analysis, providing new information about the dynamics of gene expression (Stewart, 1992; Schalling *et al.*, 1988).

In this chapter I aim to present some of the most significant developments in image analysis and specific staining techniques in the context of recent studies into changes in the peripheral nervous system during development and ageing and in disease.

Catecholamine histochemistry – methodology

The majority of blood vessels are innervated by a 2-D plexus of nerve fibres, some of which originate from postganglionic sympathetic neurones distributed in pre- and para-vertebral sympathetic ganglia. Their catecholaminergic neuro-transmitter, noradrenaline, can be demonstrated by the formaldehyde-induced fluorescence (FIF) method established by Falck, Hillarp and co-workers (Falck *et al.*, 1962). These nerves lie at the junction between the tunica media and tunica adventitia of the blood vessel wall and the plexus can be demonstrated in exquisite detail using the glyoxylic acid modification of FIF (Lindvall & Bjorklund, 1974) on whole mount stretch preparations (Cowen & Burnstock, 1980; Furness & Costa, 1975: see Fig. 1). Perivascular catecholaminergic nerve plexuses show a bewildering variety of patterns and densities in different regions and types of blood vessel. Whilst the human eye and brain are very good at pattern recognition, they are less good at discriminating between plexuses of similar pattern but different densities, resulting from changes in either mesh size or in the size of the component nerve bundles. Methods based on visual assessment have generally attempted to distinguish a maximum of four degrees of nerve density, such as sparse, medium, dense and very dense and have required checking by two independent operators (see Cowen & Burnstock, 1982).

Catecholamine fluorescence images of nerve plexuses are suited to image analysis by virtue of the high contrast between nerves and background and the lack of granularity in the staining. However, the unstable nature of fluores-cence images is a significant disadvantage. Image analysis routines have been developed to make comparisons of fluorescence images using the Quantimet 720 (Cambridge Instruments, UK: Cowen & Burnstock, 1980, 1982, 1985). The analyser was interfaced to a Zeiss photomicroscope using a plumbicon low light video camera. Image input utilized a standard averaging procedure, summing ten images and dividing by ten, in order to reduce random noise in the image. Comparisons of direct input of images from the microscope with indirect input of photographic images, via a macro imaging system (Fig. 2), showed reduced resolution in the indirect system (Cowen & Burnstock, 1982).

The mercury lamp and associated optics used in fluorescence microscopy produce non-uniform illumination of the field of view, which necessitates the use of background subtraction routines similar to those used in transmission light microscopy. However, because of the widely used epi-illumination light path, a reflective specimen has to be used to generate a background image. Initial attempts involved subtracting a de-focussed image of the specimen from a focussed image on the assumption that the de-focussed image would sum contributions from both illumination system and specimen to the uneven background. The second assumption behind this, and subsequent, background subtraction procedures is that specific, neuronal fluorescence is summed on background fluorescence.

Standard edge- or contour-enhancing image processing algorithms were used to provide an image that could be segmented with minimum subjectivity. This produced a binary image of the nerves that closely resembled the original image. However, even following background subtraction, contrast (i.e. the difference between the lowest greyvalue of nerves and highest greyvalue of background) was never sufficient to allow a constant threshold value to be used for segmenting all images. The continuing need for subjective thresholding in biological image analysis remains one of the weakest, and most underinvestigated, links in the analytic chain.

A wide range of parameters can be measured in a binary image. On nerve plexuses, two parameters have been found to be particularly useful. Field area expresses the number of pixels occupied by specific signal and is proportional to the total number or length of nerve *fibres* in the field. Intercept density represents the number of intercepts scored on an array of parallel lines and is proportional to the total number, or length, of nerve *bundles* in the field. These parameters can change independently of each other. During regeneration, for example, when nerve fibres tend to follow pathways established at the outset of the process, the area will increase whilst the intercept density will tend to remain constant.

Using this system of analysis, the effects of fading were assessed on fluorescence images during frozen storage and exposure to ultraviolet light (Cowen & Burnstock, 1982: see Fig. 3). Whilst storage and ultraviolet exposure resulted in fading of fluorescence, these experiments showed that, as far as field parameters were concerned, image analysis measurements were robust. They could compensate for the contrast lost by fading following up to three weeks of frozen storage and after at least ten minutes of exposure to ultraviolet light.

Catecholamine histochemistry – applications

Image analysis has proved valuable in studies of regional variations of nerve density (Amenta *et al.*, 1987) and in studies of degeneration and regeneration of peripheral nerves (Luthman & Hallman, 1986; Henschen & Olson, 1983). A longitudinal study of development and ageing in the noradrenergic innervation of different blood vessels at six stages in the rabbit's life cycle demonstrated the value of image analysis (Cowen *et al.*, 1982). Large numbers of specimens

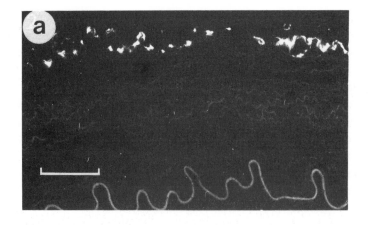

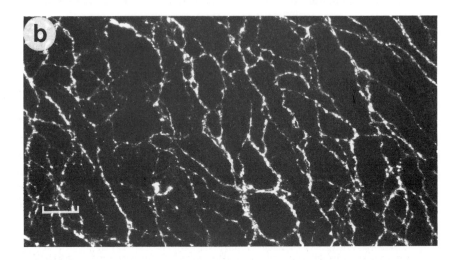

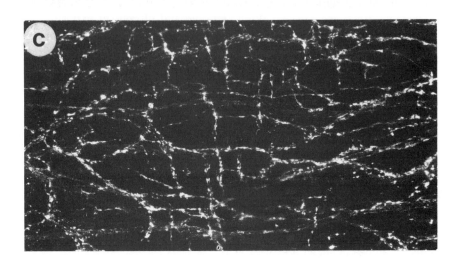

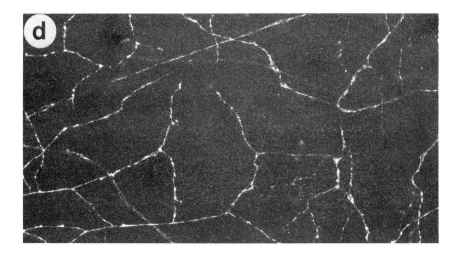

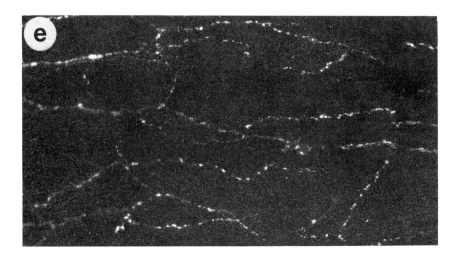

Fig. 1. Catecholamine fluorescence of nerves in different blood vessels prepared using glyoxylic acid fluorescence histochemistry. (*a*) TS; (*b*)–(*e*) whole mounts, vessel axis horizontal; scale bars represent 50 μm. (*a*) TS carotid artery. Fluorescent adrenergic nerves are arranged as a 2-D network at the adventitial–medial border in a band approximately 10 μm wide. Note the autofluorescence of the internal elastic lamina of the intima. Plastic section (3 μm). (*b*) Carotid artery. A dense plexus of adrenergic nerves with a wide range of nerve bundle size and with many varicosities, some of which form brightly fluorescent groups. (*c*) Mesenteric artery. A dense plexus of adrenergic nerves with very large brightly fluorescent nerve bundles, fine terminal regions and a few faintly fluorescent large nerves. A large number of varicosities are seen, some grouped together. (*d*) Mesenteric vein. A sparse plexus of fine adrenergic nerves, the majority of which carry varicosities. Some nerves appear to end over the smooth muscle layer. (*e*) Abdominal aorta. A sparse plexus of fine adrenergic axon bundles, most of which carry brightly fluorescent varicosities (Cowen & Burnstock, 1980).

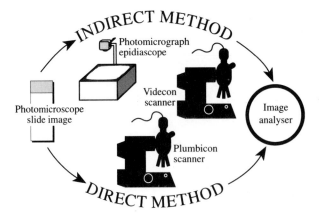

Fig. 2. Diagrammatic representation of 'direct' and 'indirect' methods of image input for image analysis (Cowen & Burnstock, 1980).

could be measured thoroughly and rapidly with methods that gave consistent results as judged by the standard deviations between successive experiments on different animals. With this level of variance, differences of 10–15% were significant indicating a resolution approximately twice that of visual methods of assessment (Fig. 4). From a biological point of view, this study showed the remarkable spatial and temporal specificity of developmental changes in nerve density, each blood vessel having a characteristic age graph of changes. It was noticeable that there was no point in the life cycle where it could be said that ageing had commenced; indeed, whilst dramatic losses of catecholamine-stained nerve fibres were seen, particularly in the renal artery, nerve plexuses in the basilar and mesenteric arteries were relatively unaffected by age, remaining apparently stable throughout maturity.

Attempts were made in this study to discriminate and count the nerve varicosities where neurotransmitter is concentrated and from where it is released, on the basis of the brighter staining of these regions of the axon. In the renal artery in old rabbits, numbers of varicosities were reduced but not to the same extent as nerve fibres (Fig. 4). These results suggested that non-varicose parts of axons, because of their lower content of noradrenaline, disappeared from view more readily than varicosities in old age. The difficulties of assessing the extent of age-related neurodegeneration from microscopical studies of this kind will be referred to later. The morphological characteristics of blood vessels with apparently non-functional nerves were compared with functionally innervated vessels using similar methods (Gallen *et al.*, 1982).

Immunohistochemistry – field measurements of nerve density

Amines

The technique of immunohistochemistry has underpinned some of the most exciting developments of the last 20 years in neuroscience, notably in the

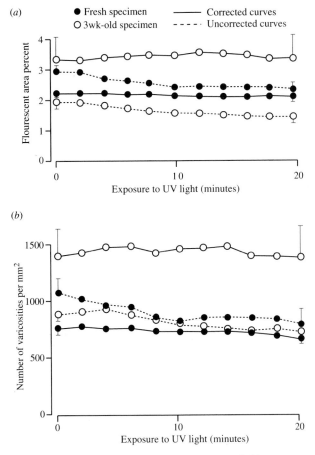

Fig. 3. Graphs showing fading of fluorescence in field measurements of nerves. Image analysis of (*a*) fluorescent area and (*b*) number of varicosities of perivascular substance P-positive nerves labelled with FITC using immunofluorescence histochemistry on stretch preparations of the guinea-pig carotid artery. Uncorrected curves (---) show fading during 20 min of exposure to ultraviolet light in fresh specimens (●) and in specimens stored for three weeks in the freezer (○). Corrected curves (——) show the ability of the image analyzer to compensate for fading on exposure to ultraviolet light in the fresh and stored specimens (Cowen, 1984).

discovery and localization of new neurotransmitter substances (Lundberg & Hokfelt, 1983; Hokfelt *et al.*, 1980). Our understanding of the role of biogenic amines in the nervous system came to include the indoleamine, 5-hydroxy-tryptamine (5-HT or serotonin), identified initially using fluorescence histochemistry (Dahlstrom & Ahlman, 1983) and then, more sensitively, using antisera raised against the small amine molecule conjugated to serum albumin (Steinbusch *et al.*, 1978). More recently, the capacity of neurones to synthesise 5-HT has been demonstrated using an antibody against the rate-limiting enzyme, tryptophan hydroxylase (Chedotal & Hamel, 1990). Previous methods of image analysis were adapted in order to study the distribution of 5-HT in

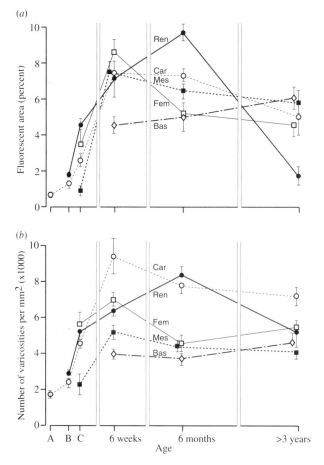

Fig. 4. Graph of age related changes in (*a*) fluorescent area (percentage of total surface area), and (*b*) numbers of varicosities ($\times 10^{-3}$ mm^{-2} surface area) of perivascular adrenergic nerves in five arteries of the rabbit. Nerves demonstrated by glyoxylic acid fluorescence histochemistry and measured by image analysis (Cowen *et al.*, 1982).

perivascular nerves using conventional indirect immunohistochemistry with fluorescence-labelled second antibodies (Coons, 1958).

Developments in image analysis technique were required to quantify immunofluorescence staining. In particular, the brightness of staining varied between antibodies, calling for methods that could cope with different levels of image contrast. New image analysers became available that allowed the development of software-driven measuring programs tailored to particular tissues. Fluctuations in the output of mercury lamps were reduced using a stabilized power supply. Lamp brightness was set and checked during and between experiments using a uranyl glass standard (Zeiss, Germany), which generated a spatially and temporally uniform output in response to ultraviolet light. A survey of different fluorescence microscopes showed considerable differences in the intensity and uniformity of fluorescence illumination (Cowen & Thrasivoulou, 1992*a*). Whilst video scanners were becoming more sensitive, it was found that the Panasonic Moonlight camera (model WV-1900) itself contributed to the non-uniformity of illumination in the system.

The achievement of a uniformly illuminated field where nerves could be reliably segmented from background therefore remained a key problem in image analysis of immunofluorescence labelling. Tissue elements and non-specific binding added to the uneven background. The principal contributors were fibrous connective tissue elements in the blood vessel wall, notably elastin, which autofluoresced at a wavelength close to that of FITC. Pontamine Sky Blue (BDH, UK) was used to stain the connective tissue selectively (Cowen *et al.*, 1985). Red fluorescence resulting from absorption of blue light over the stained areas was filtered out of the FITC-stained image using a 560 nm cutoff filter. However, counterstaining was not always able to eliminate non-specific fluorescence generated by the specimen. The increased range of image processing algorithms available with the new generation of image analysers was useful in subtracting the uneven background. On the IBAS IPS image analyser, a large matrix, low pass filter was used which included a greylevel cutoff in order to generate images of the non-specific fluorescence for each specimen that could be used for background subtraction. These images also provided some compensation for the uneven illumination produced by the optics and scanner.

Using these methods, 5-HT immunoreactive nerves supplying cerebral blood vessels were quantified. It was shown that these nerves originated in the superior cervical ganglion in the gerbil (Cowen *et al.*, 1986: see Fig. 5) and rat (Cowen *et al.*, 1987) and that the nerve supply from each ganglion was to some extent bilateral. Changes in the distribution of 5-HT immunoreactive nerves in blood vessels from ageing animals were also studied (Gale *et al.*, 1989) and it was found that 5-HT immunoreactivity declined in cerebral and other blood vessels with age in similar, but not identical ways to noradrenaline. This suggested that these substances, coexisting in the same nerves, could be differentially regulated during ageing.

Neuropeptides

Image analysis proved applicable to immunohistochemical studies of neuro-peptides such as substance P (Contestabile *et al.*, 1987; Cowen, 1984), neuro-peptide Y (Calza *et al.*, 1990) and other neuropeptides (Terenghi *et al.*, 1991). Recently, age changes in sudomotor innervation of rat and human skin have been evaluated. Using image analysis, dramatic reductions have been shown in the total numbers of nerve fibres using the general neuronal marker, PGP9.5 (Thompson *et al.*, 1983) and in the neuropeptides VIP and CGRP around sweat glands and in the skin of old rats (Abdel-Rahman & Cowen, 1993: see Fig. 6). Histochemical staining for acetyl cholinesterase was greatly reduced.

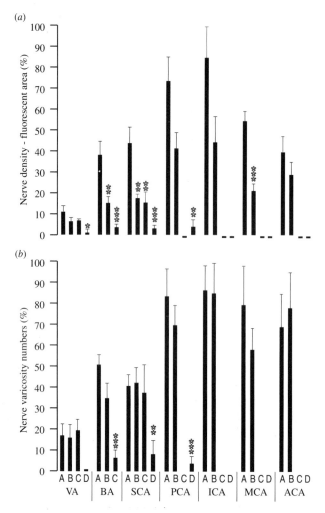

Fig. 5. Histograms showing the effects of unilateral and bilateral superior cervical ganglionectomy on the density of 5-HT-containing nerves to the vertebral (VA), basilar (BA), superior cerebellar (SCA), posterior cerebral (PCA), internal carotid (ICA), middle cerebral (MCA) and anterior cerebral (ACA) arteries of the gerbil. Histogram bins: A, control; B, right side vessels after left unilateral ganglionectomy; C, left side vessels after left unilateral ganglionectomy; D, bilateral ganglionectomy. Nerves were demonstrated on whole mount preparations using fluorescence immunohistochemistry and measured using image analysis. Values are expressed as mean percentage of maximum (±s.e.m.). (a) Nerve density expressed as mean fluorescent area. (b) Nerve varicosity numbers (Cowen et al., 1986).

Furthermore, in a previous study of ageing in human sweat glands using PGP9.5-staining and electron microscopy, evidence was found that reductions in neuropeptides were associated with loss of axon collaterals (Abdel-Rahman et al., 1992a). These studies have demonstrated that reductions in neuroactive substances observed during ageing were probably the result of both degenera-

(a)   (b)

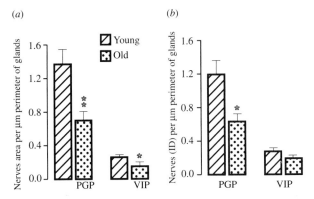

Fig. 6. Histograms showing mean nerve densities, expressed as (a) area and (b) intercept density, of PGP- and VIP-LI nerves per μm perimeter of sweat gland secretory coils in old and young rats. Error bars show s.e.m. Differences between means: *$p < 0.05$, **$p < 0.02$ (Abdel-Rahman and Cowen, 1993).

tion of axon collaterals and of reductions in intraneuronal concentrations of these substances in surviving collaterals.

The highly autofluorescent age pigment, lipofuscin, present in sweat glands from old people and rodents proved a serious problem in this study. Image analysis masking techniques were helpful in resolving the difficulty: following background subtraction, a mask delineating the outer circumference of the sweat gland acinus was drawn interactively and used to measure age changes in acinar dimensions. Lipofuscin present in the gland cells was eliminated from the image by filling the mask and setting the phase to black. Image processing could then be carried out to optimize identification of nerves, without interference of lipofuscin (Abdel-Rahman & Cowen, 1993).

Double immunolabelling

It has been found possible to quantify nerves in double-labelling studies in order to evaluate changes in different populations of nerves innervating the same tissue, or in different neuroactive substances coexisting in the same nerve fibres (Fuxe *et al.*, 1985). In the latter case, caution has to be exercised in the sequence of staining procedures because of the problem of steric hindrance where binding of one antibody can inhibit binding of subsequently applied antibodies at adjacent sites within a nerve. Trial and error determined the most sensitive sequence of staining (Webster *et al.*, 1991). When using the normal green/red combination of fluorophors, texas red was found to give reliable spectral separation from FITC fluorescence whereas the more commonly used TRITC label caused interference in the green band.

The latest generation of image analysers included algorithms (Boolean operators) which allowed the matching of different binary images. Images could be summed or compared for the degree of match or mismatch. These seemed ideally suited for quantifying the extent of coexistence of different neuronal substances in double labelling studies. However, in epi-fluorescence microscopy the position of the final image is determined by the alignment of the dichroic mirror which transmits light emitted by the specimen. The majority of microscopical systems use separate filter sets for red and green epi-fluorescence, the dichroic mirrors of which are rarely identically aligned. Misalignment results in slight displacements relative to each other of the red and green images, such that the fluorophors of truly coexisting antigens appeared not to have matched distributions. This problem is serious only where small structures such as nerve fibres are under investigation; coexistence of different antigens in nerve cell bodies are not so seriously affected (Johansson & Hallman, 1985). The problem can be resolved by using the new, multiple coated dichroic mirrors which allow dual channel fluorescence imaging with the same mirror and different absorption and excitation filters.

Despite these difficulties, double labelling studies of diabetic neuropathy were able to show that diabetes affects selected populations of mesenteric perivascular nerves, leaving others unimpaired (Webster et al., 1991). Tyrosine hydroxylase (TH), the rate-limiting enzyme in the synthesis of noradrenaline, coexists with 5-HT in the terminal plexuses of sympathetic nerves. Immuno-reactivity related to both TH and 5-HT was substantially reduced during induction of diabetes in the streptozotocin animal model of the disease, suggesting that sympathetic axonal damage may have occurred. Staining for substance P, present in presumptive afferent fibres, showed that these fibres were unaffected by diabetes. The resolution of fluorescence light microscopical images in cryostat sections or whole mount preparations rarely achieves 1 μm. Therefore, whilst it was possible to see that substance P was present in separate fibres from TH-stained nerves, even when they ran in the same nerve bundle, it was not possible to be certain that all TH-immunoreactive fibres also contained 5-HT.

This study brought into sharp focus one of the most intractable problems in interpreting this kind of data. How could changes in levels of neuroactive substances in intact nerves be distinguished from the physical degeneration of nerve fibres? Without additional experiments using structural markers for nerve fibres such as PGP9.5 or neurofilament antibodies, it is difficult to answer this question. Even then, the question remains since expression of structural markers may also be altered (see below).

Immunochemistry – densitometric measurements of neurotransmitter dynamics

The studies described above and those from other laboratories (King et al., 1989) raised the question of whether image analysis could be used to study the dynamics of neuroactive substances. In particular, it was important to investi-gate whether 5-HT was present in perivascular sympathetic nerves as a result of neuronal synthesis or uptake. Furthermore, it seemed clear that at least in some of our studies, changes were taking place in transmitter levels, or in nerve fibre number, or, perhaps, in both (see above). The question was whether the intensity of immunohistochemical staining could provide quantitative information about the intraneuronal concentration of neuroactive substances which, combined with field measurements of nerve density, could help to resolve these problems. Image analysis is able to make densitometric measurements of stain intensity that can be localized to particular populations of nerve fibres, with possible advantages over biochemical techniques involving tissue homogenates, where cellular localization is lost. Furthermore, several elements in the blood vessel wall have the capacity to take up or metabolize 5-HT, so that the capacity to localize changes to nerve fibres is essential.

Using this approach, it has proved possible to measure changes in intraneuronal 5-HT in tissue samples too small to allow detection by high pressure, liquid chromatography. To achieve this, several areas of technique had to be examined. Much of this work has been published recently (Cowen & Thrasivoulou, 1992*a*) and will only be summarized here.

Methodology – specimen preparation

Densitometric image analysis was used to optimize fixation conditions, select suitable buffers for tissue processing, evaluate antibodies and titrate dilutions and assess the rate of fading of fluorescence. In common with other studies of fixation (Polak & Van Noorden, 1986), fixation in 4% paraformaldehyde for 1.5–2 hours was found to give the most reliable preservation, although particular antibodies and tissues may benefit from treatment with, for example, Zamboni's fixative. It was found that organic buffers markedly enhance stain intensity in comparison with the more generally used phosphate-buffered saline (PBS). In particular, the use of Hepes buffer throughout immunostaining procedures can result in stain intensities 25–50% greater than PBS, (Fig. 7: Cowen & Thrasivoulou, 1992*a*). The positively charged metal ions in PBS are thought to attract antibody proteins thereby increasing non-specific staining and reducing the amount of available antibody for specific binding.

A model system using cryostat sections of gelatine containing dissolved antigen has been developed to assess specificity of binding of 5-HT antibodies (Schipper & Tilders, 1983). The same system was employed to select and titrate 5-HT antibodies against varying concentrations of antigen (Cowen & Thrasivoulou, 1992*a*). These experiments showed that monoclonal antibodies gave a more sensitive and linear response to varying concentrations of antigen compared to polyclonals (Fig. 8). However, in the case of 5-HT, detection was restricted to antigen concentrations in excess of 10^{-6} M. It was found that amplification of signal using streptavidin–biotin systems abolished any quantitative relationship between greyvalue and antigen concentration (Table 1).

As expected, densitometric assessment of fading demonstrated more serious

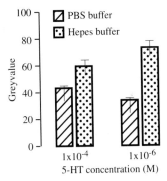

Fig. 7. Histogram demonstrating the effects of PBS and Hepes buffers on intensity of fluorescence (greyvalue). Whole mounts of rabbit mesenteric vein incubated in 10^{-4} and 10^{-6} M serotonin for 20 minutes. Tissue was subsequently processed using indirect immunohistochemistry (Cowen & Thrasivoulou, 1992a).

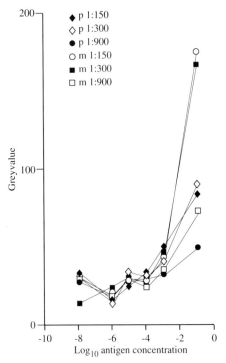

Fig. 8. Plot of stain intensity (greyvalue) against antigen concentration using mono-(m) and poly-(p) clonal antibodies at dilutions of 1:150, 1:300 and 1:900. Fixed, gelatine, vibratome (50 μm) sections containing 10^{-1}–10^{-8} M concentrations of serotonin were processed for indirect immunohistochemistry (Cowen & Thrasivoulou, 1992a).

problems than had been shown by previous experiments measuring field data (see above). Even when specimens were stored frozen, fluorescence intensity faded significantly during the first two days following preparation (Fig. 9). Thus measurements of stain intensity on different specimens should be carried out at the same time following preparation, for example, after two days.

Table 1. *Stain intensity in rabbit mesenteric veins*

Serotonin concentration (M)	Greylevel (amplified)	Greylevel (non-amplified)
10^{-4}	61 ($\pm$ 7)	57 ($\pm$ 10)
10^{-6}	63 ($\pm$ 5)	33 ($\pm$ 1)

Greylevels shown in the table are means ($\pm$ S.E.M.) in 5 animals. Samples were incubated in serotonin for 20 min and processed for normal indirect and avidin–biotin amplified fluorescence immunohistochemistry (Cowen & Thrasivoulou, 1992*b*).

(*a*)

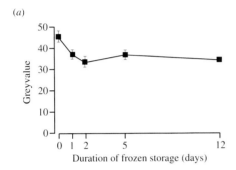

(*b*)

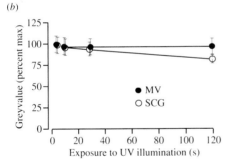

Fig. 9. Measurements of fading of FITC fluorescence using image analysis. (*a*) Effect of frozen storage on sections of rabbit superior cervical ganglion (SCG) stained using a monoclonal antibody to tyrosine hydroxylase followed by indirect labelling with FITC. (*b*) Effect of exposure to ultraviolet light on sections of SCG and whole mounts of mesenteric vein (MV) from rabbits stained using a monoclonal antibody to serotonin followed by indirect labelling with FITC (Cowen & Thrasivoulou, 1992*a*).

Unexpectedly, exposure to ultraviolet light for up to one minute after two days of frozen storage had a negligible effect on greyvalues.

Methodology – greylevel resolution

Image analysers measure intensity of staining as a greyvalue. An eight-bit processor can therefore generate 256 greylevels between black (0) and white (255), whilst a 16-bit processor produces 1024. In practice, image analysers resolve far fewer greylevels. Both the amount of image memory available and the image processing algorithms employed may reduce greylevel resolution in the final image. Methods for assessing greylevel resolution in image analysis have been developed (Cowen & Thrasivoulou, 1992*a,b*). Using these methods it has been shown that, whilst a number of factors contribute to reduced greylevel resolution, by far the most important element is the scanner used to interface the microscope to the image analyser.

Using a Panasonic Moonlight intensified video camera (model WV1900) with disabled auto-gain, mean greyvalues were measured in full field images (512 × 512 pixels) of a uranyl glass standard between 0 and 255 greyvalue using a graded series of neutral density filters interposed in the reflected light path (Fig. 10). The standard deviations indicated that the system could resolve only about five greyvalues between black and white, largely because of the spatial variation in illumination intensity. Comparison of measurements made over small frames (20 × 20 pixels) positioned at the centre and edge of the field identified uneven illumination as the principal source of variance. Comparison of different scanners showed that the scanner rather than the microscope optics was mainly responsible (Cowen & Thrasivoulou, 1992*a*). Three aspects of this problem were addressed. A background subtraction routine separate from that used for the specimen was devised in order to eliminate the central hotspot, using a low greyvalue image of the uranyl glass standard. The contribution of non-linearity of camera response was corrected using a greyvalue transformation table implemented in the image analysis software. Finally, because it seemed that these corrections needed to be applied in a non-linear fashion across the full greylevel range, additive and multiplicative methods of background subtraction were compared, the latter providing predictably lower variances (Fig. 10). As a result of these corrections, greylevel resolution was improved to about 50 greyvalues (i.e. more than fivefold) compared with the greylevel resolution of uncorrected images, although this was still substantially lower than the theoretical 256 greyvalues of the image analysis system (Cowen & Thrasivoulou, 1992*b*).

The recently available peltier cooled, solid state (CCD) scanners avoid many of these problems. Response is sensitive, spatially uniform and linear across the greyscale, and whilst high spatial resolution remains expensive, the cost per pixel is falling rapidly. These scanners allow the direct input of a digital signal to the analyser, although this is not always possible because the framegrabbers of many image analysis systems will accept only analogue signals. Greylevel resolution measured using a CCD scanner (PCO Optics Ltd) without background subtraction has shown a greylevel resolution of about 100 greyvalues, i.e. better than that shown using the fully corrected video system previously described (Cowen & Thrasivoulou, 1992*b*).

In practical applications of these methods, a two stage background subtraction procedure was adopted. In the first stage, unevenness contributed by the system was eliminated as described above using an image of the uranyl glass

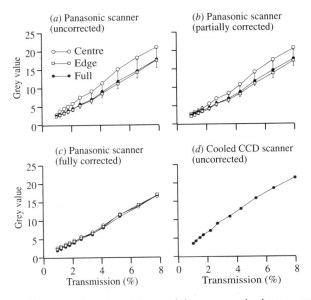

Fig. 10. Tests of densitometric resolving power in image analysis. (*a*) Uncorrected response of a Panasonic (model WV1900) low light video scanner to a range of image intensities measured over small (400 pixels) measuring frames situated at the **centre** and **edge** of the field of view and a larger (200 000 pixels), **full** measuring frame. Results are the mean of six measurements and standard deviations are the sum of spatial and temporal variation. Note the large standard deviation of the data from the **full** curve. (*b*) Response of Panasonic video scanner (as (*a*)) to the same range of image intensities used in (*a*) after additive correction for uneven illumination and non-linearity of response. Standard deviations are shown for the full frame. (*c*) Response of Panasonic video scanner (as (*b*)) after multiplicative correction for uneven illumination. Curves for the three measuring frames (see (*a*)) were virtually indistinguishable from one another. Data from the full measuring frame are shown and standard deviations ranged from 5–8% (Cowen & Thrasivoulou, 1992*b*). (*d*) Uncorrected response of a peltier cooled CCD scanner (Model VL350, PCO Optics GmbH, Germany) to the same range of image intensities used in (*a*). Curves for the three measuring frames (see (*a*)) were indistinguishable from one another. Data from the full measuring frame are shown and standard deviation ranged from 0.2–1%. Note that the field of view of the CCD camera is smaller than that of the video scanner, eliminating some peripheral unevenness generated by the microscope.

standard. Background non-specific staining contributed by the specimen was then removed using a large matrix, low pass filter set up and kept constant for particular tissues. The fully corrected image was then saved. Image processing was used to optimize the definition of nerves and to create a binary image. This was then used to create a mask which could be superimposed over the fully corrected greylevel image using a binary operator, allowing measurement of greyvalues from within the mask. Masking techniques in this and other applications (Ahrens *et al.*, 1990), have been shown to be powerful tools in biological image analysis.

Applications of densitometric image analysis

The capacity of these methods to assess neurotransmitter dynamics was evaluated in a study of 5-HT uptake into perivascular autonomic nerves. Initial experiments showed that mesenteric vessels, fixed by immersion, showed 5-HT immunoreactive nerve plexuses, whilst exsanguination and perfusion fixation caused the nerves to disappear (Cowen & Thrasivoulou, 1990; Levitt & Duckles, 1986). These results suggested that intraneuronal 5-HT was present as a result of uptake from a blood-derived source, perhaps platelets, probably employing the amine uptake pump since uptake was blocked by desmethyl-imipramine (Cowen & Thrasivoulou, 1990). Densitometric image analysis was used to analyse the timescale of uptake. Vessels were perfused with Tyrode's solution, incubated in solutions containing 10^{-6} M 5-HT for varying times and then immunostained for 5-HT. The time taken to saturate neuronal 5-HT uptake was unexpectedly long, taking 30 minutes to reach maximum (Fig. 11). These and other data suggested that a combination of low and high affinity uptake systems (Violet & Cowen, 1990) for 5-HT existed in these nerves. Some confidence in the technique was derived from the fact that intercept measurements, showing the number of stained nerve bundles, remained relatively constant after more than one minute of incubation in 5-HT despite changes in 5-HT content. However, fluorescent area was affected by stain intensity because of increased flare around each nerve bundle with increasing brightness of staining.

Recently, a study of changes in tyrosine hydroxylase (TH) in sympathetic neurones in response to cold stress and ageing in rabbits has been carried out (Andrews *et al.*, 1993). The densitometric microscopical assay system was used to estimate changes in intraneuronal TH protein levels whilst a biochemical assay was used to measure TH activity. Prolonged cold stress was found to induce increases in TH levels (Fig. 12); TH activity decreased, suggesting differential regulation of these two processes. Furthermore, old age resulted in reduction or loss of adaptive responses affecting both TH levels and activity. Surprisingly, a regulator of TH activity other than preganglionic sympathetic stimulation was identified. These results were unexpected in the light of previous studies showing that shorter periods of exposure to cold stress generate similar increases in both TH levels and activity (Thoenen, 1970; Otten & Thoenen, 1975).

Densitometry in confocal microscopy

The principle that immunohistochemical stain intensity can provide information about tissue antigen levels has recently been applied to a study of age changes in the extracellular matrix surrounding cerebral blood vessels (Gavazzi *et al.*, 1992*a*). The question was whether extracellular matrix, in particular the neurite growth-promoting molecule laminin, was involved in trophic inter-

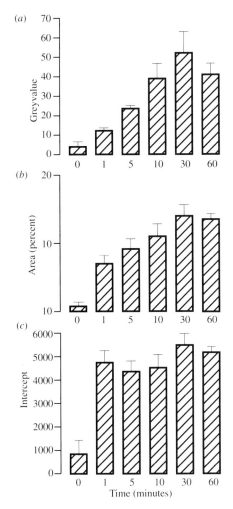

Fig. 11. Histograms demonstrating the rate of uptake of serotonin into autonomic nerves on rabbit mesenteric veins, incubated in 10^{-6} M serotonin for 0, 1, 5, 10, 30 and 60 min and subsequently processed for indirect immunohistochemistry. (*a*) Stain intensity (greylevel), (*b*) Nerve density (area %) and (*c*) Total intercept density per unit area of vessel wall (intercept). Data expressed as mean ± s.e.m.; $n = 5$ (Cowen & Thrasivoulou, 1992*a*).

actions between neurones and their target tissues and might cause age changes in neurones. Confocal microscopy is suited to studies of this kind because the digital nature of the signal precludes spatial unevenness of illumination of the kind experienced with video scanners. Furthermore, using thin optical sections (1–2 μm), the amount of non-specific background fluorescence is minimized. Measurements were made at constant gain, neutral density and aperture settings, and laser output voltages were monitored.

In the rat, the common carotid artery is not innervated, whereas cerebral arteries are densely innervated. Laminin immunoreactivity was seen surround-

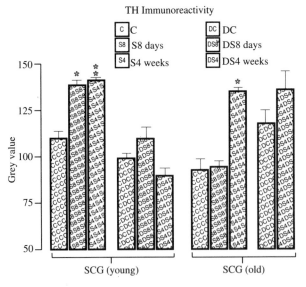

Fig. 12. Histogram showing the effect of prolonged cold exposure on intensity of TH-immunoreactivity expressed as mean greyvalue ± s.e.m. (C = control; S = cold stress; D = decentralization). Note the increase in greyvalue after 8 days of cold exposure in young animals and after 4 weeks of cold exposure in old animals (Andrews *et al.*, 1993).

ing smooth muscle cells at the adventitial–medial border of cerebral and common carotid arteries and around the Schwann cells surrounding perivascular nerve bundles. In young animals laminin immunoreactivity was less in the non-innervated common carotid artery compared with the innervated basilar artery. Densitometric measurements showed that laminin immunoreactivity was reduced by about 50% around the smooth muscle cells of old cerebral arteries compared to young ones, but showed smaller reductions around Schwann cells and in the common carotid artery (Fig. 13: Gavazzi *et al.*, 1992*a*). Other studies using light microscopy image analysis have shown reductions of about 50% in the innervation of cerebral blood vessels in old age (Cowen & Thrasivoulou, 1990; T. Andrews, unpublished observations). Consequently, there appears to be a correlation between density and age changes of innervation, on the one hand, and extracellular matrix expression on the other, although at this stage no causal relationship has been established.

Future directions

Studies have recently begun of the mechanisms regulating ageing in autonomic nerves. Using transplantation techniques, it has been shown that non-neuronal target tissues are in some way able to induce age related degenerative changes in the autonomic nerves that normally supply these tissues (Gavazzi *et al.*, 1992*b*). Furthermore, it has been shown that the nerves involved exhibit

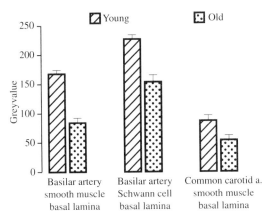

Fig. 13. Histogram showing changes with age in intensity of laminin immunostaining in smooth muscle and Schwann cell basal lamina of the basilar artery and in smooth muscle basal lamina of the common carotid artery of young (6 week) and old (24 months) rats. Intensity of fluorescence immunoreactivity was measured using confocal laser scanning microscopy. Note the substantial reductions in intensity of laminin immunostaining in old vessels, particularly in smooth muscle basal laminae (Gavazzi *et al.*, 1992).

unimpaired plasticity in old age when transplanted into contact with young target tissues (Gavazzi & Cowen, 1993). This work suggests strongly, and perhaps unexpectedly, that causes of neuronal ageing should be looked for in target tissues rather than within the nerves themselves. The work has been extended to study the influence of target tissues on age changes in neuronal phenotypes and it has been found that targets influence neurotransmitter expression as well as neuronal morphology during ageing in sweat glands (Abdel-Rahman *et al.*, 1992*b*).

These, and other studies of neurotrophic effects (Matsumoto *et al.*, 1990), have depended on light microscopical image analysis to compare differences in the distribution of nerves and other substances and in neurotransmitter content of nerves in minute samples of transplanted tissues (approximately 0.5 mm^3), weighing less than 1 mg. Conventional assay techniques would not be sufficiently sensitive to analyse such small samples, nor could they provide comparable information regarding the morphology of nerves and cellular localization of neuroactive substances. The improved spatial and greylevel resolution of the latest generation of image analysers and scanners, with more sophisticated image processing and analysis facilities, will undoubtedly further improve the quality of data, although our present inability to avoid subjective thresholding of images remains a problem.

There are also outstanding biological problems within this field. Light microscopy cannot resolve the individual axons that make up a nerve bundle. The majority of peripheral nerves consist of bundles of more than one, and often many, axons. Consequently, the field parameters, area and intercept, used by light microscopical image analysis to quantify density of nerve fibres, provide information that is only relative to the actual number and length of the constituent axons. Whilst electron microscopy can resolve individual axons, the restricted sampling and difficulty of applying image analysis make this approach laborious and unsatisfactory. Quantitative immunocytochemistry has proved difficult to extend to the ultrastructural level. Confocal laser scanning light microscopy can achieve a resolution in the x,y plane of about 0.25 μm and can thus resolve even small, unmyelinated axons. Furthermore, tissue antigenicity is preserved and initial experiments indicate that quantitative immunocytochemistry is compatible with confocal microscopy. Currently data from light, confocal and electron microscopy are being compared regarding age changes in peripheral axons in an attempt to arrive at quantitative measures of the changes in axon length and number.

In order to understand the regulatory mechanisms underlying these changes, measures of total nerve fibre numbers need to be supplemented by quantification of individual nerve groups identified by their transmitter phenotype or by some other marker. It is to be hoped that the high resolution and preserved tissue antigenicity of specimens viewed in confocal microscopy may help to answer some of these questions, perhaps in combination with the sampling capacity and analytic power of image analysis and conventional light microscopy.

Innervated tissues are often supplied by several different populations of nerves, distinguished by their nerve cells of origin. In addition, particular populations of, for example, parasympathetic nerves may exhibit local variations in neurotransmitter phenotype (Gibbins, 1990, 1991). Developmental changes and experimental manipulations affect particular groups of nerves differently, often with reciprocal changes in nerve density and/or in transmitter content. For example, sympathetic cerebrovascular nerves decline in density during ageing whilst parasympathetic and sensory fibres and their associated neuropeptides may increase (Mione et al., 1988). Equally, sympathectomy may result in an increase in expression of non-sympathetic neuropeptides such as substance P (Kessler et al., 1983) and NPY (Mione et al., 1990).

In order to understand the regulatory mechanisms underlying these changes, measures of total nerve fibre numbers need to be supplemented by quantification of individual nerve groups identified by their transmitter phenotype or by some other marker. It is to be hoped that the high resolution and preserved tissue antigenicity of specimens viewed in confocal microscopy may help to answer some of these questions, perhaps in combination with the sampling capacity and analytic power of image analysis and conventional light microscopy.

References

Abdel-Rahman, T. A. & Cowen, T. (1993). Reductions of nerve density in sweat glands and skin of aged rats. *Journal of the Autonomic Nervous System* (in the press).

Abdel-Rahman, T. A., Collins, K. J., Cowen, T. & Rustin, M. (1992a). Immunohistochemical, morphological and functional changes in the peripheral sudomotor neuro-effector system in elderly people. *Journal of the Autonomic Nervous System*, **37**, 187–98.

Abdel-Rahman, T. A., Thrasivoulou, C. & Cowen, T. (1992b). Sweat glands from adult rats become reinnervated following transplantation in oculo. *Neuroscience Letters*, Supplement **42**, S12.

Agnati, L. F. & Fuxe, K. (1984). Computer-assisted morphometry and microdensitometry of transmitter-identified neurons with special reference to the mesostriatal dopamine pathway. *Acta Physiologica Scandinavica*, Supplement **532**, 1–66.

Agnati, J. F. & Fuxe, K. eds. (1985) *Quantitative Neuroanatomy in Transmitter Research; Wenner-Gren Center Symposium Series*, Vol. 42. London: Macmillan.

Ahrens, P., Schleicher, A., Zilles, K. & Werner, L. (1990). Image analysis of Nissl-stained neuronal perikarya in the primary visual cortex of the rat: automatic detection and segmentation of neuronal profiles with nuclei and nucleoli. *Journal of Microscopy*, **157**, 349–65.

Amenta, F., Bronzetti, E., Cavallotti, C. & Felici, L. (1987). Quantitative image analysis of the density and pattern of adrenergic innervation of blood vessels of rat spinal cord. *Journal of the Autonomic Nervous System*, **18**, 261–4.

Andrews, T., Lincoln, J., Milner, P., Burnstock, G. & Cowen, T. (1993). The effects of prolonged cold exposure and ageing on tyrosine hydroxylase and neuropeptide Y in sympathetic neurones from the rabbit. *Brain Research* (in the press).

Calza, L., Giardino, L., Zanni, M., Velardo, A., Parchi, P. & Marrama, P. (1990). Daily changes of neuropeptide Y-like immunoreactivity in the suprachiasmatic nucleus of the rat. *Regulatory Peptides*, **27**, 127–37.

Chedotal, A. & Hamel, E. (1990). Serotonin-synthesizing nerve fibers in rat and cat cerebral arteries and arterioles: immunohistochemistry of tryptophan-5-hydroxylase. *Neuroscience Letters*, **116**, 269.

Contestabile, A., Villani, L., Fasolo, A., Franzoni, M. F., Gribaudo, L., Oktedalen, O. & Fonnum, F. (1987). Topography of cholinergic and substance P pathways in the habenulo-interpeduncular system of the rat. An immunocytochemical and microchemical approach. *Neuroscience*, **21**, 253–70.

Coons, A. N. (1958). Fluorescent antibody methods. In *General Cytochemical Methods*, ed. Danielli, J. F., pp. 399–422. New York: Academic Press.

Cowen, T. (1984). Image analysis of FITC-immunofluorescence histochemistry in perivascular substance P-positive nerves. *Histochemistry*, **81**, 609–10.

Cowen, T., Alafaci, C., Crockard, H. A. & Burnstock, G. (1986). 5-HT-containing nerves to major cerebral arteries of the gerbil originate in the superior cervical ganglion. *Brain Research*, **384**, 51–9.

Cowen, T., Alafaci, C., Crockard, H. A. & Burnstock, G. (1987). Origin and postnatal development of 5-HT-containing nerves supplying major cerebral arteries of the rat. *Neuroscience Letters*, **78**, 121–6.

Cowen, T. & Burnstock, G. (1980). Quantitative analysis of the density and pattern of adrenergic innervation of blood vessels. *Histochemistry*, **66**, 19–34.

Cowen, T. & Burnstock, G. (1982). Image analysis of catecholamine fluorescence. *Brain Research Bulletin*, **9**, 81–6.

Cowen, T. & Burnstock, G. (1985). Image analysis of catecholamine fluorescence and immunofluorescence in studies on blood vessel innervation. In *Quantitative Neuroanatomy in Neurotransmitter Research; Wenner-Gren Center Symposium* No. 42, ed. Agnati, L. F. & Fuxe, K., pp. 213–30. London: Macmillan.

Cowen, T., Haven, A. J., Wen Qin, C., Gallen, D. D., Franc, F. & Burnstock, G. (1982). Development and ageing of perivascular adrenergic nerves in the rabbit. A quantitative fluorescence histochemical study using image analysis. *Journal of the Autonomic Nervous System*, **5**, 317–36.

Cowen, T., Haven, A. J. & Burnstock, G. (1985). Pontamine sky blue: a counterstain for background autofluorescence in fluorescence and immunofluorescence histochemistry. *Histochemistry*, **82**, 205–8.

Cowen, T. & Thrasivoulou, C. (1990). Cerebrovascular nerves in old rats show reduced accumulation of 5-hydroxytryptamine and loss of nerve fibres. *Brain Research*, **513**, 237–43.

Cowen, T. & Thrasivoulou, C. (1992*a*). Methods of image analysis for the measurement of densitometric data on immunofluorescence-stained preparations of nerves. In

Quantitative Methods of Neuroanatomy, ed. Stewart, M. J., pp. 85–94. Chichester: J. Wiley.

Cowen, T. & Thrasivoulou, C. (1992*b*). A 'microscopical assay' using a densitometric application of image analysis to quantify neurotransmitter dynamics. *Journal of Neuroscience Methods*, **45**, 107–16.

Dahlstrom, A. & Ahlman, H. (1983). Immunocytochemical evidence for the presence of tryptaminergic nerves of blood vessels, smooth muscle and myenteric plexus in the rat small intestine. *Acta Physiologica Scandinavica*, **117**, 589–91.

Falck, B., Hillarp, N.-A., Thieme, G. & Torp, A. (1962). Fluorescence of catecholamines and related compounds condensed with formaldehyde. *Journal of Histochemistry and Cytochemistry*, **10**, 348–54.

Furness, J. B. & Costa, M. (1975). The use of glyoxylic acid for the fluorescence histochemical demonstration of peripheral stores of noradrenaline and 5-hydroxytryptamine in whole mounts. *Histochemistry*, **41**, 335–52.

Fuxe, K., Agnati, L. F., Zoli, M., Harfstrand, A., Grimaldi, R., Bernardi, P., Camurri, M. & Goldstein, M. (1985). Development of quantitative methods for the evaluation of the entity of coexistence of neuroactive substances in nerve terminal populations in discrete areas of the central nervous system: evidence for hormonal regulation of cotransmission. In *Quantitative Neuroanatomy in Neurotransmitter Research; Wenner-Gren Center Symposium* No. 42, ed. Agnati, L. F. & Fuxe, K., pp. 157–74. London: Macmillan.

Gale, J. D., Alberts, J. C. J. & Cowen, T. (1989). A quantitative study of changes in old age of 5-hydroxytryptamine-like immunoreactivity in perivascular nerves of the rabbit. *Journal of the Autonomic Nervous System*, **28**, 51–60.

Gallen, D. D., Cowen, T., Griffith, S. G., Haven, A. J. & Burnstock, G. (1982). Functional and non-functional nerve-smooth muscle transmission in the renal arteries of new born and adult rabbit and guinea pig. *Blood Vessels*, **19**, 237–46.

Gardette, R., Mallet, A. & Bisconte, J. C. (1981). Automatic recognition of nervous structures by image analysis. A pattern recognition method applied to the study of mouse cerebellum. *Journal of Neuroscience Methods*, **3**, 233–46.

Gavazzi, I., Andrews, T. J., Thrasivoulou, C. & Cowen, T. (1992*a*). Influence of target tissues on their innervation in old age using a transplantation model. *Neuroreport*, **3**, 117–20.

Gavazzi, I., Boyle, K. S. & Cowen, T. (1992*b*). Influence of age-related alterations in the target tissues on their pattern of reinnervation following transplantation. *European Journal of Neuroscience*, Supplement **5**, 98.

Gavazzi, I. & Cowen, T. (1993). Autonomic neurones whose axons show impairments in old age show no reductions in neurite outgrowth following transplantation into young hosts. *Experimental Neurology* (in the press).

Gibbins, I. L. (1990). Target-related patterns of co-existence of neuropeptide-Y, vasoactive intestinal peptide, enkephalin and substance-P in cranial parasympathetic neurons innervating the facial skin and exocrine glands of guinea pigs. *Neuroscience*, **38**, 541.

Gibbins, I. L. (1991). Vasomotor, pilomotor and secretomotor neurons distinguished by size and neuropeptide content in superior cervical ganglia of mice. *Journal of the Autonomic Nervous System*, **34**, 171–83.

Henschen, A. & Olson, L. (1983). Hexachlorophene-induced degeneration of adrenergic nerves: application of quantitative image analysis to Falck-Hillarp fluorescence histochemistry. *Acta Neuropathologica (Berlin)*, **59**, 109–14.

Hokfelt, T., Johansson, O., Ljungdahl, A., Lundberg, J. M. & Schultzberg, M. (1980). Peptidergic neurons. *Nature*, **284**, 515–21.

Johansson, O. & Hallman, H. (1985). Image analysis of transmitter identified neurons using the IBAS system. In *Quantitative Neuroanatomy in Transmitter Research; Wenner-Gren Center Symposium* No. 42, eds. Agnati, L. F. & Fuxe, K., pp. 231–50. London: Macmillan.

Kessler, J. A., Bell, W. O. & Black, I. B. (1983). Interactions between the sympathetic and sensory innervation of the iris. *Journal of Neuroscience*, **3**, 1301–7.

King, M. A., Hunter, B. E., Reep, R. L. & Walker, D. W. (1989). Acetyl-cholinesterase stain intensity variation in the rat dentate gyrus: a quantitative description based on digital image analysis. *Neuroscience*, **33**, 203.

Levitt, B. & Duckles S. P. (1986). Evidence against serotonin as a vasoconstrictor neurotransmitter in the rabbit basilar artery. *Journal of Pharmacology and Experimental Therapeutics*, **238**, 880–5.

Lindvall, O. & Bjorklund, A. (1974). The glyoxylic acid fluorescence histochemical method: a detailed account of the methodology for the visualization of central catecholamine neurons. *Histochemistry*, **39**, 92–127.

Lundberg, J. M. & Hokfelt, T. (1983). Co-existence of peptides and classical neurotransmitters. *Trends in Neuroscience*, **6**, 325–33.

Luthman, J. & Hallman, H. (1986). Quantitation of noradrenaline nerve density in mouse iris by computer-assisted image analysis. *Acta Physiologica Scandinavica*, **128**, 167–74.

Matsumoto, T., Oshima, K., Miyamoto, A., Sakura, M., Goto, M. & Hayashi, S. (1990). Image analysis of CNS neurotrophic factor effects on neuronal survival and neurite outgrowth. *Journal of Neuroscience Methods*, **31**, 153.

Mione, M. C., Cavanagh, J. F. R., Lincoln, J., Milner, P. & Burnstock, G. (1990). Long-term chemical sympathectomy leads to an increase of neuropeptide Y immunoreactivity in cerebrovascular nerves and iris of the developing rat. *Neuroscience*, **34**, 369–78.

Mione, M. C., Dhital, K. K., Amenta, F. & Burnstock, G. (1988). An increase in the expression of neuropeptidergic vasodilator, but not vasoconstrictor, cerebrovascular nerves in aging rats. *Brain Research*, **460**, 103–13.

Otten, U. & Thoenen, H. (1975). Circadian rhythm of tyrosine hydroxylase induction by short term cold stress: modulatory action of glucocorticoids in newborn and adult rats. *Proceedings of the National Academy of Sciences of the USA*, **72**, 1415–9.

Polak, J. M. & Van Noorden, S. eds. (1986). *Immunocytochemistry: Modern Methods and Applications*. Bristol: John Wright.

Schalling, M., Dagerlind, A., Brene, S., Hallman, H., Djurfeldt, M., Persson, H., Terenius, L., Goldstein, M., Schlesinger, D. & Hokfelt, T. (1988). Coexistence and gene expression of phenylethanolamine *N*-methyltransferase, tyrosine hydroxylase and neuropeptide tyrosine in the rat and bovine adrenal gland: effects of reserpine. *Proceedings of the National Academy of Sciences of the USA*, **85**, 8306–10.

Schipper, J. & Tilders, F. J. H. (1983). A new technique for studying specificity of immunocytochemical procedures: specificity of serotonin immunostaining. *Journal of Histochemistry and Cytochemistry*, **31**, 12–18.

Steinbusch, H. W. M., Verhofstad, A. A. J. & Joosten, H. W. J. (1978). Localisation of serotonin in the central nervous system by immunohistochemistry: description of a specific and sensitive technique and some applications. *Neuroscience*, **3**, 811–19.

Stewart, M. J. (ed.) (1992). *Quantitative Methods in Neuroanatomy*. Chichester: Wiley.

Terenghi, G., Bunker, C. B., Liu, Y.-F., Springall, D. R., Cowen, T., Dowd, P. M. & Polak, J. M. (1991). Image analysis quantification of peptide-immunoreactive nerves in the skin of patients with Raynaud's phenomenon and systemic sclerosis. *Journal of Pathology*, **164**, 245–52.

Thoenen, H. (1970). Induction of tyrosine hydroxylase in peripheral and central adrenergic neurones by cold-exposure of rats. *Nature*, **228**, 861–2.

Thompson, R. J., Doran, J. F., Jackson, P., Dhillon, A. P. & Rode, J. (1983). PGP 9.5 – a new marker for vertebrate neurons and neuroendocrine cells. *Brain Research*, **278**, 224–8.

Violet, J. & Cowen, T. (1990). Changes in uptake of serotonin into sympathetic perivascular nerves in old age. *Journal of Anatomy*, **173**, 220P.

Wallen, P., Carlsson, K., Liljeborg, A. & Grillner, S. (1988). Three-dimensional reconstruction of neurons in the lamprey spinal cord in whole-mount, using a confocal laser scanning microscope. *Journal of Neuroscience Methods*, **24**, 91–100.

Webster, G. J. M., Petch, E. W. A. & Cowen, T. (1991). Streptozotocin-induced diabetes in rats causes neuronal deficits in tyrosine hydroxylase and 5-hydroxytryptamine specific to mesenteric perivascular sympathetic nerves and without loss of nerve fibers. *Experimental Neurology*, **113**, 53–62.

Zoli, M., Fuxe, K., Agnati, L. F., Harfstrand, A., Terenius, L., Toni, R. & Goldstein, M. (1986). Computer-assisted morphometry of transmitter-identified neurons: new openings for the understanding of peptide-monoamine interactions in the mediobasal hypothalamus. In *Neurohistochemistry: Modern Methods and Applications*, pp. 137–72. New York: Alan R. Liss, Inc.

21

Automated grain counting as applied to *in situ* hybridization histochemistry

J. A. CHOWEN

Introduction

The vast number of image analysis systems and computer programs available to the investigator indicates the rising demand for such systems. Most commercially available systems are designed to be multifunctional, able to perform various different kinds of analyses and therefore capable of being used in a wide range of different experimental situations. This increased diversity often decreases the power or specificity of each individual application, so that there are also programs that have been specially designed to do one particular type of analysis. Therefore, before choosing an image analysis system or program, one must first know what type of data are to be gathered, not only immediately, but in the near future. In this chapter, I present data from a computer based image analysis system designed to perform a specific function, the determination of the number of silver grains overlying individual cells.

The mechanics of image analysis are described in preceding chapters. However, the best image analysis system, even if it were designed to address the particular question on hand, is useless without proper experimental controls and conditions. Furthermore, each experiment should be designed so that it yields the maximum quantity of useful information from the image analysis. These questions are discussed below. Particular attention is paid to how poor experimental design and minor technical errors in performing an assay can give erroneous results. The example chosen is the application of computer aided image analysis to the technique of *in situ* hybridization histochemistry to detect relative levels of specific messenger RNAs (mRNAs) for hypothalamic neuropeptides. Each step of this procedure is discussed with regard to the technical points that must be addressed in order to obtain the best possible results with respect to efficiency, reproducibility and, of course, the maximum quantity of reliable data.

In situ hybridization histochemistry

Overview

Radioactively labelled riboprobes are prepared by *in vitro* transcription (Green *et al.*, 1983). The *in situ* hybridization methodology, as outlined in Fig. 1, has been described in detail elsewhere (Rogers *et al.*, 1987). Briefly, fresh frozen tissue should be lightly fixed and then rinsed several times in phosphate buffer. These rinses should be stirred so that the paraformaldehyde is thoroughly removed from the tissues. The slides are pretreated with 0.25% acetic anhydride in 0.1 M triethanolamine (pH 8.0) to neutralize surface charges. The slides are then delipidated and dehydrated before application of the probe mixture to the tissue. Parafilm coverslips are applied to each slide and sealed with rubber cement. The slides are then placed in a moist chamber and

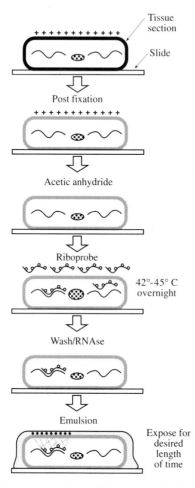

Fig. 1. An overview of the steps involved in performing *in situ* hybridization histochemistry.

incubated overnight. On the following day, the coverslips are removed and the slides are passed through a treatment with RNAse A and a series of washes of increasing stringency to decrease the non-specific binding. After being de-hydrated, the slides are dipped in photographic emulsion and allowed to dry before being placed in lightproof boxes containing desiccant. They are then exposed for the desired length of time, developed and counterstained.

Potential problems and solutions

Tissue preparation

The choice of tissue fixation depends on the type of tissue to be used and whether another procedure (e.g. immunocytochemistry) is to be done in conjunction with the *in situ* hybridization. For *in situ* hybridization of rat brain tissue, fresh frozen tissue is the most convenient and gives results comparable to perfused tissue. Since tissue preparation for image analysis has been addressed in detail in a previous chapter (Chapter 8), only brief comments will be made about the points which are relevant to semiquantitative *in situ* hybridization.

Because mRNA levels are of interest and mRNA is rapidly degraded at room temperature, tissues must be removed and frozen as quickly as possible. However, if rat brain is frozen too rapidly, for example by freezing in liquid nitrogen, artefacts often occur. Even more dramatically, the brain can crack. These freezing artefacts can interfere with the assay and its analysis since the radioactively labelled probes used in these procedures tend to accumulate in the various crevices. Taking both points into consideration, the following technique is recommended to obtain fresh frozen tissue. The animal should be asphyxiated with carbon dioxide generated from dry ice and then decapitated. The brain should be removed rapidly, placed on aluminum foil which has been set on a solid block of dry ice, and a small plastic or glass cap (just large enough to enclose the brain) placed over it to facilitate freezing. After it is frozen, the brain should be wrapped in the foil and stored at −80 °C until processed for *in situ* hybridization. This method of freezing is also used for perfused tissue.

Whether perfusing or post-fixing fresh frozen tissue, 4% paraformaldehyde is used. This fixative does not interfere with the *in situ* hybridization protocol. However, if a stronger protein cross-linker (e.g. glutaraldehyde) is used, a step may be needed to increase penetration of the riboprobe into the tissue. Proteinase K (PK) treatment can be used for this purpose; however, Triton X-100 or sodium dodecylsulphate may also be employed. The concentration of PK will change depending upon the type of tissue, the thickness of the tissue slices, and the manufacturer or lot number of the PK. A titration curve should be done when any of these variables has changed in order to determine the concentration of PK that allows maximum probe penetration while maintaining satisfactory tissue morphology.

In situ *hybridization assay*

The assay conditions should be standardized individually for each type of probe that is to be used, with the aim of attaining the highest possible ratio of specific signal to background noise. This involves adjusting incubation temperatures and wash stringencies according to the theoretical melting temperature of the mRNA:mRNA (or DNA:mRNA) hybrid in question. Furthermore, care should be taken to preserve tissue morphology and thoroughly to remove from the tissue any of the reagents that may interfere with the subsequent autoradiography. For example, residual paraformaldehyde may react with subsequent solutions and cause a slight browning of the tissue, which ultimately interferes with the image analysis process. (See Angerer *et al.*, 1987 for a review of this technique.)

Autoradiography

It is important to use fresh photographic emulsion with each assay since the emulsion loses sensitivity after repeated melting and cooling. It is therefore helpful to make aliquots of the diluted emulsion so that only the desired amount of emulsion is melted with each assay. After the slides have been dipped in the photographic emulsion, they are placed in a vertical slide holder to dry. A thin even layer of emulsion is desirable since the thickness of the emulsion can greatly influence the radiographic signal obtained. As the emulsion dipped slide dries, the emulsion becomes slightly thicker at the bottom (Fig. 2). If two consecutive sections of tissue are placed on different portions of the slide, different signal levels for a peptide can be obtained due to differences

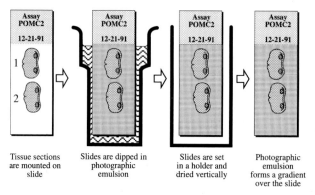

Fig. 2. The process of dipping slides into photographic emulsion and then standing them vertically to dry. As the slides dry, the emulsion becomes thicker at the bottom of the slide. Therefore tissue section 2 has a slightly thicker layer of emulsion than section 1.

in emulsion thickness (Fig. 3). Hence care should be taken to ensure that the tissue to be analysed is placed on the slide in approximately the same location in every experimental group and that the emulsion coat is as even as possible.

Exposure time

The exposure time of each assay depends on the specific activity (SA) of the probe, the presumed abundance of the message to be detected and the desired grain density. The desired grain density should be high enough that positively labelled cells are easily detectable both by eye and by the image analysis system, but low enough that the silver grains do not overlap so that they cannot easily be distinguished from one another. It is also important to control the exposure period so that the radiographic emulsion does not become saturated.

In order to determine the exposure time necessary to obtain the desired autoradiographic signal, the SA of the probe must be known. First, the current SA of the ^{35}S-alpha-thio-uridine-5'-triphosphate (UTP) must be determined. This information is supplied by the manufacturer. The SA of the labelled riboprobe (dpm/μg of probe) is then calculated as follows:

$$S_r = S_{UTP} \cdot c_1 \cdot p_r \cdot f_{UTP} \cdot c_2$$

where S_{UTP} is the current SA of the UTP in Ci/mM,

  c_1 is a constant, 2.22×10^{12} dpm/Ci, representing the rate of radioactive decay (n.b. if S_{UTP} is measured in Bq/mM, $c_1 = 60$ dpm/Bq),
  p_r is the percentage of radiolabelled UTPs in the probe,
  f_{UTP} is the number of UTPs in probe/number of bases in probe,
  c_2 is a constant, mM/3.1×10^5 μg, used to convert the results to μg.

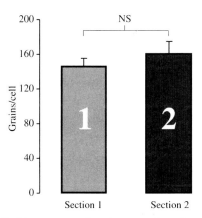

Fig. 3. Two consecutive tissue sections from the same animal were placed on a series of slides and processed for *in situ* hybridization histochemistry for pro-opiomelanocortin. The mean number of grains/cell for sections 1 and 2 (in Fig. 2) are shown. Although the mean number of grains/cell were not significantly different, there is a tendency for those tissue sections with a slightly thicker layer of emulsion (section 2) to have a higher autoradiographic signal.

The percentage of radiolabelled UTPs in the probe (p_r) is determined by the experimenter, by adjusting the ratio of radiolabelled UTPs/unlabelled UTPs used in the *in vitro* transcription reaction. In order to calculate the ratio of UTPs to the total number of bases in the probe (f_{UTP}) the base sequence of the cDNA must be known. This allows the determination of the percentage of the molecular weight of the probe which is contributed by the UTPs.

The exposure period for each new probe can be estimated from its SA, the presumed abundance of the message in question and the desired grain density. Once a satisfactory result has been obtained, all subsequent exposure periods for that probe can be determined as follows.

During the correct exposure period, a proportion of the label decays:

$$e^{-\lambda t}$$

where λ is the decay constant of the radioisotope ($\lambda = 0.693/T_{1/2}$, i.e for ^{35}S, $\lambda = -0.008$/day) and

t is the exposure period (days).

Therefore the emulsion is exposed to:

$$S_1(1 - e^{-\lambda t_1}),$$

where S_1 is the initial SA.

If the SA of the new probe is S_2, then for similar exposure of the emulsion:

$$S_1(1 - e^{-\lambda t_1}) = S_2(1 - e^{-\lambda t_2}),$$

where t_2 is the exposure period to be determined.

Thus:

$$t_2 = (-\ln x)/\lambda,$$

where:

$$x = 1 - \frac{S_1}{S_2}(1 - e^{-\lambda t_1}).$$

For the purpose of reproducibility, a three day exposure period is the practical minimum. This is because if the exposure period is too short (e.g. one day), a variation in a couple of hours of exposure from one assay to the next can seriously affect the results. This problem will arise only when assaying for messages that are very abundant. To obtain a longer period of exposure, the riboprobe can be labelled using a mixture of unlabelled and radioactive UTP. For example, a three day exposure period for somatostatin (SS) is obtained by adjusting the percentage of radioactive UTPs in the reaction to 15–20%. This practice not only helps to make exposure periods more uniform, but it is also much more economical.

Slide development

Fresh developer and fixer should be used with each assay to avoid the precipitants that can form on the tissue if old solutions are used. The developing solutions should be cooled to 15 °C to develop the emulsion more slowly and obtain finer, more homogeneous silver grains. After developing, it is important to ensure that slides are thoroughly rinsed since any residual fixer will react with the subsequent staining procedure and make reliable image analysis virtually impossible. Slides can be counterstained with cresyl violet, dehydrated and a coverslip applied to the tissue. The choice of stain varies between experimenters and does not seem to be important. However, the intensity of the stain is critical since intense staining will interfere in the analysis process.

Control experiments

Before attempting to perform semiquantitative *in situ* hybridization studies, a number of control experiments should be completed. First, as with all quantitative studies, the assay must be performed under saturating conditions. Therefore, a probe-saturation curve must be obtained. Furthermore, it should be verified that the probe used in the assay is binding specifically to the mRNA species in question. To address these questions, the following control experiments should be performed.

Saturation curve

Saturation curves are performed to demonstrate that the binding of a probe is saturable, and therefore specific, as well as to determine the optimum concentrations of probe for subsequent assays. If the number of binding sites of the probe is limited, incubation with increasing concentrations of labelled probe should result in increasing signal levels until the binding sites are saturated. Background, or non-specific binding, should increase linearly with increasing probe concentrations. Therefore, it is important not only to use enough probe to saturate all binding sites, but also not to use excess quantities of probe, as this will increase the non-specific binding. To perform a saturation curve, the quantity of labelled probe obtained from the transcription reaction must be determined. This can be calculated by measuring a small aliquot of the probe in a scintillation counter to determine its radioactivity concentration. The yield (y) can then be calculated:

$$y = r \cdot v/(\varepsilon \cdot S)$$

where r is the radioactivity concentration (cpm/μl of probe),
  v is the total volume of labelled probe (μl),
  ε is the efficiency of the scintillation counter (cpm/dpm) and
  S is the SA of the probe (dpm/μg).

Knowing the total quantity of probe (in μg) the appropriate dilutions can then be made in hybridization buffer. The saturation curve should be run on tissue from the experimental model where the highest level of mRNA is expected.

Furthermore, data analysis should be performed separately in all anatomical locations of importance. For example, to construct a saturation curve for pro-opiomelanocortin (POMC) probe, labelled probe was applied to brain slices from an intact male rat in concentrations ranging from 0.0925 μg/ml to 9.25 μg/ml (Chowen-Breed *et al.*, 1989). Fig. 4 illustrates the effect of increasing concentrations of POMC probe on specific and non-specific binding in neurones of the arcuate nucleus. These data suggest that specific binding of POMC mRNA is saturable and attained in this tissue at a probe concentration of approximately 0.278 μg/ml. As expected, non-specific binding increased linearly as probe concentration increased. To ensure that saturation is obtained under all experimental conditions, a standardized concentration of 0.55 μg/ml is used in the POMC *in situ* hybridization assay.

Assay specificity

Control experiments should also be performed to verify the specificity of an *in situ* hybridization assay. Although no single control is ideal for this purpose, a few of the following in combination will strengthen the case for specificity. First, a non-complementary RNA probe can be used during the hybridization procedure. Second, tissue can be pretreated with RNAse to destroy all mRNA in the section. Lack of binding in this assay strengthens the case that the probe is binding specifically to mRNA. Third, tissue can be incubated with the normal quantity of labelled probe in the presence of excess unlabelled probe. If the binding of the probe is specific, the unlabelled probe should displace the labelled probe. Fourth, a Northern Blot analysis can be performed to verify that the probe recognizes only RNA species of the appropriate size or sizes.

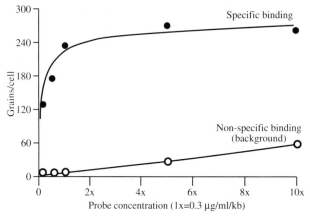

Fig. 4. Effect of increasing POMC cRNA probe concentration on the specific binding and non-specific binding. Probe concentrations were between 0.0925 μg/ml (0.1 ×) to 9.25 μg/ml (10 ×). The specific binding saturates at approximately 1 ×, whereas the non-specific binding continues to increase linearly. (Modified from Chowen-Breed *et al.*, 1989).

Further support for probe specificity can be gathered from the anatomical mapping of positive cells. Comparisons between the general anatomical distribution of peptide-containing cells, as determined by immunocytochemistry, and mRNA containing cells, as determined by hybridization histochemistry, can be carried out. It is also possible to combine *in situ* hybridization to detect the mRNA of a peptide, with immunocytochemistry for that peptide in a single tissue section. Using this approach it is often possible to demonstrate that neurones detected by a cRNA probe also contain the peptide product.

Measurement of autoradiographic silver grains

Overview of data analysis process for in situ *hybridization*

After an *in situ* hybridization assay has been completed, there are a number of tissue sections to be analysed with a computer aided image analysis system. The aim of this process is to determine the relative amount of mRNA for the neuropeptide of interest which is contained in the cells of the different experimental groups. To determine the number of silver grains which are associated with individual cells a specially designed image analysis system has been employed (Chowen *et al.*, 1991).

In each tissue section, the silver grains over every identifiable and isolatable cell contained within the nuclei of interest are counted. Under bright field optics, a cell is identified by the presence of a cresyl-stained nucleus associated with a cluster of dark silver grains. To qualify for analysis, a cell must have an isolated cluster of silver grains and be free of artefacts, which could include fixation and staining artefacts, as well as the presence of debris. The grain counting is performed with a ×50 objective on clusters of grains that lie over isolated cells. Dark field illumination is used so the grains appear as bright points of light over a relatively uniform black background. First the centre of the grain cluster is located and a threshold level is determined by the computer program. This threshold is set based on the greylevel histogram of the background grains outside the grain cluster. The grains within the viewing field are then identified and the number of grains in the background as well as the number of grains that appear over the cell are counted.

Performance of grain counting system

Performance checks will be illustrated with reference to the system described by Chowen *et al.* (1991).

Variations in illumination

Fluctuations in light intensity can markedly influence the results obtained with image analysis systems. This problem is often addressed by performing a calibration step at the beginning of each analysis session. Systems should be designed so that they are as insensitive as possible to variations in light intensity. To test the system described above, a single cell was analysed at various levels of illumination. It was found that the grain counts remained essentially constant over a twofold change in lamp voltage.

Photometric uniformity

Another problem with most tube-type image sensing devices is that their photometric response is not uniform across the entire video field. The extent of this problem will vary depending upon the video system used. However, the operator should be aware of the potential problems that this variation may cause. The performance of the grain counting system described above has been evaluated as a function of image position by counting the same cell at five different positions in the video field. This resulted in significantly different grain counts. To minimize these effects, each image to be analysed should be positioned in the same region of the video field.

System stability

Ageing of system components and environmental fluctuations can lead to longterm drift in system performance. The temporal stability of the grain counting system described above was verified by measuring the number of grains associated with two cells. The cells were measured twice a day on 13 different days over a period of three months. Fluctuations in the measured number of grains per cell appeared to be random. There was no trend in the data over the three month period. This suggests that the system is relatively stable, even in the absence of any formal calibration or standardization procedure.

Proper slide preparation

Before grain counting is undertaken, preliminary steps must be taken to avoid the introduction of systematic errors. First, the slides must be thoroughly cleaned since any traces of emulsion left on the non-tissue side of the slide may interfere with the analysis. Second, the slides should be anatomically matched across experimental groups and then coded so that the slides can be read without the person doing the analysis being aware of their experimental group. These two steps are essential to ensure that relevant comparisons are made and to avoid biased results.

   Even if they produce the same neuropeptide, not all neurons throughout the brain, or even within the same anatomical nucleus, can be expected to respond identically to the same stimulus. Therefore, if 16 tissue sections are analysed per animal, they should represent approximately the same 16 planes of section through the nucleus in all animals. The slides should be matched by using a level of magnification at which the anatomical structures can be easily discerned, but the labelling of the positive cells cannot, so that bias can be avoided in choosing tissue sections. To ensure objectivity in the measurements, all of the slides of the assay can then be assigned a random alphabetical code. Information concerning the study name, group, animal number, slide number, and the code should be stored for later decoding and data analysis. Following assignment of codes, the operator can organize the slides into alphabetical order by code and measure them in a blinded fashion.

Interpretation of results

By using the system described above results can be obtained in units of grains/cell or mean number of grains/cell. Because various steps in the procedure are non-linear, these data can only be semiquantitative and will only reflect relative quantities of messenger RNA. Many investigators have begun to calculate the amount of radioactivity in each sample (or cell) by simultaneously running standards of known radioactivity with each assay. These standards commonly consist of commercially prepared ^{14}C embedded polymer squares of different activities or individually prepared standards of homogenated brain to which known quantities of a radioisotope are added. A standard curve can then be generated with each assay and the amount of radioactivity/cell or area can then be determined. This practice can help the experimenter to determine if their assay is on the linear portion of the emulsion's response to the radioactivity, as well as to increase the apparent differences between experimental groups.

Comparison of quantitative analysis by in situ *and solution hybridization*

To obtain an indirect assessment of the relationship between grain counts and somatostatin (SS) mRNA copy number, *in situ* hybridization and solution hybridization have been performed on transfected baby hamster kidney (BHK) cells which express the SS gene at different levels. Dr Richard Palmiter at the University of Washington transfected these cells with a construct containing the structural genes for SS and dihydrofolate reductase attached to the metallothionein promoter. To select for various levels of expression of this construct, these cells were then grown in different concentrations of methotrexate (2 μM, 20 μM or 500 μM). Because dihydrofolate reductase imparts resistance to the toxin methotrexate, cells surviving in a higher concentration of methotrexate necessarily express the construct at a higher level. After the selection process, solution hybridization (Durnam & Palmiter, 1983) was performed to determine the average number of copies of SS mRNA/cell and *in situ* hybridization was performed (as described above) to determine the average number of autoradiographic grains/cell. The results are shown in Fig. 5.

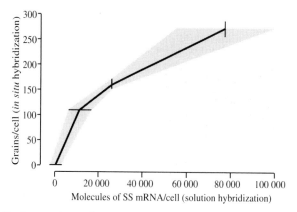

Fig. 5. Comparison of *in situ* and solution hybridization measured variables. Somato-statin (SS) mRNA levels in transfected baby hamster kidney (BHK) cells, which express the SS gene at different levels, were analyzed by both methods. Both methods detected an increase in the measured variables when there was an increase in gene expression. However, the degree of increase differed between the two methods with solution hybridization detecting a relatively greater change in gene expression. (Modified from Argente *et al.*, 1990).

These results indicate a direct relationship between the variables measured by *in situ* and solution hybridization (i.e. autoradiographic grains/cell increase as the number of copies/cell of SS mRNA increase). Furthermore, it appears that a change in the number of grains/cell may underestimate the actual change in the number of copies of mRNA/cell. Hence, a small difference in the number of grains/cell as detected by semiquantitative *in situ* hybridization may actually reflect a much larger change that has occurred at the molecular level.

Application to *in situ* hybridization histochemistry

The primary advantage of using the *in situ* hybridization technique, as opposed to other RNA detection methods (e.g. Northern Blots, solution hybridization or dot blots) is the preservation of anatomical specificity. Within the central nervous system, one neuropeptide may be involved in the modulation of numerous physiological functions. It follows that the neurones serving these different physiological systems may be divided into functionally related subsets, each responding to different modulators. Hence, if only a fraction of the neuronal population responds to a certain stimulus, analysing all neurons together may obscure an important change in the gene expression of that select subset. *In situ* hybridization histochemistry allows the investigator to analyse separately neurones within specific nuclei or anatomical locations. This concept is illustrated in Figs. 6 and 7. In this experiment, the effects of the sex steroid environment on signal levels of POMC mRNA was assessed by *in situ* hybridization. Adult male rats were castrated and immediately received silastic capsules that contained either testosterone, dihydrotestosterone (DHT), or

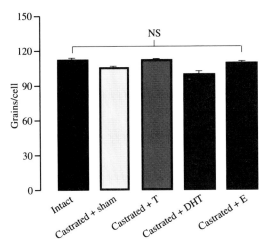

Fig. 6. The relative level of POMC mRNA, as reflected in the number of grains/cell, in the arcuate nucleus of five groups of male rats: (*a*) intact, (*b*) castrated, (*c*) castrated testosterone-replaced, (*d*) castrated dihydrotestosterone-replaced, and (*e*) castrated estradiol-replaced. Approximately 200 cells were analyzed in each animal. (NS = not significant). (Modified from Chowen *et al.*, 1990).

estradiol, or an empty sham capsule. Intact controls were sham castrated. All animals were sacrificed four days following surgery and *in situ* hybridization for POMC mRNA was performed as described above. After developing the slides, 16 tissue sections were anatomically matched throughout the arcuate nucleus so that the same levels of this nucleus were analysed in each animal. Approximately 200 positive neurones in each animal were analysed by using the image analysis system described above. Fig. 6 demonstrates that with this type of analysis no significant difference between experimental groups was detected.

However, in order to determine if this population of neurones is heterogeneous in its response to manipulation of sex steroids, another experiment was performed where the arcuate nucleus was arbitrarily divided into four segments anteroposteriorly and four tissue sections from each area were analysed. As can be seen in Fig. 7, analysis in this manner revealed that castration resulted in a significant reduction in the levels of the POMC mRNA signal in neurones of the most anterior portion of the arcuate nucleus. Furthermore, whereas replacement with testosterone and estradiol prevented this decline, DHT did not. In contrast, POMC mRNA levels in the posterior three-quarters of the nucleus were not detectably modified by any of these steroid manipulations. This suggests that POMC neurones of the anterior arcuate nucleus respond to modulation by testosterone and that this effect is most likely to be mediated by the estrogen receptor.

The afferent and efferent projections of this portion of the nucleus differ from those of the posterior arcuate (Chronwall, 1985), suggesting that this population of neurones may be functionally distinct from the POMC neurones in the posterior portion of the same nucleus. This concept is further supported

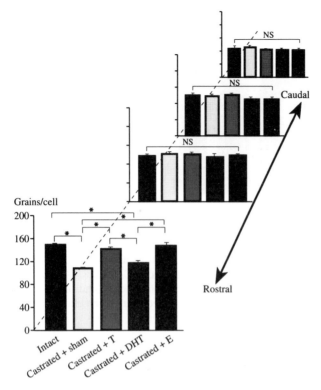

Fig. 7. The relative level of POMC mRNA, as reflected in the number of grains/cell, throughout the arcuate nucleus of five groups of rats (as for Fig. 6). Four anatomical divisions of the arcuate nucleus are represented by the four fields of view, with area A being the most anterior division and continuing posteriorly to area D. In each field of view the *y*-axis range is from 0 to 200 grains/cell. (NS = not significant, * = $p < 0.05$). (Modified from Chowen *et al.*, 1990).

by the fact that the mean level of POMC mRNA, as shown by the number of grains/cell, is different in the anterior portion of the arcuate nucleus of the intact male rat as compared to those neurones in the posterior portion of this nucleus (Fig. 8). These examples emphasize the need to understand the specific circumstances, in this case the physiology and anatomy, of the question at hand in order to gather the most data when applying image analysis techniques.

Another advantage of *in situ* hybridization is that subsets of neurons can be further identified by using double-labelling techniques. For example, a select population of SS neurones in the periventricular nucleus (PeN) have been shown to contain androgen receptors (Burton *et al.*, 1990), allowing the possibility of analysing these neurones as a separate subpopulation. The power of this technique is that it affords the experimenter the opportunity to define and analyse individual neurones on the basis of their anatomical location and, if used in conjunction with other techniques, the presence of other neuronal markers such as receptors or enzymes. However, there are some technical problems that must be considered when doing double-labelling techniques.

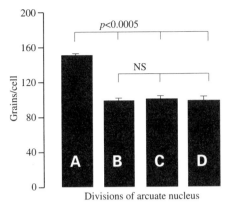

Fig. 8. POMC mRNA levels, as reflected in the number of grains/cell, in four anatomical regions of the arcuate nucleus of intact male rats. The arcuate nucleus was
arbitrarily divided into four regions of approximately the same length, with area A
representing the most anterior portion of the arcuate nucleus and continuing posteriorly
to area D. There is a significant gradient in the amount of POMC mRNA in individual
neurons throughout the arcuate nucleus of the intact male rat with neurons of the most
anterior region containing significantly more message than those of the posterior
regions. (NS = not significant, * = $p < 0.05$). (Modified from Chowen *et al.*, 1990).

Most double-labelling procedures involve the use of a radioactively labelled
probe plus another that will be detected with some form of chromogen. The
combination of these two procedures can result in the loss of specific signal;
hence, semiquantitative analysis may be difficult. Furthermore, the combination of the two products, the silver grains and colour reaction product, may
make it difficult to analyse one product without the interference of the other.
This can be circumvented by proper adjustment of the illumination during the
analysis.

Conclusion

Although a number of powerful image analysis programs and systems are
available to the researcher today, the value of each system depends on the way
that it is applied to each individual experiment. The system used to analyse the
experiments presented in this chapter was designed specifically for the task of
counting silver grains over individual cells after *in situ* hybridization had been
performed. Therefore, many of the potential problems of this process were
taken into consideration when the system was designed. Regardless of this fact,
there still exist a number of steps in the image analysis process where errors
can be introduced. Many of these possible sources of error have been identified
and have been minimized. For example, since the photometric response of the
system was not uniform over the entire video field, cells are always analysed in
approximately the same region of the video field. However, for every experimenter the first step in the process of image analysis must be to identify the
possible sources of variation within the system being used.

Minor variations in sample preparation or experimental technique can lead to erroneous results. Slight differences in photographic emulsion thickness, insufficient rinsing of tissue and non-saturating probe concentrations are all common occurrences that can greatly affect the image to be analysed, although they can easily be remedied. Furthermore, as shown above, important results can often be missed if questions of physiology or biology are overlooked when designing experiments and analysing data. In other words, a well designed and technically well run experiment is as important as a powerful image analysis system.

References

Angerer, L. M., Cox, K. H. & Angerer, R. C. (1987). Demonstration of tissue-specific gene expression by *in situ* hybridization. *Methods in Enzymology*, **152**, 649–61.

Argente, J., Chowen-Breed, J. A., Steiner, R. A. & Clifton, D. K. (1990). Somatostatin messenger RNA in hypothalamic neurons is increased by testosterone through activation of androgen receptors and not by aromatization to estradiol. *Neuroendocrinology*, **52**, 342–9.

Burton, K. A., Steiner, R. A., & Clifton D. K. (1990). Colocalization of the androgen receptor and somatostatin messenger RNA in neurons in the periventricular nucleus. (Abstract) Society for Neuroscience.

Chowen, J. A., Argente, J., Vician, L., Clifton, D. K. & Steiner R. A. (1990). Pro-opiomelanocortin messenger RNA in hypothalamic neurons is increased by testosterone through aromatization to estradiol. *Neuroendocrinology*, **52**, 581–8.

Chowen, J. A., Steiner, R. A. & Clifton, D. K. (1991). Semiquantitative analysis of cellular somatostatin mRNA levels by *in situ* hybridization histochemistry. In *Methods in Neuroscience*, vol. 5, ed. P. M. Conn, pp. 137–58. New York: Academic Press.

Chowen-Breed, J. A., Fraser, H. M., Vician, L., Damassa D. A., Clifton D. K. Steiner, R. A. (1989). Testosterone regulation of proopiomelanocortin messenger ribonucleic acid in the arcuate nucleus of the male rat. *Endocrinology*, **124**, 1697–702.

Chronwall, B. M. (1985). Anatomy and physiology of the neuroendocrine arcuate nucleus. *Peptides*, **6**, 1–11.

Durnam, D. M. & Palmiter, R. D. (1983). A practical approach for quantitating specific mRNAs by solution hybridization. *Analytical Biochemistry*, **131**, 385–93.

Green, M. R. Maniatis, T. Melton, D. A. (1983). Human β-globin pre-mRNA synthesized in vitro is accurately spliced in xenopus oocyte nuclei. *Cell*, **32**, 681–6.

Rogers, K. V., Vician, L, Steiner, R. A. & Clifton, D. K. (1987). Reduced preprosomatostatin mRNA in the periventricular nucleus of hypophysectomized rats determined by quantitative *in situ* hybridization. *Endocrinology*, **121**, 90–3.

22

New interpretation techniques to aid automatic quantification of pathology

J. ALDRIDGE

Introduction

Image analysis provides a wide range of sophisticated measurement techniques. Even so, it is often difficult to analyse histological and cytological preparations automatically as in many cases standard detection methods simply do not interpret the image well enough on their own to find the regions to be measured.

The issue of recognition is complex. The interpretation of an image often depends on background information about the sample. Show the same image to a metallurgist and a biologist and in the absence of additional data they are likely to identify the sample in wildly different ways.

However, important changes in the approach adopted by manufacturers of image analysis equipment are promising advances. The first is a shift away from developing general purpose analysis software and towards developing analysis software which will solve particular problems in interpreting types of images. The second is a realization that image analysis is only the end point of a wider experiment, and that contextual information should be taken into account when designing the image analysis experiment.

To develop software to solve problems of interpreting specific image types, it is necessary to define generic rule sets to which all images of the particular genre conform. The power of the rule sets is that they allow the software engineer the freedom to adopt new approaches and to tailor the software to an extent that would otherwise be impossible.

In this chapter, I describe two new software packages that were developed by Seescan plc (Cambridge) that are now commercially available. They were written specifically for cellular level analysis of radiolabelled *in situ* hybridization and receptor autoradiography and for differential counting of immuno-labelled cells in sections or cytospins. The functions are novel in that they make use of analysis algorithms that were not written to provide general purpose tools. Instead, they perform defined and specific recognition tasks on relatively narrow sets of images and, in fact, employ pattern recognition algorithms to form the basis of the interpretation process.

Cellular level analysis of radiolabelled sections

The binding sites of radiolabelled mRNA transcripts in *in situ* hybridization and ligands in receptor autoradiography studies can be localized to the cellular level if the appropriate radioactive isotope is used. If quantification is required, the results of binding are normally visualized by apposing a coverslip coated with a photographic emulsion to the section as it is easier to achieve an even coating of emulsion on a coverslip than by the alternative technique of dipping the section into photographic emulsion. After a period of exposure, the emulsion is developed. Where levels of radioactivity in the section were higher than a minimum value, grains of silver halide form in the emulsion layer.

Sections have usually first been counterstained to reveal the histological structure of the sample so the silver halide grains are seen superimposed on the counterstained cells using bright field microscopy at an appropriate magnification.

However, quantification often proves difficult. Low levels of labelling can easily be assessed by eye simply by counting the numbers of silver halide grains superimposed on a single cell or on groups of cells. When grains become more dense, clumping occurs and clumps are hard to assess visually. However, even at low levels, the sheer volume of grain counting needed in many experiments to generate statistically valid data is daunting if the work has to be done by eye.

Attempts to use automatic image analysis to quantify the extent of radio-labelling on counterstained sections have been confounded by the difficulty of thresholding the grains. Although the grains are easy to see, a threshold level that detects grains on lightly counterstained regions of the image will usually overdetect grains on heavily counterstained cells, and will often even detect the cells themselves. This is thought to be caused by optical diffraction effects due to the small (submicron) size of individual grains, and by video bandwidth limitations arising from basic camera design and from filtering the video at the input to the image analysis system to meet Nyquist's theorem. A further problem arises from the relative thickness of the sample. At the highest magnifications, it is not normally possible to select a single focal plane in which both the counterstained cells and the grains are adequately focussed. In fact, the thickness of the emulsion layer in which grains can form is usually greater than the depth of focus at high magnifications.

Two analysis methods have been developed to overcome some of these problems and enable automatic image analysis to be used to quantify grain density. The first method uses dark field microscopy. The counterstain information disappears from the image, while the grains appear as bright dots on a black background. This technique is commonly used in receptor autoradiography and *in situ* hybridization. Its main disadvantage is that grain density can no longer be related to histological structure unless the bright field image is also referred to, involving swapping regularly between dark field and bright field images of the same field of view.

In the second method, the section is counterstained so lightly that a single threshold can be chosen which properly detects all grains and does not pick up the counterstain. This technique is commonly used in the unscheduled DNA synthesis assay for assessing chemical compounds for genetic toxicity. The disadvantage is that in practice, the counterstain often proves so light that it can be difficult to make out the histological structure of the sample. Morever, to avoid problems of video bandwidth limitations hindering thresholding, analyses are normally performed using a ×100 oil immersion objective, which results in the need to change the plane of focus regularly and analyse multiple fields of view. In many autoradiographic applications, this would slow down analysis considerably.

It is desirable to quantify radiolabelling on bright field images of samples that have been counterstained to make their morphology easy to recognize and at magnifications that maximise the depth of focus while allowing grains to be well resolved.

The following assumptions were made to form the basis of the rule set. First, the silver halide grains would be as well focussed as possible and the magnification would be set so that single grains were as small as possible on the screen, commensurate with their being well resolved. Second, the counterstained cells would tend to be less well focused than the grains. Third, there would be a contrast difference between grains and their local background. Fourth, unless there were large clumps of grains, the size of counterstained objects would be significantly larger than that of the grains. Fifth, grains would either be single or clumped. These assumptions were backed up by a set of images providing typical examples.

Software was developed that detected single grains, small and large clumps of grains using pattern recognition techniques and relative density information and would work on images captured using either a ×20 or ×40 objective, the choice depending on the grain size. The software was optimized by checking its results using a routine which, on a keypress, switched on or off a yellow or green overlay superimposed on the image to show the results of the detection over the original image.

An early observation was that it is necessary for the user to be able to vary the severity with which algorithms are applied to adapt for different grain sizes. The problem of assessing clumps was addressed by measuring the total area covered by grains within a region of interest, and then expressing the grain cover either per unit area or per cell. A count estimate was derived for comparison with visual counts by dividing the area of grain cover by the average area of a single grain.

Initial studies showed that these algorithms gave better than 99% repeatability on the same image, and also showed that the data were more immune to variations in lighting than data produced by the standard method involving quantifying the dark field image. Dr Jonathan Seckl's team at the University of Edinburgh performed validation studies comparing the data acquired automatically with counts made by eye. At low densities, a correlation of 98% was reported. At higher densities the correlation was not so good; 87% was reported. This was thought to be because the difficulty of assessing grain density visually increases as the labelling becomes heavier. Tests were performed using commercially available ^{32}P and ^{35}S standards (Amersham, Bucks) apposed to emulsion coated coverslips. A 97% correlation was shown between the nominal radioactivity values of the standards and the grain densities measured using the new technique. It was felt that this indicated the validity of the measurement technique and that it supported the hypothesis that at higher densities visual assessment is less accurate than automatic assessment. The graph of nominal versus measured values also showed the start of the typical non-linearity at higher radioactivity levels experienced in autoradiography due to saturation of the emulsion.

A software program was written using these algorithms specifically for *in situ* hybridization and receptor autoradiography. It allowed the operator to set up and execute an experiment by defining and then implementing a protocol. The protocol definition included an experimental description, including identifying the sections to be analysed and the regions to be analysed for each section. The protocol setup also included optimizing the grain detection algorithms at the beginning of the analysis so that the detection method was identical throughout the experiment. The user could specify whether grain density should be assessed per cell or per unit area, and how data were to be corrected, if at all, for variations in background labelling. A range of calibration algorithms could be used to convert image analysis data to the units used in calibration standards.

Another application for this type of pattern recognition algorithm has been found in the quantitation of immunogold labelling visualized using transmission electron microscopy. The image analysis problem is analogous to the problem of quantifying cellular level autoradiography on bright field images described above. The pattern recognition algorithms have been modified to produce a routine which simply locates and counts all particles with the right size and shape characteristics. At the time of writing, the software cannot discriminate between particles of different sizes, and is really best suited to locating and counting particles of a particular size. It is envisaged that the next logical step, the adaptation of the pattern recognition techniques to locate particles of two size classes, will be completed in the near future.

Differential cell counting

The end point of many immunohistochemical experiments is a sample in which the number of cells for which there has been a positive reaction must be counted and expressed as a percentage of the total number of cells. As an example, a standard preparation could be counterstained using haematoxylin with a subset of cells immunolabelled using a horseradish peroxidase reaction.

This type of image presents problems that often defy automation using standard image analysis routines. Moreover, this type of image is not just arduous to quantify visually, it can often be difficult to get a repeatable count on samples that have a high background as the eye is not good at maintaining constant a fine intensity threshold to discriminate between positive and negative cells.

It is important that the cell counting process is based only on morphological characteristics and is separate from the process of determining for each cell whether or not it is stained positive; otherwise the results may be biased. Often, monochrome images produced using coloured filters do not provide an obvious separation of the counterstain and immunolabel. It was found that the best way to achieve this separation was to capture red, green and blue coloured images and then to deconvolve to produce two new monochrome images: one in which immunostaining information is suppressed, retaining simply the morphological information revealed by the counterstain for identifying the cells and marking their positions, and a second in which the counterstain information is suppressed to allow the immunostaining levels to be quantified. Special colour processing techniques have been developed by Seescan plc (Cambridge) providing a wide range of software tools for converting colour images to monochrome.

This type of image can be difficult to count using standard image analysis software because the cells often touch and are stained to different intensities; as a result it is difficult to find a single adequate threshold. These two characteristics were built into the rule set defining the image genre for the purposes of developing recognition software to identify and locate the centres of cell nuclei. The other assumptions in this rule set were that nuclei would be stained most densely in the centre, that nuclei would have an aspect ratio of no more than 1.5, that in the same image the nucleus diameter would not change by more than 100% and that each time the software was used, the magnification would be selected so that the apparent size of cells on the screen would always be similar.

Besides this rule set, a group of example images was collected to illustrate the problem. The first sample presented to define the image analysis problem was cultured breast cells, and in the first instance, the counting software was developed specifically to analyse this type of image. Pattern recognition techniques were used again. Subsequently, the software was tested and adapted on intestinal lymph tissue and on brain sections with immunostained neurones. The software returned a count of all cells, and put a coloured overlay showing the results of testing onto the image for visual checking.

The next step was to build in a test for positivity referencing information about the immunological stain. The second monochrome image that had been generated from the colour image held information about the local intensity of the immunological stain. A threshold was used on this image to discriminate between positive and negative staining; the normal methodology being to set up the threshold on a control section. The counting software was then adapted to reference this second image each time it found a cell so that if there was staining above the positivity threshold within a maximum distance from the centre of the cell, the cell would be counted as positive. Again, the results of the analysis were displayed by superimposing dots and crosses on cells found to be negative or positive using a coloured overlay which could be toggled on and off over the original image. The differential counting process took about ten seconds per image, with up to 1000 cells in a single image.

At the time of writing, this software is going into use in about 40 laboratories in the UK. Initial trials show good repeatability of counting; however, repeatability of positivity discrimination depends on the stability of the intensity and colour of the illumination. Initial trials and discussions with scientists indicate widespread applications and a great deal of enthusiasm.

Conclusion

The application of pattern recognition algorithms designed to work with images meeting a well-defined and relatively extensive rule set has allowed some of the more difficult recognition problems in histology to be automated. The analysis of radio-labelled sections has been successfully developed to such an extent that, in this case no further major development of the analysis algorithms appears to be needed. The cell counting application is more open ended, simply because of the diversity of potential applications for the type of software. Ultimately, the goal must be to produce software which learns its recognition task through the user showing it example cells.

23

Quantitative pathology

D. R. SPRINGALL, S. M. GENTLEMAN,
G. TERENGHI and J. M. POLAK

Introduction

The human eye and brain form the basis of an extremely versatile system for the collection and analysis of visual images, using a combination of highly developed pattern recognition skills and previously accumulated experience. Pathologists are able to view a microscope slide and come to a conclusion which in some way classifies what can be seen on the slide, but the accurate and reproducible quantification of the components of an image requires a computer image analysis system, which is far better at extracting quantitative data from images. (These important concepts have been discussed in many of the chapters of this book.)

Two examples of the possible application of image analysis in solving pathological problems are described below, illustrating the power of image analysis to derive quantitative information from histological preparations.

Quantitative histopathology in Alzheimer's disease

The use of image analysis as an aid to pathological investigation is well illustrated by some recent work carried out on the changes in the brain associated with Alzheimer's disease, a progressive dementing condition affecting between 5 and 10% of the population over the age of 65 (Katzman, 1986). The disease is characterized neuropathologically by a regional loss of neurons in the cerebral cortex and by the occurrence of neurofibrillary tangles and extracellular amyloid (βA4)-containing plaques (Fig. 1). The plaques are one of the diagnostic features of the disease and as such have been the focus of extensive research, particularly with respect to their potential role in aetiology. A number of attempts have been made to correlate the number of plaques seen at post mortem with the severity of the dementia observed *in vivo* (Blessed *et al.*, 1968; Wilcock & Esiri, 1981) in order to help determine their role in the pathogenesis of the disease. These studies have been based on conventional silver staining and manual counting techniques and have produced equivocal results.

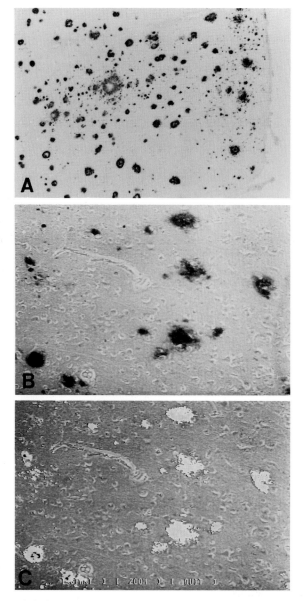

Fig. 1. (A) βA4-immunoreactive plaques in a section of temporal cortex from a patient with Alzheimer's disease. (B) By capturing a high magnification image of the stained section (B), and thresholding on the basis of greylevels, an estimate of βA4 'load' can be obtained (C).

More recently, immunostaining with an antiserum to βA4 protein has been shown to be far more effective than standard silver staining in detecting the full extent of plaque deposits in the brains of control and Alzheimer's disease patients. Furthermore, the high contrast nature and specificity of the immuno-staining makes it eminently suitable for quantitative studies in which computer image analysis techniques can be employed (Gentleman *et al.*, 1989). Before the discovery and isolation of βA4 (Glenner & Wong, 1984), senile plaques were seen as discrete structures which could be classified according to their morphology (Wisniewski & Terry, 1973) and could be counted individually with relative ease. However, the introduction of sensitive immunostaining techniques for the detection of βA4 has revealed a further population of βA4 deposits. In addition to the morphological subtypes previously described, large numbers of diffuse or pre-amyloid deposits have been found in the brains of demented patients (Ikeda *et al.*, 1988; Probst *et al.*, 1987; Yamaguchi *et al.*, 1988). These deposits are not detected by the majority of silver staining methods which probably explains the equivocal results obtained in previous quantitative studies (Blessed *et al.*, 1968; Wilcock & Esiri, 1981). The diffuse nature of the deposits causes problems for manual counting methods because it is no longer possible to define with any degree of certainty what is and what is not a discrete lesion. To overcome this problem a new means of quantifying the plaques has been devised based on the estimation of a total βA4 'load' within the cerebral grey matter (Cairns *et al.*, 1991; Gentleman *et al.*, 1992).

The latter study describes how this method has been used to reveal differences in the distribution and amount of βA4 protein between the frontal and temporal lobes of Alzheimer's disease patients (Gentleman *et al.*, 1992). In brief, paraffin sections were incubated overnight with a monoclonal antiserum raised against residues 8–17 of the βA4 sequence (Allsop *et al.*, 1986). They were then stained using an avidin–biotin-complex technique and analysed. At the beginning of each analysis session the first image to be captured was that of the background illumination which was then used in the analysis of all the subsequent images in that session. By subtracting this image from the section images, the effects of defects in the lighting and microscope optics were eliminated to a large extent. All images were captured using the ×10 objective on the microscope and the green gun of a colour video camera. The green channel was used in preference to the red or blue channels because its spectral response most closely resembles that of the human eye and the image was generally of better contrast than the others. To minimize random noise in the video signal the image was captured as the average of 16 frames. The sampling of each section was started at a random point in the cortical ribbon and then every tenth frame was analysed around the perimeter of the section. Each sample site was designated as either sulcal or gyral and because approximately two-thirds of the cortical surface area lies within the sulci there were generally more measurements made in sulci than there were in gyri. As far as it was possible by rotating the microscope stage, all sampling was done perpendicular to the pial surface of the brain.

Interactive thresholding of the image produced a binary image from which automatic area determinations could then be performed. The percentage of the cortical grey matter covered by βA4 deposits in the Alzheimer's disease sections was determined by adding the highlighted pixels from all fields at a particular site and dividing by the total grey matter area (in pixels) at that site. Using this technique it was found that there was more deposition of βA4 at the base of the cortical sulci than there was on the crests of the gyri ($p < 0.05$). In addition there was a consistently higher level of deposition of βA4 in the frontal as opposed to the temporal cortical tissue in any given case.

In this study the use of image analysis achieved two things. Firstly it was able to confirm previous anecdotal reports from neuropathologists that there are more plaques to be found in the depths of the sulci than on the gyral crests. More importantly, however, it provided the novel finding that there are a significantly greater number of βA4 plaques in frontal rather than temporal cortex. This had not been previously reported and the phenomenon would have gone unnoticed without the use of this technique. The same method of quantifying βA4 has subsequently been used to show that there is a significant correlation between the βA4 load in certain areas of the temporal cortex and the severity of Alzheimer-type dementia seen *in vivo* (Gentleman *et al.*, 1991).

Although the determination of the βA4 load has produced some interesting and valuable results, it remains a relatively straightforward application of the image analysis procedure. Having established that the distribution of βA4 protein is heterogeneous within the cortex, further investigations have been made into its pattern of distribution (Bruce *et al.*, 1992). In this study, tissue sections were immunostained, images were analysed using greylevel threshold-ing and a mathematical model based on a Fourier analysis was used to describe both the amount and pattern of distribution across the cortex. As with the simple load determination technique this more sophisticated analysis has provided new insights into the differential distribution of βA4 in the brains of demented patients. Edwards *et al.* (1992) have taken the sophistication of the image analysis of βA4 deposits one stage further by actually making the computer distinguish between two distinct morphological subtypes of deposit. This is achieved by segmenting an image of an immunostained section by greylevel thresholding and then further segmenting the image on the basis of size, texture and the presence or absence of an internal area in individual deposits. This analysis is currently being used in an attempt to determine the role played by plaques of differing morphology in the development of Alzheimer's disease.

It should be noted that, although all of the investigations described above have been aimed at shedding further light on the pathogenic processes underly-ing Alzheimer's disease, the techniques are easily adaptable and may have a wide range of applications in solving of many other pathology-based research problems.

Neurovascular skin pathology

Regulatory peptides are abundantly present in nerve fibres of the skin, fibres that can be visualized by immunocytochemistry (Wallengren *et al.*, 1987;

Karanth *et al.*, 1991). The best morphological results are obtained using the indirect immunofluorescence technique, which gives the maximum contrast even for very small or weakly positive fibres. However, quantification of fluorescence staining has been hampered by some problems, such as fading with exposure to light and background autofluorescence, that are intrinsic to the staining method. Recently, it has been possible to overcome some of these problems and to use image analysis to evaluate these preparations quantitatively and thereby measure changes in disease (Gale *et al.*, 1989; Terenghi *et al.*, 1991: see Chapter 20).

One example of this work is the assessment of changes in the spectrum or concentrations of neuropeptide in patients with Raynaud's phenomenon or systemic sclerosis. Raynaud's phenomenon is characterized by episodic digital ischemia subsequent to cold or emotional stimuli, and it could be primary to or associated with other conditions such as systemic sclerosis. Intravenous calcitonin-gene-related peptide (CGRP) has been used successfully to treat patients with Raynaud's phenomenon (Bunker *et al.*, 1989), which is consistent with a decrease of CGRP-immunoreactive nerves around the capillaries of the papillary dermis in patients with either primary Raynaud's phenomenon or systemic sclerosis (Fig. 2) (Bunker *et al.*, 1990; Terenghi *et al.*, 1991). These changes could be observed on subjective microscopical examination. However, using image analysis quantification it was possible to demonstrate changes in nerves detected with antisera to protein gene product 9.5 (PGP), a pan neuronal marker (Gulbenkian *et al.*, 1987; Dalsgaard *et al.*, 1989), and vasoactive intestinal polypeptide (VIP), which had not been detected by visual screening (Fig. 3: Terenghi *et al.*, 1991).

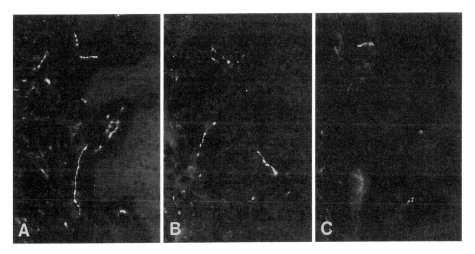

Fig. 2. CGRP-immunoreactive nerves in the same area of comparative sections of human skin from (A) control, (B) primary Raynaud's phenomenon, and (C) systemic sclerosis patients. Note the progressive decrease of CGRP immunoreactivity from control to systemic sclerosis samples. Indirect immunofluorescence method.

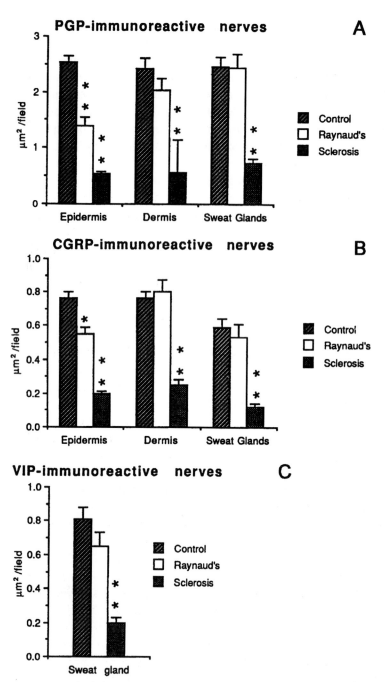

Fig. 3. Histograms showing the total field fluorescence area (μm^2) of (A) PGP-, (B) CGRP- and (C) VIP-immunoreactive nerves, expressed as mean values with the standard errors of the means, represented by error bars, in different areas of the skin of controls and patients with Raynaud's phenomenon and systemic sclerosis. $^*p = 0.005$; $^{**}p < 0.0001$.

Another example is diabetic neuropathy. Sensory and autonomic cutaneous nerve fibres are severely affected by diabetes, contributing to the development of neuropathy. Semiquantitative studies have demonstrated that in human skin there is a depletion of specific neuronal subpopulations as characterized by the presence of different neuropeptides (Levy *et al.*, 1989). In further studies, quantitative immunocytochemical measurements were made in order to define precisely the changes according to the duration of diabetes and to the severity of the neuropathy. The immunocytochemical findings were compared with the results of neurophysiological tests reflecting the function in both large and small nerve fibres.

When patients were divided into two groups according to the duration of diabetes, there was an increase of PGP- and VIP-immunoreactive nerves around the sweat glands of patients that had suffered diabetes for up to three years (Fig. 4A). This was followed by a significant decrease in immunoreactivities, which progressed with the duration of the disease. In the subepidermal layer, there were similar duration-related changes for PGP- and CGRP-immunoreactive nerves (Fig. 4B) (Properzi *et al.*, 1992). However, no correlation could be found between quantification data and neurophysiological tests. Neural immunostaining in the skin relates to small peripheral fibres, which might show alterations at early stages of diabetes, whereas functional tests are indicative of damage to large nerve fibres, which occurs late during the disease. Hence, quantitative immunocytochemistry can give a reliable assessment of nerve changes at earlier stages than is possible with functional tests.

A comparison was also carried out between long-term diabetic patients with normal small fibre function (non-neuropathic) and those with abnormal small fibres function (neuropathic). When comparing control, non-neuropathic and neuropathic, there was a progressive reduction of PGP- and CGRP-immunoreactive nerves in epidermal and subepidermal layers, and of VIP-immunoreactive fibres in sweat glands (Fig. 5) (Levy *et al.*, 1992). Also, a statistically significant association was found between sweat gland measurements and acetylcholine-stimulated sweat output or sympathetic skin response.

Nodular prurigo is characterized histologically by acanthosis and by cutaneous nerve proliferation. However, there is some controversy as to whether the increase of nerves is specific for a given subpopulation or is a generalized phenomenon. Using immunocytochemistry and image analysis, a significant increase of PGP-immunoreactive nerves was found in the dermal papillae of all nodular prurigo cases. Characterization of these nerves showed that they were mainly reactive for CGRP and substance P whereas the densities of other neuropeptide-immunoreactive nerves were similar in controls and nodular prurigo patients (Abadia Molina *et al.*, 1992). These results indicate that in nodular prurigo the increase in numbers of nerves is related to the sensory component of the nervous system, and it might be related to the intense feeling of itch observed in this disease.

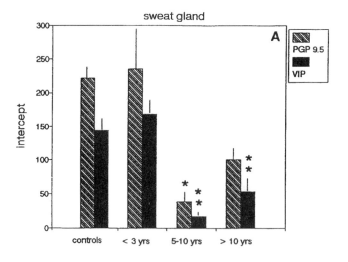

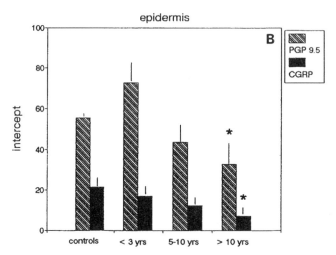

Fig. 4. Histograms showing intercept counts of PGP-, CGRP- and VIP-immunoreactive nerves, expressed as mean values and standard errors of the means (bars), in (A) sweat glands and (B) epidermal and subepidermal layer of control and diabeticpatients divided according to duration of the disease. $*p < 0.05$; $**p < 0.004$.

Conclusions

The application of image analysis has added greatly to the amount of information that can be obtained from morphological studies. Although quantitative pathology is still in its infancy, the availability of user-friendly image analyses and specific and suitable programmes makes the future of quantitative pathology a real and exciting task. The added dimension of computerised morphometry to descriptive pathology makes it into an exacting and essential discipline.

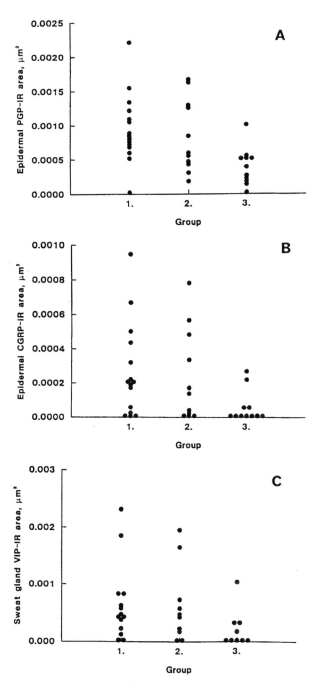

Fig. 5. Dot plots of (A) PGP- and (B) CGRP-immunoreactive nerve area (μm^2) in epidermal and subepidermal layers, and of (C) VIP-immunoreactive nerve area in sweat glands. All nerve types show a progressive reduction through the three groups (1, controls; 2, non-neuropathic diabetics; 3, neuropathic diabetics). The depletion was statistically significant ($p < 0.05$) for PGP and CGRP immunoreactivities in the neuropathic group 3 versus age-matched normal subjects.

References

Abadia Molina, F., Burrows, N. P., Russell Jones, R., Terenghi, G. & Polak, J. M. (1992). Increased sensory neuropeptides in nodular prurigo: a quantitative immunohistochemical analysis. *British Journal of Dermatology*, **127**, 344–51.

Allsop, D., Landon, M., Kidd, M., Lowe, J. S., Reynolds, G. P. & Gardner, A. (1986). Monoclonal antibodies raised against a subsequence of senile plaque core protein react with plaque cores, plaque periphery and cerebrovascular amyloid in Alzheimer's disease. *Neuroscience Letters*, **68**, 253–56.

Blessed, G., Tomlinson, B. E. & Roth, M. (1968). The association between quantitative measures of dementia and of senile changes in the cerebral grey matter of elderly subjects. *British Journal of Psychiatry*, **114**, 797–811.

Bruce, C. V., Clinton, J., Gentleman, S. M., Roberts, G. W. & Royston, M. C. (1992). Quantifying the pattern of βA4 amyloid protein deposition in Alzheimer's disease by image analysis. *Neuropathology and Applied Neurology*, **18**, 125–36.

Bunker, C. B., Foreman, J. C., O'Shaughnessy, D., Reavly, C. & Dowd, P. M. (1989). Calcitonin gene-related peptide in the treatment of severe Raynaud's phenomenon. *British Journal of Dermatology*, **121**, 43–44.

Bunker, C. B., Terenghi, G., Springall, D. R., Polak, J. M. & Dowd, P. M. (1990). Deficiency of calcitonin gene-related peptide in Raynaud's phenomenon. *Lancet*, **336**, 1530–1533.

Cairns, N. J., Chadwick, A., Luthert, P. J. & Lantos, P. L. (1991). β-Amyloid protein load is relatively uniform throughout neocortex and hippocampus in elderly Alzheimer's disease patients. *Neuroscience Letters*, **129**, 115–18.

Dalsgaard, C. J., Rydh, M. & Haegerstrand, A. (1989). Cutaneous innervation in man visualized with protein gene product 9.5 (PGP 9.5) antibodies. *Histochemistry*, **92**, 385–9.

Gale, J. D., Alberts, J. C. J. & Cowen, T. (1989). A quantitative study of changes in old age of 5-hydroxytryptamine-like immunoreactivity in perivascular nerves of the rabbit. *Journal of the Autonomic Nervous System*, **28**, 51–60.

Gentleman, S. M., Bruton, C., Allsop, D., Lewis, S. J., Polak, J. M. & Roberts, G. W. (1989). A demonstration of the advantages of immunostaining in the quantification of amyloid plaque deposits. *Histochemistry*, **92**, 355–358.

Gentleman, S. M., Perry, R. M. & Roberts, G. W. (1991). Correlations between β-amyloid protein (βAP) load and mental test scores in Alzheimer's disease. *Neuropathology and Applied Neurobiology*, **17**, 531.

Gentleman, S. M., Allsop, D., Bruton, C. J., Jagoe, R., Polak, J. M. & Roberts, G. W. (1992). Quantitative differences in the deposition of β/A4 protein in the sulci and gyri of frontal and temporal isocortex in Alzheimer's disease. *Neuroscience Letters*, **136**, 27–30.

Glenner, G. G. & Wong, C. W. (1984). Alzheimer's disease: initial report of the purification and characterization of a novel cerebrovascular amyloid protein. *Biochemical and Biophysical Research Communications*, **120**, 885–90.

Gulbenkian, S., Wharton, J. & Polak, J. M. (1987). The visualization of cardiovascular innervation in the guinea pig using antiserum to protein gene product 9.5 (PGP 9.5). *Journal of the Autonomic Nervous System*, **19**, 581–93.

Ikeda, S., Allsop, D. & Glenner, G. G. (1988). Morphology and distribution of plaque and related deposits in the brains of Alzheimer's disease and control cases: an immunohistochemical study using amyloid β-protein antibody. *Laboratory Investigation*, **60**, 113–22.

Karanth, S. S., Springall, D. R., Kuhn, D. M., Levene, M. M. & Polak, J. M. (1991). An immunocytochemical study of cutaneous innervation and the distribution of neuropeptides and protein gene product 9.5 in man and commonly employed laboratory animals. *American Journal of Anatomy*, **191**, 369–83.

Katzman, R. (1986). Alzheimer's disease. *New England Journal of Medicine*, **314**, 964–73.

Levy, D. M., Terenghi, G., Gu, X-H., Abraham, R. R., Springall, D. R. & Polak, J. M. (1992). Immunohistochemical measurements of nerves and neuropeptides in diabetic skin-relationship to tests of neurological function. *Diabetologia*, **35**, 889–897.

Levy, D. M., Karanth, S. S., Springall, D. R. & Polak, J. M. (1989). Depletion of cutaneous nerves and neuropeptides in diabetes mellitus: an immunocytochemical study. *Diabetologia*, **32**, 427–433.

McKenzie, J. E., Gentleman, S. M., Royston, M. C., Edwards, R. J. & Roberts, G. W. (1992). Quantification of plaque types in sulci and gyri of the medical frontal lobe in patients with Alzheimer's disease. *Neuroscience Letters*, **143**, 23–26.

Probst, A., Brannschweiler, H., Lautenschlager, C. & Ulrich, J. (1987). A special type of senile plaque, possibly an initial stage. *Acta Neuropathologica*, **74**, 133–41.

Properzi, G., Francavilla, S., Poccia, G., Aloisio, P., Gu, X-H., Terenghi, G. & Polak, J. M. (1993). Early increase precedes a depletion of VIP and PGP 9.5 in the skin of insulin-dependent diabetics – correlation between quantitative immunohistochemistry and clinical assessment of peripheral neuropathy. *Journal of Pathology*, **328**, 595–603.

Terenghi, G., Bunker, C. B., Lui, Y-F., Springall, D. R., Cowen, T., Dowd, P. M. & Polak, J. M. (1991). Image analysis quantification of peptide immunoreactive nerves in the skin of patients with Raynaud's phenomenon and systemic sclerosis. *Journal of Pathology*, **164**, 245–52.

Wallengren, J., Ekman, R. & Sundler, F. (1987). Occurrence and distribution of neuropeptides in the human skin. *Acta Dermatologia Venereologia*, **67**, 185–92.

Wilcock, G. K. & Esiri, M. M. (1981). Plaques, tangles and dementia – a quantitative study. *Journal of Neurological Science*, **56**, 343–356.

Wisniewski, H. M. & Terry, R. D. (1973). Reexamination of the pathogenesis of the senile plaque. In *Progress in Neuropathology*, vol. 2, ed. H. M. Zimmerman, pp. 1–26. New York: Grune & Stratton.

Yamaguchi, H., Hirai, S., Morimatsu, M., Shooji, M. & Ihara, Y. (1988). A variety of cerebral amyloid deposits in the brains of the Alzheimer-type dementia demonstrated by β-protein immunostaining. *Acta Neuropatholica*, **76**, 541–9.

Index

Abbe's formula   180
Accept   85
accuracy
    image registration   283–4
    input digitization   16
    measurement   93, 94
acousto-optic deflection (AOD)   155, 160
acquisition, image   5, 25–6
    3-D reconstructions   304–6, 309–10,
        314–15, 318
    colour images   45–6, 223–4
    electron microscopy   198
affine transformations   265, 266
agarose beads   348, 349
ageing
    5-HT immunoreactive nerves   363, 364
    neurotransmitter dynamics   372–4, 375
    noradrenergic nerves   357–60, 362
    peptidergic nerves   363–5
aliasing 224, 327
alignment, see registration
Allium cepa   200
alpha blending   294–5
amines, biogenic   360–3
amplifier   213
analogue-to-digital convertor (ADC)   51
analysis of variance, nested   100
Analyze   65, 66
animation, 3-D images   332
anti-aliasing   320, 321, 327–8
apochromatic objectives   140
architectures, computer   26–7, 28–9, 54
arcuate nucleus   393–4, 395
aspect ratio, $x{:}y{:}z$ 318–19
autofluorescence   175–6, 363
autoradiograms
    development   386–7
    emulsion dipped   131, 132, 384–5
    film type   130–1
autoradiography   146–7
    in situ hybridization   128, 384–7
    receptor, see receptor autoradiography
avidin–biotin complex (ABC) method   129,
    344

baby hamster kidney (BHK) cells   391–2
back-to-front alpha blending   294–5
background
    cleaning   76
    fluorescence   314, 363
bi-linear transformation   266
bias
    allocation   90–1
    assessment   91
    systematic, stereological estimators   96–7
Bigbee effect   341
binary images   56–7, 58–9, 71
    confocal microscopy   189
    connected components analysis   242–3
    editing   85
    formation   76, 77, 199–200, 242–3
    processing operations   76–9, 200, 243–4
Binary Space Partitioning (BSP) tree   324
biotin   128
bitmapped image files   55–61
blinding   91
blur removal, see haze removal
bodipy   169, 172
body, image   61
Boltzmann machines   30
Boolean operations   77–9
boundaries
    derived from images from scanning
        systems   306
    detection, see edge detection
    digitization, 3-D reconstructions   305–6
brightness
    adaptation   10
    adjustment, light microscope   139
    fluorescence microscopy   146

calcitonin gene-related peptide (CGRP)
    agarose beads   348, 349
    pulmonary endocrine cells   344, 346, 347,
        350–1
    sudomotor nerves   363, 365
calcium concentration sensitive fluorescent
    dyes   170–1
cameras, see video cameras

capture, image, *see* acquisition, image
case-control studies   88, 90
catecholamine histochemistry   355
  applications   357–60
  methodology   356–7
cathode ray tubes (CRTs)   46–8, 49
Cavalieri's principle   101–2, 104, 112
CCD cameras, *see* charge coupled device
  cameras
CCIR video system   39, 51
CD-ROM   20, 53–4
cell(s)   124
  differential counting   400–2
  fixation   125–6
  images, boundary detection   245–6
  living, confocal microscopy   165–9
  organelles   200–7
CGRP, *see* calcitonin gene-related peptide
charge coupled device (CCD; solid state)
  cameras   25, 33, 35–6, 212
  attachment to microscope   219–20
  biological applications   220–1, 222
  colour imaging   46, 223–4
  cooled   40, 222
  dark current and noise   40
  dynamic range   41
  frame transfer type   35, 36
  gamma ratio   40
  integrating   222
  interline transfer type   35, 36
  neurotransmitter densitometry   370, 371
  signal generation/errors   212
charge coupled devices (CCDs)   25, 34
chromatic aberration
  confocal microscopy   184–5
  light microscopy   140, 148–9
chromatin patches   200–2, 203
classification   13–14, 15, 21–4
  3-D visualization   319–20
cliff boundaries   246, 248
clinical trials   88–9
closing   79, 244
cloud motion   263–4
CMY colour system   42, 43
CMYK colour system   42–3, 45
co-occurrence method,
  segmentation   229–30, 231
coordinate transformations, 3-D
  displays   320, 321–2
cold stress   372, 374
colloidal gold probes   203, 206–7
colour cameras   45–6, 223–4
  signals   39–40
  single chip   223–4
  three chip   223
colour filters, light microscopy   142–3
colour images
  capture   45–6, 223–4
  deconvolution   292, 293–4
  digitization   71
  file formats   59–61
  systems for producing   11, 41–5, 66
colour printers   49–50

compact disk, read only memory
  (CD-ROM)   20, 53–4
compactness (*P2A*)   13, 14
compositing approach, volume
  rendering   330–1
compression, image files   66–7
computer(s)   3–5
  architectures   26–7, 28–9, 54
  electron microscope image analysis   207–8
  host   19, 26–7
  vision   23–4
computerized tomography (CT)
  scanning   300, 301, 308, 309
condenser lens   136, 137
  adjustment   138–9
conditioning   241–2
  examples   251, 253
cones   10
confocal microscopy   151–91, 293–4, 355
  3-D reconstructions   155, 186, 189, 300
    data acquisition   306, 309–10, 314–15
    x:y:z aspect ratio   318–19
  biomedical applications   162–79
  and deconvolution   295–7
  edge detection algorithm   248–9
  extended focus or range images   185
  fluorescence mode   160–1, 163, 183, 191,
    314–15
    autofluorescence and negative
      fluorescence   175–6
    fluorescent stains   173–5
    ion concentration sensitive dyes   169–71
    live cells   167–9
    prepared, fixed specimens   171–6
    vital fluorescent dyes   169
  historical development   152–6
  immunohistochemical
    densitometry   372–4, 375
  limits   180–7
  living tissues   163–71
  optical thickness of a slice   315
  prepared, fixed specimens   171–9
  principle   151–2
  reflection   182–3
    coatings   177–9
    interference contrast, cells on flat
      substrates   165–7
    live cells   167, 168
    live tissues   164–5
    prepared, fixed specimens   176–9
    stains   176–7
  resolution   180–1
  serial section production   308–9
  spatial grid technique   116–17
  stereo imaging   185–6
  stereology/other uses of image
    processing   188–9
  surface mapping   186–7, 188
confocal scanning laser microscope (CSLM)
  axial chromatic aberration   184–5
  choosing type   189–91
  history   153–6
  magnification calibration   182

confocal scanning laser microscope (CSLM)
    (Continued)
    objective lenses   183–4
    real time, direct view, laser
            illuminated   162
        biomedical applications   163, 171–3
    signal strength, absorption, scattering and
            depth   182–3
    single beam, slow scan, digital imaging
            laser   159–60
        biomedical applications   167–9, 171–3
        mirror beam scanning   160
        stationary beam, on-axis
                scanning   159–60
    type I and type II scanning   190–1
    types   156–62
    video rate (VRCSLM)   155, 160, 190
        biomedical applications   163, 165–6
        stereo imaging   185
    video rate, video output, laser
            scanning   160–2
    see also tandem scanning microscope
            (TSM)
confounding   91–2
conjugate planes
    aperture set   137, 138
    field set   135, 137
connected components analysis   242–3
    examples   248, 251, 254, 257–8
connectivity   305–6
consistency   17
ContextVision computer system   4–5
contour based 3-D models   306–8, 310
contour data, 3-D reconstructions   305–6,
        318
contrast
    differential interference   143
    discrimination, video cameras   215–16
    expansion   74, 75, 199
    light microscopy   142
    phase   143
control (fiducial; registration) points   265–7,
        302–3
    laser-created   302
    location   267, 273–4
controls   90
convolution masks (filters)   80–4
    high pass   82, 83
    low pass averaging   82–4
cooled CCD cameras   40, 222
correspondence problem   274
counterstaining   387, 398, 399, 400–1
counting
    differential cell   400–2
    grain, *see* grain counting
    point   220
    quantitative immunocytochemistry   341
coverglass thickness   141, 183
cross-correlation coefficients   269–70, 303
CSLM, *see* confocal scanning laser
        microscope
cubic convolution   282

dark current noise   40, 222
dark ground (field) microscopy   144, 398
DASPMI   169, 171, 172, 173
deconvolution   289, 290–2
    3-D volumetric rendering and   294–5
    choice of technique   297
    and confocal microscopy   295–7
    in true colour   292, 293–4
deformation, *see* distortion
degradation, image   288
dendritic tree length   118, 119
densitometry, *see* microdensitometry
dental restorations/implants   172–3
depth
    aberrations, confocal microscopy   309
    cues, 3-D displays   316–17, 332
    image   56, 57–9
    resolution, confocal microscopy   180–1,
            182–3
    shading   325–6
design
    quantitative immunocytochemical
            studies   340
    study   87–94
deterministic similarity criteria (DSC)   271–2
development, *in situ* hybridization
        autoradiograms   386–7
diabetic neuropathy   366
diaminobenzidine (DAB)   177
dichroic mirror   145–6, 366
difference image   283
differential interference contrast   143
diffraction   140
digital-to-analogue convertors (DACs)   51
digitization   26, 51, 70–1
    boundaries, for 3-D reconstructions   305–6
    precision and accuracy   16
digitized image   5–6, 33
    basic processing operations   69–85
    editing   85
    frame processing operations   84–5
    group processing operations   80–4
    point processing operations   72–9
digitizing tablets   148, 305, 306
digoxigenin   128
dilation   78–9, 244
disks   9, 52–4
    magnetic Winchester   20, 52
    optical   20, 52–4
display, image   10, 46–50
dissector   105
    optical   105–6
distortion
    geometric correction   22–3
    image alignment and   265–7, 303
    light microscopy   141
dithering   49–50
dividing-cubes algorithm   329
double labelling techniques   365–6, 394–5
draw files   55
drawing system (tube), projection   147–8,
        305

dye-sublimation printing 50
dynamic range, video cameras 40–1, 216–17

edge detection 22, 241–60
  3-D reconstructions 306
  algorithms for microscopic images 246–60
  cell images 245–6
  facet model 244–5
  gradient magnitude 244–5
  mathematical morphology 243–4
  thresholding and connected
    components 242–3
editing, image 85
electron microscopy, transmission 197–208
  3-D reconstructions 302
  biosynthetic machinery 204–5
  chromatin patches 200–2, 203
  colloidal gold probes 206–7
  hardware and software 207–8
  image processing 198–200
  immunogold particle quantification 400
  nucleolar components 202–4
  quantification of cell organelles 200–7
  secretory granules and lysosomes 205–6
embedding media 126
emulsion dipped autoradiograms 131, 132,
  384–5
endoplasmic reticulum 203, 204–5
endothelin-1 (ET-1) 131, 132
enhancement, image 17, 288
  3-D reconstructions 319
  electron microscopy 199–200
enlargement 84
entropy method, thresholding 228–9, 230
eosin 176
epifluorescence microscopy 145–6
erosion 78–9, 244
ethidium 169
Evans blue 169
experimental studies 88–9
exposure time, *in situ* hybridization
  autoradiography 385–6
extended focus/range images, confocal
  microscopy 185
extracellular matrix 372–4, 375
eye, confocal microscopy 163
eyepiece, light microscope 135

facet edge detection 244–5, 247
  examples 251, 256
fast Fourier transform (FFT) 189, 269
feature extraction 23, 235–8, 239
fiducial points, *see* control points
field density, nerve plexuses 357
field of view, flatness 141
files, image 55–68
  bitmapped 55–61
  compression 66–7
  formats 62–6
  structure 61–2

vector 55
Fill 85
film autoradiograms 130–1
film recorders 50
films, negative 198
fixation 124–6
  autofluorescence and 175–6
  in situ hybridization 383–4
  neurotransmitter immunochemistry 367
flatness, field of view 141
floating point images 59
fluorescein 175
fluorescein dextran 169
fluorescein isothiocyanate (FITC) 363, 365,
  369
fluorescence
  background 314, 363
  confocal microscopy, *see* confocal
    microscopy, fluorescence mode
  fading 176
    minimizing 146, 315
    nerve/neurotransmitter studies 357,
      361, 367–9
  negative 175–6
fluorescence microscopy 144–7
  nerves/neurotransmitters 356–63, 365–6,
    367–9
  video cameras 222–3
fluorescent dyes
  ion concentration sensitive 169–71
  prepared, fixed tissues 173–5
  stability, *see* fluorescence, fading
  vital 169
footer 61–2
footprints 279
formaldehyde 125, 175–6
formaldehyde-induced fluorescence (FIF)
  method 356
  glyoxylic acid modification 356, 359
four-dimensional (4-D) datasets 315–16
fractionator 101, 102
frame buffer (store) 26, 71
frame processing operations 84–5
frame processors 52, 53
framegrabber 5, 26, 51–2
freezing 126, 383
front-to-back ray tracing technique 295
frozen sections 125, 126
full width at half maximum (FWHM) 319
Fullman method of metallurgical grain
  sizing 99–100

gamma ratio 40, 216–17
geometric correction 22–3
GIF (graphics interchange format) 63, 65
glutaraldehyde 125, 175–6
glyoxylic acid fluorescence method 356, 359
gold probes, colloidal 203, 206–7
Golgi complex 203, 204, 205
Golgi preparations 177, 178, 179
Gouraud shading 326

grain counting
  automated 389–95, 398
    applications 394–5
    in situ versus solution
        hybridization 391–2
    interpretation of results 391
    overview 389
    performance checks 389–92
    photometric uniformity 390
    proper slide preparation 390–1
    system stability 390
    variations in illumination 389–90
  by eye 398
grains
  density measurement 398–400
  metallurgical, Fullman method of
      sizing 99–100
granules, secretory 205–6
graphics interchange format (GIF) 63, 65
greylevel histograms 74, 75, 76
greylevel resolution 6, 7–8, 57
  neurotransmitter densitometry 369–71
greylevel trace 74, 76
greyscale images 57
  electron microscopy 198–200, 201
grid, spatial 114–17
group processing operations 80–4

hard copy 10
hardware 3–5, 19–31
  electron microscope image analysis 207–8
  see also computer(s); confocal scanning
      laser microscope; light microscope;
      scanners; video cameras
haze removal 288–97
  factor (*k*) 290–1, 293
  in-focus 289–90
  out-of-focus 290–2, 295–7
header, image 61
height, image 56
Hepes buffer 367, 368
hidden feature removal 320, 323, 329
high definition television (HDTV) 48
high level image processing 21–3
histograms
  greylevel 74, 75, 76
  scalar 235–7
  stretching 199
  vector 235–7
HLS colour system 43–4, 45
holograms 317
horizontal data entry 305
host computer system 19, 26–7
Hough transform technique 277, 278
HSV colour system 44, 45
5-HT, *see* 5-hydroxytryptamine
hybridization
  in situ, *see in situ* hybridization
  solution 391–2
5-hydroxytryptamine (5-HT; serotonin)
  dynamics, densitometry 366–72, 373
  immunohistochemistry 361–2

measurements of nerve density 363, 364,
    366
hypothalamic hormones 205, 206, 348

I-measure 235–7
illuminated field diaphragm (IFD) 137–8,
    139
illuminating aperture diaphragm (IAD) 137,
    138, 139
illumination
  automated grain counting and 389–90
  dark ground microscopy 144
  epifluorescence microscopy 145–6
  light microscopy 136–40
  quantitative immunocytochemistry 347,
      362–3
  sensing by video cameras 213, 216–17,
      223
  stability 16
  uniformity 16, 199, 390
image analysis
  common pitfalls 16–17
  principle steps 11
image processing
  3-D image 319
  advantages 17–18
  basic elements 3–5
  basic operations 69–85
  classification 21–4
  confocal microscope images 189
  definition 3
  electron microscope images 198–200
  high level 23–4
  low level 21–3
  major system components 24–5
  software 9
IMG format 65, 66
immersion media 146, 184, 315
immersion objectives 135, 141
  confocal microscopy 177–9, 183–4
  fluorescence microscopy 146
immunocytochemistry/immunohistochemistry
    123
  differential cell counting 400–2
  immunostaining methods 128, 129
  quantitative 339–53, 355
    counting or measuring structures 341
    double immunolabelling 365–6
    measuring intensity of
        immunoreactivity 342–51
    microdensitometry 342–8
    nerve density measurement 360–6
    neurotransmitter dynamics 366–74
    Sternberger technique 351–3
    study design 340
    supraoptimal dilution technique 342,
        350–1
    techniques 340–1
immunofluorescence, quantitative 340
immunogold techniques 147, 177
  particle quantification 400
impact printers 49

in situ hybridization   123, 356, 381–96
  assay conditions   384
  assay specificity   388–9
  autoradiography   128, 384–7
    control experiments   387
    exposure time   385–6
    slide development   386–7
  grain counting   389–95
    applications   392–5
    overview of process   389
    system performance   389–92
  grain density measurement   398–400
  overview   127–8, 382–3
  saturation curve   387–8
  tissue preparation   383–4
infra-red-blocking filters   46, 219–20
inkjet printers   49
input, image   5, 33–46
intensifers, image   222–3
intercept density, nerve plexuses   357
interlaced scanning   37, 38
interphase nuclei, chromatin patches   200–2,
    203
interpolation, 3-D reconstruction   308, 319
interpretation
  3-D images   332
  automatic techniques   397–402
invariant moments   272–3
inverse Laplacian filters   82
inversion   72, 73, 199
ion concentration sensitive fluorescent
    dyes   169–71
isotropic directions, generation   106–9
isotropic, uniform random (IUR)
    sections   106–7, 108
  length density estimation   110
  orientator and   106–7
  particle sizing   113, 114
  spatial grid technique   115, 116
  surface density estimation   109–10

Kirsch operator   84
Köhler illumination   136–8
  setting up   138–40

labelling   242
lag, image   41
laminin   373–4, 375
Landsat images   264
Laplacian filters, inverse   82
laser printers   49–50
length
  density   99, 110–12, 117–18
  total, from total vertical
      projections   117–19
lens
  aberrations   140–1
  condenser   136, 137, 138–9
  lamp collector   136, 137
  objective, *see* objective/objective lens

light microscope   134–50
  electronic image representation   213–14
  illuminating system   136–8
  imaging system   135
  optical system defects   140–1
  setting up   138–40
  stand   147
  video camera attachment   140, 148–50,
      218–20
light microscopy   134–50
  colour filters   142–3
  contrast   142
  dark ground (field)   144, 398
  differential interference contrast   143
  drawing tube   147–8, 305
  fluorescence, *see* fluorescence microscopy
  images, edge detection algorithms   253–60
  phase contrast   143
  resolution   180–1
  see also confocal microscopy
light sensors   213–14
line matching   277
line rendering   329–30
linearity, video cameras   216–17
lipofuscin   365
liquid crystal displays (LCDs)   48–9
liquid nitrogen cooled cameras   222
lissamine rhodamine   169
living tissues/cells, confocal
      microscopy   163–71
longitudinal data entry   305
longitudinal slices   316
lookup tables (LUT)   10, 51–2, 60–1, 71, 72
  background cleaning   76
  binary image formation   76, 77
  contrast expansion   74, 75
  image inversion   72, 73
lossy compression   66, 67
low level image processing   21–3
lysosomes   205–6

machine vision   23–4
magnetic resonance imaging (MRI)   300,
      308, 309
magnetic tape   9
magnetic Winchester disks   20, 52
magnification   16, 149
  calibration, confocal microscope   182
mapping
  3-D displays   320
  surface, confocal microscopy   186–7, 188
masks, convolution, *see* convolution masks
mathematical morphology   243–4, 247
maximum point projection   295
measurements   13–14, 123–4
  3-D models   310
  absolute versus relative   17, 99
  electron microscope images   200
  morphological   220–1
  optical density   221–2
  stained area   14–16, 341
median filter   80–1

messenger RNA (mRNA)   127–8
microdensitometry   355
    immunocytochemical   342–8
        antigen–antibody reactions   344–5
        enzymatic reactions   345, 346
        general approach   343
        morphometry and   345–7
        standards   347–8, 349
    neurotransmitter dynamics   366–74
        applications   372–4
        confocal microscopy   372–4
        greylevel resolution   369–71
        specimen preparation   367–9
micrographs   305
microscopy, *see* confocal microscopy; electron
        microscopy, transmission; light
        microscopy
MicroTome   290–1
MIMD processors   29
minimum spanning trees (MSTs)   275
MISD processors   29
moat boundaries   246, 251, 253
modulation transfer function (MTF)   216,
        221
modulation transfer ratio   216
monitors   10, 20, 46–9
    cathode ray tube (CRT)   46–8, 49
    non-CRT   48–9
    raster scanning   38
monochrome cameras
    biological applications   220, 221
    signals   38–9
morphology, mathematical   243–4, 247
motion parallax   317
mounting media   141, 176
MRC image format   64
mRNA   127–8
multiplanar reformatting   316

Nearest Neighbour Algorithm (NNA)   290,
        291–2, 296, 297
negative films   198
nerves   355–76
    catecholamine histochemistry   356–60
    field area   357
    field measurements of density   360–6
    in situ hybridization histochemistry   392–5
    intercept density   357
nested analysis of variance   100
networks
    artificial neural   29–30
    computer   21
neural networks   29–30
neuroendocrine cells, pulmonary   344, 346,
        347, 350–1
neuropeptide Y (NPY)   363, 376
neuropeptides   363–5, 376, 392–3
neurotransmitters   355–76
    dynamics   366–74
    nerve density measurements   360–6
nile red   169
nitrocellulose strips   348, 349

noise   16
    dark current   40, 222
    removal   22
noradrenaline   356, 357–60, 362
Northern blotting   127
NTSC colour TV system   39
nucleator   113, 114
nucleolar components   202–4
numerical aperture (NA)   135, 136, 289

objective/objective lens   135
    changing to higher/lower power   139–40
    chromatic correction   140, 148–9
    confocal microscopes   183–4
    dry   135, 141, 183
    flatness of field of view   141
    fluorescence microscopy   145, 146
    focusing   138
    immersion, *see* immersion objectives
    numerical aperture (NA)   135, 136, 289
    tubelength correction   141
observational studies   88, 89
octree   324
opening   78–9, 244
optical density (OD)   216–17
    measurements   221–2
    see also microdensitometry
optical disks   20, 52–4
optical dissector   105–6
orf virus   295
organelles, cellular   200–7
orientator   106–7
Ostu's thresholding method   228, 229, 230
output, image   10, 46–50

paint (bitmapped) image files   55–61
painter's algorithm   324
PAL video system   39, 51
Panasonic Moonlight video camera   370, 371
paraffin wax   126
paraformaldehyde   383, 384
parallel-group studies   88–9
parallel processing   29, 30
parallel projection   321
paraxial slices   316
particle sizing   99–100, 112–14
    direct methods   112–14
    indirect methods   112
pattern recognition algorithms   402
    differential cell counting   401–2
    grain detection   399–400
peltier cooled cameras   222
perimeter to area ratio (*P2A*)   13, 14
periventricular nucleus (PeVN)   394
peroxidase–antiperoxidase (PAP)
        method   129, 341, 344
perspective projection   316, 321
PGP9.5   363, 364–5
phase contrast   143
Phong shading   326
phosphate-buffered saline (PBS)   367, 368
photoelectric sensors   213–14

photographic film recorders 50
photographic prints 198
photomicrographs 305
photomultipliers 222
physical 3-D models 300, 313
pinhole, virtual 291
pituitary cells 201, 203, 204–5, 206
pituitary hormones 348
pixel (bitmapped) image files 55–61
pixels 5, 33, 56, 70–1
  representation 6
placebo effect 91
plastic embedding media 126
plotter files 55
plumbicon camera 34, 35
point counting 220
point dependent segmentation
  techniques 227, 228–9, 230
point-pattern matching 275–7
point processing operations 72–9
point rendering 328–9
point sampled intercept 112–13
point spread
  in-focus 289–90
  out-of-focus 290–2, 295–7
point spread function (PSF) 288–9, 290–1,
  297
  full width at half maximum (FWHM) 319
polymethylmethacrylate (PMMA) 176
polynomial coefficients, estimation 280–2
Pontamine Sky Blue 363
positional formatting method 62
positron emission tomography (PET) 300,
  308
power, study 92
precision
  input digitization 16
  stereological estimators 96–7
preparation methods 123–32, 198
  in situ hybridization 383–4
primary image 135
principal axis transformation 303
printers, colour 49–50
priority algorithms 323–4
pro-opiomelanocortin (POMC) 385, 388,
  392–4, 395
proteinase K (PK) 383–4
protocol, study 88
pseudocolour images 72–3
publications, image processing 3, 4
pulmonary neuroendocrine cells 344, 346,
  347, 350–1

quality, image 8–9, 47
quantification 17, 123–4
  electron microscope images 200–7
  immunocytochemical, *see*
    immunocytochemistry/immunohisto-
    chemistry, quantitative
  nerves and neurotransmitters 355–76
  see also measurements
quantization 6, 7–8, 33, 57

radioimmunoassay (RIA) 128, 339
radiolabelled ligand binding 128–31
random access memory (RAM) 9, 51
random sampling, uniform 98, 100–1, 102–3
randomization 90–1
raster graphics devices 329
raster (bitmapped) image files 55–61
raster scanning 37–8, 214
ratio method, shading correction 73
ray casting 324, 331
ray tracing 295, 324
re-mapping, image 280–2
receptor autoradiography 123, 129–31
  grain density measurement 398–400
reconstruction, image 288
reduced instruction set chips (RISC) 26, 54
reduction 84
reference volume 99
reflection confocal microscopy, *see* confocal
  microscopy, reflection
reflective coatings 177–9
region based matching 280
region dependent segmentation
  techniques 227–38
region growing scheme 248, 256–7, 259
registration (alignment) 262–84
  2-D slices for 3-D reconstructions 302–3
  accuracy 283–4
  history 262–4
  image re-mapping 280–2
  image resampling 282
  line matching 277
  local methods 282–3
  location of control points 267, 273–4
  overview 265–7
  point-pattern matching 275–7
  points, *see* control points
  region based matching 280
  shape matching 277–80
  similarity estimators 269–73
  template matching 267–9
  template search strategies 273
Reject 85
relaxation method, segmentation 230–2, 233
rendering algorithms 294–5, 328–32
repeatability 94
resampling, image 282
residual 282
resin embedding media 126
resolution
  confocal and conventional light
    microscopy 180–1
  depth, confocal microscopy 180–1
  greylevel, *see* greylevel resolution
  horizontal 215
  lateral, confocal microscopy 180, 181
  spatial 6–7, 33, 47, 70–1, 215
  vertical 215
RGB colour system 11, 41–2, 44, 60
  conversion between formats 42, 43, 45
  signal digitization 51
Rhodamine B 169

rigid transformations   266, 267
Roberts filter   84
rods   10–11
rotations
   3-D space   322
   image   84, 265, 266
RS-170 video system   39
rubber sheet deformations   84–5, 282–3
run-length encoding (RLE)   67

samples, preparation methods   123–32, 198
sampling
   frequency, serial sections   301–2, 308
   unbiased   100–1, 102–3
   uniform random   98, 100–1, 102–3
satellite imaging   263–4, 266
saticon camera   35
saturation curves   387–8
scalable files   55
scan conversion, 3-D visualization   321,
   324–5
scanline algorithms   323
scanners   5, 25–6, 33, 34, 211–24
   flying spot   211–12
   history   211–12
   see also video cameras
scanning
   interlaced   37, 38
   raster   37–8, 214
scanning systems
   boundary data extraction   306
   data acquisition   309–10
   sampling frequency   308
   serial section production   308–9
   see also confocal microscopy
SECAM colour TV system   39
secretory granules   205–6
sections   97–8
   fixation   124–5
   isotropic, uniform random, *see* isotropic,
      uniform random (IUR) sections
   preparation methods   124–6
   processing   126
   serial, *see* serial sections
   staining   126–31
   thickness   16, 199, 347
   uniformity   16, 199
   vertical, *see* vertical sections
Seescan plc   397–402
segmentation   11–13, 23, 227–39
   3-D visualization   319–20
   co-occurrence method   229–30, 231
   entropy method   228–9, 230
   multiple homogeneous region   232–4
   Ostu's method   228, 229, 230
   point dependent techniques   227, 228–9,
      230
   region dependent techniques   227–38
   registration using   280
   relaxation method   230–2, 233
   texture regions   234–8, 239
   using region and boundary
      information   232–4

Wang & Haralick method   232
selection, subject   89–90
selector   113
sequential similarity detection algorithm
   (SSDA)   270–1, 273
serial sections   301–4
   alignment for 3-D reconstruction   262–3,
      302–3
   data acquisition from   304–6
   estimating separation   303–4
   from scanning systems   308–9
   sources of error   301–2
serotonin, *see* 5-hydroxytryptamine
servers   19, 20–1
sex steroids   392–3
shading
   3-D visualization   316–17, 320, 321, 325–7
   constant   326
   correction   73–4, 199
   density gradient   327
   distance gradient   326–7
   distance-only/depth   325–6
   Gouraud   326
   Phong   326
shadow generation   316–17
shape matching   277–80
sharpening, image   199
signal-to-noise ratio (SNR), video
   cameras   218
signed images   59
silver grain counting, *see* grain counting
silver staining, confocal microscopy   177,
   178–9
SIMD processors   29
similarity criteria
   deterministic (DSC)   271–2
   stochastic (SSC)   271–2
similarity estimators   269–73
   cross-correlation coefficients   269–70, 303
   invariant moments   272–3
   sequential similarity detection algorithm
      (SSDA)   270–1
   sum of differences   270
simplicity, study design   93
SISD (von Neumann) architecture   26–7,
   28–9, 54
skeletal implants   172–3
skeletonization   79, 80
slides
   changing, light microscopy   140
   preparation, *in situ* hybridization   390–1
   see also autoradiograms; sections
Small Computer System Interface (SCSI)   52
Sobel filters   84
software   5, 21–4
   assessment   27–8
   automated interpretation   397–402
   choosing   28
   electron microscope image analysis   207–8
somatostatin (SS)   386, 391–2, 394
spatial grid technique   114–17
spatial resolution   6–7, 33, 47, 70–1, 215
specific activity (SA)   385–6

speckle 22
speed, computerized image processing 17
spherical aberration 140–1
splatting approach 331
spot size 47
stained area, measurement 14–16, 341
staining 126–31, 142
  colour and uniformity 16
  receptor binding sites 128–31
  reflection confocal microscopy 176–7
  stored products 128
  synthetic machinery 127–8
  see also counterstaining; fluorescent dyes
stand, light microscope 147
standards
  automated grain counting 391
  immunocytochemical
    microdensitometry 347–8, 349
star volume estimator 114, 115
stereo imaging, confocal microscopy 185–6
stereology 96–119
  Cavalieri's principle 101–2, 104
  confocal microscopy 187–9
  dissector 105–6
  generation of isotropic directions 106–9
  length density estimation 110–12
  model/design based approaches 99–100
  nested analysis of variance 100
  particle sizing 112–14
  ratios and densities 99
  sectioning 97–8
  spatial grid 114–17
  surface density estimation 109–10
  systematic bias and precision 96–7
  total length from total vertical
    projections 117–19
  unbiased sampling strategies 100–1,
    102–3
  volume density 104
stereoscopy, 3-D visualization 317
steric hindrance,
  immunocytochemistry 344–5
Sternberger technique 351–3
stochastic similarity criteria (SSC) 271–2
storage media 9, 20, 52–4
  electron microscope images 198
stratification 92–3
study
  design 87–94
  developing new image processing
    applications 93–4
  organization and structure 89–93
  protocol 88
  simplicity of design 93
  size and power 92
  types 88–9
sub-regioning 319
subjects
  number required 92
  selection 89–90
substance P 363, 366, 376
subtraction technique, shading correction 73
sulphaflavine 176, 177

sum of differences 270
summed voxel projection method 331–2
Sun rasterfiles 64
SunVision 66
supraoptimal dilution technique 342, 350–1
surface area
  3-D models 310
  particle 112
  spatial grid technique 114–16
surface density 99, 109–10
surface mapping, confocal 186–7, 188
surface models, 3-D 301, 306–8
surface rendering 295, 328, 330
synchronizing (sync) pulse 39, 214

tag image file format (TIFF) 62–3, 65
tandem scanning microscope (TSM) 154,
  156–9, 162
  biomedical applications 163, 164–5, 172–3
  choice 190–1
  chromatic aberration 184
  one-sided disc scanning (1sTSM) 154, 159
  stereo imaging 186
  video rate, video output, laser
    scanning 160
television (TV) 48, 49
  cameras, *see* video cameras
  high definition (HDTV) 48
  signals 38–40
template
  matching 267–9
  search strategies 273
Texas Red 365
texture based segmentation 234–8, 239
TGA format 64, 65
thermal wax printers 50
three-dimensional (3-D; volume)
  datasets 309–10, 315–16, 318
three-dimensional (3-D) images,
  true 317–18
three-dimensional (3-D) models 300–11
  2-D slice alignment 262–3, 302–3
  confocal microscopy, *see* confocal
    microscopy, 3-D reconstructions
  construction 306–8, 318–19
  contour based 306–8, 310
  data acquisition
    from 2-D images 304–6
    from volumetric data 309–10, 314–15
  deconvolution and 294–5
  physical 300, 313
  quantitative measurements 310
  serial sections
    from scanning systems 308–9
    physical 301–4
  surface 301, 306–8
  types 300–1, 313
  visualization, *see* three-dimensional (3-D)
    visualization
  volume 301, 308
three-dimensional (3-D)
  visualization 313–32

three-dimensional (3-D)
  visualization   313–32 *(Continued)*
  approaches   314
  creating illusion of solidity   316–18
    depth cues   316–17
    true 3-D images   317–18
  image interpretation   332
  multidimensional
      datasets/manipulation   315–16
  principles of computer graphics
      display   321–8
    anti-aliasing   327–8
    co-ordinate transformation   321–2
    scan conversion   324–5
    shading   325–7
    visible object determination   322–4
  rendering algorithms   328–32
  stages in process   318–20
thresholding   12–13, 228–9, 230, 242–3, 247
  entropy method   228–9, 230
  examples   248, 251
  Ostu's method   228, 229, 230
TIFF (tag image file format)   62–3, 65
tissues   124
  fixation   124–5
  living, confocal microscopy   164–5
  processing   126
  staining, *see* staining
toluidine blue   177, 180, 181
trailer, image   61–2
transverse slices   316
triangulation   307–8, 319, 330
tryptophan hydroxylase   361–2
tubelength correction   141
two-and-a-half dimensional ($2\frac{1}{2}$-D)
      images   314, 316–17
tyrosine hydroxylase (TH)   348, 349, 366,
      372, 374

unbiased 2-D counting frame (USF)   101,
      103, 110–12
unbiased 3-D sampling brick   101, 103
unsigned images   59

variance, nested analysis of   100
varifocal mirror   317–18
vasoactive intestinal polypeptide (VIP)   363,
      365
vector graphics devices   329
vector image files   55
vertical data entry   305
vertical sections   107–9, 110
  particle sizing   113, 114
vibrating mirror   317–18
video cameras   5, 25, 211–24, 305
  attachment to light microscope   140,
      148–50, 218–20
  biological applications   218–24
    colour imaging   223–4
    fluorescence microscopy   222–3
    morphological measurements   220–1
    optical density measurements   221–2

point counting   220
choosing   224
contrast discrimination   215–16
dark current and noise   40
dynamic range   40–1, 216–17
electronic image representation   212–14
gamma ratio   40, 216–17
history   154, 156, 211–12
image lag   41
linearity   216–17
neurotransmitter densitometry   370–1
performance   215–18
resolution   215
scanning and synchronization   214
signal generation/errors   38–40, 212
signal-to-noise ratio   218
solid state/charge coupled device, *see*
      charge coupled device (CCD; solid
      state) cameras
vacuum/thermionic
      tube/photoconductive   25, 33, 34–5,
      212
  biological applications   220, 221
  see also vidicon cameras
video images
  edge detection   249–52
  nerves   355–6
  recording, confocal microscopy   164,
      165–7
vidicon cameras   25, 34–5, 211
  point counting   220
viewing, 3-D displays   320
virtual pinhole   291
virtual reality   317
visible object determination   320, 321, 322–4
vision
  computer/machine   23–4
  human   10–11
visualization, 3-D, *see* three-dimensional
      visualization
visualization file format (VFF)   64, 65
void   114, 115
volume
  3-D models   310
  of an object, total   101–2, 104
  particle   112–14
  reference   99
volume (3-D) datasets   309–10, 315–16, 318
volume density   99, 104
volume models, 3-D   301, 308
volume rendering   330–2
volumetric compositing   330–1
von Neumann (SISD) architecture   26–7,
      28–9, 54
voxels   309–10, 318–19

wall boundaries   246
Wang & Haralick method, segmentation   232
warping, image   84–5, 265–7
width, image   56
wire frame images   329

WISARD 30
within-subject studies 88, 89
workstations 20, 26
write once, read many (WORM)
  devices 52–3

x,y translations 84, 265, 266
$x:y:z$ aspect ratio 318–19

z-buffer algorithms 323
zooming 84